WORLD HEALTH ORGANIZATION
MONOGRAPH SERIES
No. 53

THE ASSESSMENT OF THE NUTRITIONAL STATUS OF THE COMMUNITY

THE ASSESSMENT
OF THE NUTRITIONAL STATUS
OF THE COMMUNITY

(with special reference to field surveys in
developing regions of the world)

DERRICK B. JELLIFFE, M.D., F.R.C.P.,
F.A.P.H.A., F.R.S.H., F.A.A.P.

*Director, Caribbean Nutrition Institute, Jamaica; Visiting Professor of Tropical Medicine,
Tulane University School of Medicine, New Orleans, USA; formerly Professor of Paediatrics
and Child Health, Makerere Medical School, Kampala, Uganda*

Prepared in consultation with twenty-five specialists
in various countries

WORLD HEALTH ORGANIZATION

GENEVA

1966

CONTENTS

1 Introduction

In large areas of the world today, malnutrition, especially that affecting young children, is one of the principal public health problems.

In some countries energetic attempts to improve the situation are already under way. These require to be intensified and more accurately and logically guided, so that the most appropriate preventive methods can be applied where the need is greatest.

This can be done, and the results of the chosen methods properly evaluated, only if adequate information is available at the outset. Here, as with other aspects of public health, numerical measurements are required to act as a base-line, from which progress can be gauged and any changes, planned or unplanned, assessed.

The principal aim of the nutritional assessment of a community is, then, to map out the magnitude and geographical distribution of malnutrition as a public health problem, to discover and analyse the ecological factors that are directly or indirectly responsible, and, where possible, to suggest appropriate corrective measures, preferably capable of being applied with continuing community participation.

In addition, factual evidence of the incidence of malnutrition in the community, and of its often complex factors, is needed in order to make the public, and especially the fund-controlling administrators and politicians, realize the extent of the problem, and so ensure financial support for such preventive programmes as may be required.

In short, the nutritional assessment of a community should aim at discovering facts and guiding action intended to improve nutrition and health.

Standardization

It has long been apparent that there is a considerable need for an agreed standardization of the methods, techniques and procedures employed, such as the definition of clinical signs and suggested anthropometric standards of reference, and of the presentation and interpretation of results, so that some degree of uniformity and comparability can be attained between studies carried out in various parts of the world or at different times.

This need was recognized by the WHO Expert Committee on Medical Assessment of Nutritional Status (1963), which recommended as follows:

> There is an urgent need for a standard guide which would give detailed instructions about planning and conducting nutrition surveys, and the reporting of results, and which would contain information of assistance to the correct interpretation of results. The Committee strongly recommends that WHO undertake the preparation of a manual to meet this need.

With this recommendation in mind, the present publication is concerned with methods that can be employed for assessing the nutritional status of a community, especially by means of prevalence surveys, and in particular, the clinical, anthropometric, biochemical and dietary procedures that can be employed in the difficult circumstances often found in developing regions of the world.

Orientation

The present monograph is principally directed to the field worker, and especially to the medical officer, the nutritionist and the public health nurse faced with the practical problems of attempting the assessment of the nutritional state of a community in a less developed tropical country.

Malnutrition has recently been defined as a pathological state resulting from a relative or absolute deficiency or excess of one or more essential nutrients, this state being clinically manifested or detected only by biochemical, anthropometric or physiological tests. Four forms should be distinguished:

(a) *Undernutrition*—the pathological state resulting from the consumption of an inadequate quantity of food over an extended period of time. Marasmus and inanition are synonymous with severe undernutrition; starvation implies the almost total elimination of food, and hence the rapid development of severe undernutrition, marasmus or inanition.

(b) *Specific deficiency*—the pathological state resulting from a relative or absolute lack of an individual nutrient.

(c) *Overnutrition*—the pathological state resulting from the consumption of an excessive quantity of food, and hence a caloric excess, over an extended period of time.

(d) *Imbalance*—the pathological state resulting from a disproportion among essential nutrients, with or without the absolute deficiency of any nutrient as determined by the requirements of a balanced diet (Scrimshaw, Taylor & Gordon, in press).

This monograph is mainly concerned with those problems of malnutrition which are often substantial causes of illness and death in developing regions of the world—those due to undernutrition, specific deficiency and imbalance. Problems of overnutrition are touched on only briefly, although it is realized that they are responsible for increasing morbidity and mortality in the better-fed parts of the world.

The methods suggested are often somewhat crude. They are, however, attempts to translate laboratory research findings into simple and practical, if usually approximate, methods. They are not necessarily suitable for individual diagnoses, but they are adapted to field work and useful for obtaining broad, outline levels of information aimed at the nutritional diagnosis of the population groups making up the community.

Simplicity and practicability are therefore paramount considerations. The aim is always to obtain the maximum of useful information, using a minimum of staff, inexpensive equipment and uncomplicated techniques that can be analysed easily.

Obviously, the complex laboratory procedures, the detailed, time-consuming clinical examinations and the mathematically guided anthropo-metry sometimes practicable in major hospitals and centres are seldom appropriate, although it is largely from this type of work that the basic information that can be used in simple field tests is derived. By these means, for example, the principal clinical signs of a particular form of malnutrition come to be recognized, and subsequently can be suggested as possible nutritional indicators in field surveys.

Although it is hoped that the present publication will be of interest and some practical usefulness to all workers in the field of public health nutrition, the main emphasis is given to the nutritional problems of " vulnerable groups " in developing regions of the world, in particular to those of early childhood. This is right and proper, as the magnitude of the problem of protein-calorie malnutrition of early childhood dwarfs all others on the present-day nutritional world stage.

2   Direct Nutritional Assessment of Human Groups *

CLINICAL SIGNS

Clinical examination has always been, and remains, an important practical method for assessing the nutritional status of a community.

Essentially, the method is based on examination for changes, believed to be related to inadequate nutrition, that can be seen or felt in superficial epithelial tissues, especially the skin, eyes, hair and buccal mucosa, or in organs near the surface of the body, such as the parotids and thyroid glands. Occasionally, this may be supplemented in the field by certain physical tests, with or without instrumental aids, such as the testing of ankle jerks.

This method of assessment, based on the recognition of certain physical signs, has the advantage of relative inexpensiveness, as neither elaborate field equipment nor a costly laboratory is needed. Also, with very careful training and continuing supervision, junior personnel can be taught to recognize certain crucial clinical signs.

Clinical assessment of a community can give valuable, if approximate, objective information to the public health worker, especially in regions of the world where malnutrition, and hence more clear-cut nutritional stigmata, are widespread. The value of the method decreases as the nutritional plane of the community improves.

However, even in some tropical communities, actual clinical signs of malnutrition may be uncommon, although anthropometry may show malnutrition to be widespread, while in certain nutritional disorders, such as acute infantile beriberi, clinical examination plays little or no part in the assessment of prevalence (Wadsworth, 1963).

The cheapness and relatively easy organization of nutritional assessment by means of clinical examination have sometimes led to the assumption that the method is simple, quickly mastered by the beginner, and yields

---

* Discussion in this chapter is much influenced by previous work on this subject (Bigwood, 1939; Darby et al., 1953; Jolliffe et al., 1958; Plough, 1962; Rao, 1961; Sinclair, 1948; ICNND, 1963; Sebrell et al., 1959; WHO Expert Committee on Medical Assessment of Nutritional Status, 1963), and by descriptions in standard works (Jolliffe, 1962; Davidson & Passmore, 1963). The survey reports of the ICNND (1959a, 1959b, 1960a, 1960b, 1961a, 1961b, 1962a, 1962b, 1962c, 1962d) have also been most useful for this chapter and throughout the monograph.

results that are easy to interpret. This is not the case. Like any other form of assessment, the method has its own limitations, which must be known if the full benefit is to be obtained from its application. Certain common problems, difficulties and potential " non-sampling " errors, due to procedural error and observer bias, which are often inadequately appreciated, need to be emphasized.

Lack of Specificity of Clinical Signs

While a few physical signs are pathognomonic of certain specific nutritional deficiency syndromes, as with the " flaky-paint " dermatosis in kwashiorkor, this is usually not the case.

Various non-nutritional environmental influences can sometimes be responsible for identical appearances. For example, the clinical picture of angular stomatitis, often incorrectly considered pathognomonic of ariboflavinosis, can result in India from the excessive chewing of betel nut preparations *(pan)* containing large amounts of irritant lime. Again, generalized dryness of the skin, especially of the legs, with a similar appearance to xerosis, can occur in very hot, dry, windy regions; probably solely as a result of these climatic factors.

Furthermore, it is now appreciated that almost all the signs usually recorded lack nutrient specificity. Bitot's spots, classically considered as pathognomonic of vitamin-A deficiency, can sometimes be due to other causes, possibly including chronic conjunctival trauma from smoke, dust, glare and eye infections (Darby et al., 1960; Rodger et al., 1963; McLaren, 1963). Glossitis can be seen in niacin, folic acid, vitamin-B_{12}, or riboflavin deficiencies.

In fact, most signs of malnutrition are not specific to lack of one nutrient, and can often be produced by various non-nutritional factors. Frequently, they have a complex etiology, with the nature of some of the underlying factors and interrelationships still unknown (Beaton, 1964). They cannot be pigeon-holed under a single cause as can some signs found in certain infectious diseases, as with Koplik's spots in measles.

A few signs may be " two-directional " in that they can occur both in deficiency or during recovery. For example, parotid enlargement, hepatomegaly and gynaecomastia, are seen occasionally in the course of treatment of protein-calorie malnutrition, as well as in malnourished subjects (Oomen, 1957a).

The association of these signs with biochemical and other tests may help to identify the lacking nutrient or nutrients responsible for a given lesion, but the commonly found simultaneous deficiency of many nutrients in diets may render the final specific diagnosis difficult. It is in such instances that double-blind therapeutic trials on a small scale may be useful, if carried out under strictly controlled conditions.

Nutritional Relevance of Commonly Recorded Signs

In the past, a large number of ill-defined signs have often been recorded in the course of clinical nutritional surveys. More recent experience in different parts of the world has suggested that many of these are, in fact, not related to malnutrition at all. The report of the WHO Expert Committee on Medical Assessment of Nutritional Status (1963) suggests the classification of signs often recorded into the following three groups:

Group 1. Signs that are considered to be of value in nutritional assessment, as, according to present evidence, they indicate with considerable probability deficiency of one or more nutrients in the tissues in the recent past;

Group 2. Signs that need further investigation, but in whose causation malnutrition, sometimes of a chronic nature, may play some part, together with other factors. They are found more commonly in people with low standards of living than among more privileged groups;

Group 3. Signs not related to nutrition, according to present knowledge, but which, in some instances, have to be differentiated from signs of known nutritional value (Group 1).

This type of classification (Table 1) can help the field worker to choose the most useful selection of signs to record in a particular survey, whether

TABLE 1. CLASSIFIED LIST OF SIGNS USED IN NUTRITION SURVEYS *

	Group 1: Signs known to be of value in nutrition surveys	Group 2: Signs that need further investigation	Group 3: Some signs not related to nutrition
1. Hair	Lack of lustre Thinness and sparseness Straightness Dyspigmentation Flag sign Easy pluckability		Alopecia Artificial discoloration
2. Face	Diffuse depigmentation Naso-labial dyssebacea Moon-face	Malar and supra-orbital pigmentation	Acne vulgaris Acne rosacea Chloasma
3. Eyes	Pale conjunctiva Bitot's spots Conjunctival xerosis Corneal xerosis Keratomalacia Angular palpebritis	Conjunctival injection Conjunctival and scleral pigmentation Corneal vascularization Circumcorneal injection Corneal opacities and scars	Follicular conjunctivitis Blepharitis Pingueculae Pterygium Panr.u₃
4. Lips	Angular stomatitis Angular scars Cheilosis	Chronic depigmentation of lower lip	Chapping from exposure to harsh climates
5. Tongue	Oedema Scarlet and raw tongue Magenta tongue Atrophic papillae	Hyperaemic and hypertrophic papillae Fissures Geographic tongue Pigmented tongue	Aphthous ulcer Leucoplakia

TABLE 1. CLASSIFIED LIST OF SIGNS USED IN NUTRITION SURVEYS (*continued*)

	Group 1: Signs known to be of value in nutrition surveys	Group 2: Signs that need further investigation	Group 3: Some signs not related to nutrition
6. Teeth	Mottled enamel	Caries Attrition Enamel hypoplasia Enamel erosion	Malocclusion
7. Gums	Spongy, bleeding gums	Recession of gum	Pyorrhoea
8. Glands	Thyroid enlargement Parotid enlargement	Gynaecomastia	Allergic or inflammatory enlargement of thyroid or parotid
9. Skin	Xerosis Follicular hyperkeratosis, types 1 and 2 Petechiae Pellagrous dermatosis Flaky-paint dermatosis Scrotal and vulval dermatosis	Mosaic dermatosis Thickening and pigmenta- tion of pressure points Intertriginous lesions	Ichthyosis Acneiform eruptions Miliaria Epidermophytoses Sunburn Onchocercal dermatosis
10. Nails	Koilonychia	Brittle, ridged nails	
11. Sub- cutaneous tissue	Oedema Amount of subcutaneous fat		
12. Muscular and skeletal systems	Muscle wasting Craniotabes Frontal and parietal bossing Epiphyseal enlargement (tender or painless) Beading of ribs Persistently open anterior fontanelle Knock-knees or bow-legs Diffuse or local skeletal deformities Deformities of thorax (selected) Musculo-skeletal haemorrhages	Winged scapulae	Funnel chest
13. Internal systems: (*a*) Gastro- intestinal	Hepatomegaly		Splenomegaly
(*b*) Nervous [a]	Psychomotor change Mental confusion Sensory loss Motor weakness Loss of position sense Loss of vibratory sense Loss of ankle and knee jerks Calf tenderness	Condition of ocular fundus	
(*c*) Cardio- vascular	Cardiac enlargement Tachycardia	Blood pressure	

* Adapted from WHO Expert Committee on Medical Assessment of Nutritional Status (1963).

[a] Both lathyrism (Patwardhan, 1961) and the group of "tropical neuropathies" described by Cruickshank (1947, 1961), Money (1959), Latham (1964) and others are probably part of nutritional etiology. If they are sought in community surveys, further neurological tests will be required.

the survey be limited in scope and aimed at rapid clinical screening of the community, or consist of a research project, possibly including an evaluation of less certain signs (Group 2). Recognition and elimination of signs unrelated to nutrition (Group 3) will obviate confusion in interpretation and save considerable time and effort.

As a generalization, it is usually better to limit the list of signs sought for in a survey to those considered essential. Experience suggests that accuracy and reliability are often inversely proportional to the number of signs included.

Future investigations may, of course, show that the significance of some of the signs listed may have to be reappraised. Similarly, newly recognized signs considered to be related to malnutrition will be described in the future and will have to be included in the appropriate group. If they are used in surveys, they must be carefully defined, both before the actual field work and in the subsequent report.

Definition and Standardization

The physical signs recorded must always be defined as precisely as practicable. Otherwise, as has often happened in the past, the meaning of data from various parts of the world is in doubt, and comparability between the results of different observers or between the findings of the same investigator at different times is impossible.

Standardization of definition of commonly employed physical signs is obviously especially necessary for international comparison, and a descriptive list is therefore given in the present section of the report. It is based on the 1963 report of the WHO Expert Committee on Medical Assessment of Nutritional Status, but has been expanded to give fuller descriptive detail.

As well as careful written definitions, clear unambiguous photographs are needed. Those given in the present monograph are intended both for training purposes and also as a standard practical guide for use during actual field work.

The definitions of the signs to be used need to be available in *written* form for team members. Before undertaking a survey, the team must be given instruction and practical visual training in their recognition in order to ensure uniformity of judgement and understanding. The use of colour transparencies and, in some instances, a preliminary pilot field study can be most valuable in this respect. Staff members working under close supervision can have their techniques and results tested and compared.

With this in mind, the Inter-departmental Committee on Nutrition for National Development (ICNND) recommends planned standardization sessions before, and at intervals during, the survey. At these, each examiner independently records his clinical findings on 100 persons. Further spot checks are also valuable at intervals during the course of the survey, employing the written definitions agreed upon. Results are compared and inconsistencies investigated (ICNND, 1963).

At the same time, it is well recognized that the appearances of some nutritional signs are difficult to describe with scientific precision and objectivity, and these, for the most part, should not be employed in survey work. Thus, " diffuse depigmentation of the skin " can represent, in less marked instances, no more than a subjective judgement, based on experience and local genetic possibilities. In particular, the general grading of subjects into " good ", " fair ", or " poor " by physical inspection is even more difficult to assess objectively, based as it is on numerous factors, such as the amount of muscle and subcutaneous fat present, posture, pallor and behaviour; and it is often influenced subconsciously by the examiner's own body build, his recent experiences in the field of nutrition, and the cultural concept of a desirable physique in his own community. Still less possible is the assessment of the nutriture of schoolchildren by such indefinite subjective features as " carriage—erect, slack or slovenly ".

Another well-documented, serious difficulty is that the observer is subconsciously prone to interpret signs on the spot, and to change his own criteria from time to time, depending on the group he is examining. If, for example, a sign is found to be common in a certain group, but rare in the one previously examined, there is a tendency to alter the diagnostic criteria and to record grosser degrees of the sign (Sinclair, 1948). For example, physicians are inclined to alter their standards of judgement of normal physique rather rapidly if they are constantly studying a lean or an obese population (ICNND, 1963).

The problem of standardization can be aggravated by ill-advised attempts to grade the signs recorded into different degrees of positiveness (e.g. 0 to $+++$). Under field circumstances, and with some exceptions (such as the estimation of thyroid enlargement), it is usually not only impossible, but also time-consuming, frustrating and pseudo-scientific, to attempt to differentiate *degrees* of severity of the physical signs noted. A record of a positive or a negative is usually the best that can be achieved.

Theoretically, certain signs can be estimated quantitatively and objectively using objective mechanical instruments. For example, the gums may be tested for bleeding by the use of a spring-loaded probe that can exert a standard pressure (Sinclair, 1948), or a special apparatus can measure tendon jerks quantitatively (ICNND, 1962a). Similarly, an apparatus might be devised to test for oedema. In practice, however, these procedures are usually manually performed without special equipment.

In addition to the standardization of definition, it is important that the technique of examination should be described. The skin of the whole body should be examined, as some lesions are found most commonly on the buttocks or perineum; if this is not practicable, a note should be made to this effect. Clinical assessment must always be carried out with good illumination, preferably with indirect sunlight.

Descriptive List of Selected Clinical Signs

The following descriptive list of physical signs is based on the 1963 report of the WHO Expert Committee on Medical Assessment of Nutritional Status, but has been expanded slightly to include some additional comments and fuller explanation. It is given as an aid towards achieving uniformity of terminology and the standardization of results obtained by different investigators.

Most of the signs given are believed to be of value in the clinical assessment of malnutrition (Group 1). A few are included which are of uncertain significance nutritionally (Group 2); others are probably not nutritionally significant, but require to be differentiated (Group 3).

In this list, no attempt is usually made to link particular signs with specific nutrient deficiencies. Suggested groupings of signs in relation to specific deficiencies are given later (see p. 43).

The order of arrangement of the list of signs also follows the WHO Expert Committee's report, and is related to the common practice of examining subjects from head to foot.

1. Hair

Group 1

Lack of lustre. The hair is dull and dry. As with all hair changes, comparison has to be made with local normal standards in healthy subjects. The effect of scalp disease, such as extensive fungus infection or impetigo, of certain cultural practices, especially the use of oil on the hair, and of some environmental factors, such as exposure to salt water and a very hot dry atmosphere, must also be taken into account.

Thinness and sparseness (Fig. 1 (*a*) and (*b*)). The hair may become thin —that is, fine and silky in texture—and sparse—that is, covering the scalp less abundantly and completely, and with wider gaps between hairs. Allowance must be made for local practices in the treatment of hair; as, for example, with the sparseness that can result in adult women in parts of Africa from the tight braiding of hair into many short pigtails, with resultant " tension alopecia ". A similar frontal baldness appears to occur in older Chinese women, possibly as a result of the traditional combed-back hair style.

Straightness. In some ethnic groups, with normally curly hair, malnutrition may produce pathological straightness. This is especially noticeable in negro children, for whom normal healthy hair is in thick tight curls. Colour changes of some degree and easy pluckability are usually also present.

FIG. 1. THIN SPARSE HAIR

(a) Adult   (b) Pre-school child

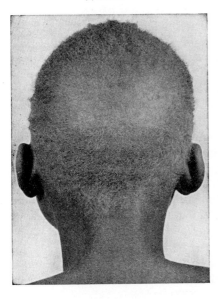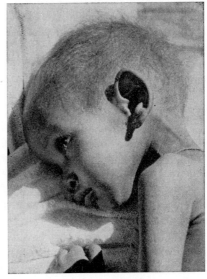

FIG. 2. DYSPIGMENTED HAIR   FIG. 3. FLAG SIGN IN HAIR

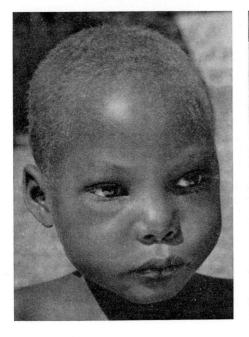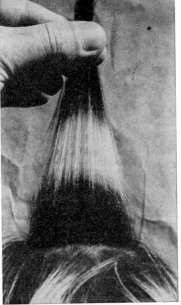

Dyspigmentation of the hair (Fig. 2). The hair shows a distinct lightening of its normal colour, most usually evident distally. Again, normal standards will vary with the particular ethnic group; sometimes the mother, if well nourished, may be immediately available as a living colour standard for her children. The sign is a common feature of some forms of protein-calorie malnutrition in young children, and is due to disturbance in melanogenesis. Normal hair colour returns following protein feeding. The term " dyspigmentation " is employed rather than " hypochromotrichia ", as there may be, in some instances, an abnormal pigmentation, as well as a lightening of colour.

Various changes of colour may be found. In subjects with normally black hair, the changes usually seen in decreasing order of frequency are dark brown, light brown, red-brown, blonde and grey. Difficulties with precise estimations of shade of hair are related to observer error and to the occurrence of a gradation of colour changes. Mechanical grading may be possible with hair samples, using a reflectometer (Harrison et al., 1964).

It is not usually necessary to group the different types of colour change seen. Where this is required—as it may be for research purposes—attempts have been made to grade the hair colours seen with colour charts used by paint manufacturers, artists, wool firms and even beauty salons. None has been found to be satisfactory, as the colours displayed do not approximate to those seen in malnutrition. It may be more satisfactory to prepare a local hair-colour guide made up of clear-cut specimens of the most usual shades of dyspigmented hair seen. These can be stuck to a piece of white cardboard with transparent cellotape, and used on the survey.

Numerous problems arise in the assessment of dyspigmented hair. It may be customary for children of one or both sexes to have their hair cut short or shaved, so that the hair colour is not apparent. Local factors may be important, such as dyeing, the effect of sunshine, salt-spray and dust, genetic factors and the habitual use of oil.

Confusion has arisen between different workers because some have recorded this sign as positive when only the tips of the hair or the fringe of scalp hair (" fair frontal fringe " or " halo effect ") are affected.

It is suggested that dyspigmentation should be noted only if all the area of the scalp is affected, including the middle third of a lock in the parietal area (Falkner, 1960). If lesser degrees are recorded, the exact definition should be given.

Flag sign (Fig. 3). This hair change, found in young children and first reported from South America as *signa de bandera*, is usually uncommon. It is characterized by alternating bands of light and dark colour along the length of the hair, and reflects alternating episodes of protein-calorie malnutrition and cure. It has been described in Arab children, and especially in South and Central America. It does not appear to be seen commonly elsewhere.

Easy pluckability. In this sign, a small clump or tuft of hair can be easily pulled out with moderate force and without pain. In extreme examples, this looseness of the hair is a striking finding, easily demonstrated. In less advanced cases, it is often most marked in the temporal region, but is a difficult sign to judge objectively, as it plainly depends on the force applied to the clump of hair by the examiner's thumb and forefinger.

It is usually accompanied by other hair changes, such as dyspigmentation, thinness, and sparseness, and occurs in kwashiorkor and other forms of protein-calorie malnutrition in early childhood. The easy pluckability and the sparseness are both related to a looseness of hairs in their follicles.

2. Face

Group 1

Diffuse depigmentation (Fig. 4). A general lightening of colour of the pigment of the skin of the face can occur, and may sometimes be exaggerated by associated underlying anaemia. In protein-calorie malnutrition, it is usually first and most easily noticeable on the face, centrally rather than laterally. As usual with estimations of colour change, lesser degrees are difficult to determine precisely, while genetic influences may sometimes be relevant. Its etiology is probably similar to that of dyspigmented hair—that is, interference with melanogenesis. Both are found in protein-calorie malnutrition in young children, especially in kwashiorkor, in which condition the skin slowly darkens following treatment with protein foods.

Naso-labial dyssebacea (Plate I A). The lesion consists of dry greasy filiform excrescences, greyish, yellowish or pale in colour, most commonly located in the naso-labial folds. They may also be seen in the bridge of the nose, eyebrows and back of the ears. They are produced by plugging of the ducts of the enlarged sebaceous glands by retained sebum, which accounts for the scaly greasiness produced.

Moon-face (Fig. 5). This is a peculiar rounded prominence of the cheeks, which protrude over the general level of the naso-labial folds. The mouth presents a pursed-in appearance. The condition is encountered mostly in the pre-school child with protein-calorie malnutrition of the kwashiorkor type. Pitting on pressure does not occur.

3. Eyes [1]

Eye signs have to be considered in relation to the possible effects of chronic ocular trauma from a combination of bright sunlight, dust, wind, smoke and infection.

---

[1] The definitions are based on descriptions given by McLaren (1963), Oomen, McLaren & Escapini (1964), and McLaren, Oomen & Escapini (1966).

FIG. 4. DEPIGMENTED SKIN, COMPARED WITH NORMAL CHILD

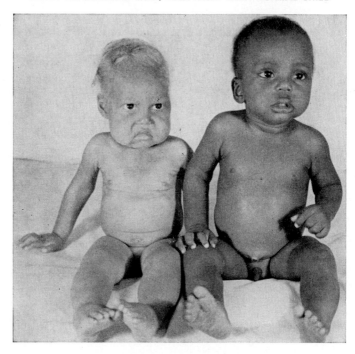

FIG. 5. MOON-FACE

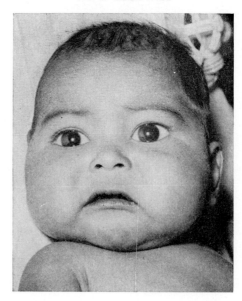

Group 1

Pale conjunctiva. This sign is positive if there is pallor of the conjunctival and buccal mucosae. It is principally a clinical reflection of severe anaemia.

Conjunctival xerosis (Plate I B). This condition is characterized by dryness, thickening, pigmentation and lack of lustre and transparency of the bulbar conjunctiva of the exposed part of the eyeball. A few seconds' exposure by drawing back the lids will aid in its identification.

Small, more or less vertical, dry folds of the conjunctiva can best be demonstrated by rucking up the loose temporal conjunctiva against the outer canthus with the eye in full external movement. The xerotic conjunctiva is not wetted by tears.

The process is due to keratinization affecting the cells of the conjunctival epithelium.

Bitot's spots (Fig. 6).[1] These are usually well-demarcated, superficial, dry, greyish, silvery or chalky-white foamy plaques, often triangular or irregularly circular in shape, more often confined to the regions lateral to the cornea and rarely overlying it. They are usually bilateral, and are composed of keratinized epithelial debris, which can be removed by firm wiping, revealing a xerotic conjunctival bed with a rough surface.

Bitot's spots may accompany the generalized conjunctival xerosis described above. They are then usually part of the ocular manifestations of vitamin-A deficiency, and the subject is most commonly a pre-school child or infant. However, Bitot's spots are also frequently observed, usually in school-age children and adults, as isolated and often minimal lesions in subjects with no evidence of vitamin-A deficiency.

Corneal xerosis (Plate I C). The cornea is hazy or opaque, frequently with a bluish milky appearance, usually most marked in the lower central area. It is due in part to cellular infiltration of the corneal stroma. Corneal xerosis is usually accompanied by conjunctival xerosis. Both corneae usually show change, sometimes to a widely varying degree. Photophobia, pain and inflammatory congestion are not usually present.

Keratomalacia (Plates I C and II A; Fig. 7). This consists of a characteristic softening (colliquative necrosis) of the entire thickness of part or more often the whole of the cornea, leading to perforation and iris prolapse.

Keratomalacia is usually bilateral, but often with unequal involvement of the two eyes. Xerosis of the conjunctiva is usually, though not invariably, present. The condition is essentially quiet and insidious, with no pain or other complaints, and no secretion or discharge. It can occur " behind closed eyelids " (McLaren, 1966).

The process is a rapid one, the corneal structure melting into a cloudy gelatinous mass, which may be dead-white or dirty-yellow in colour.

---

[1] Also known in the Russian literature as Iskerskii's patches (Shevalev, 1962).

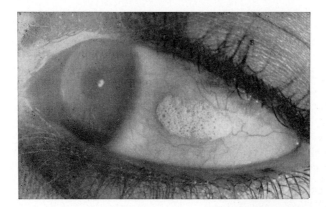

FIG. 6. BITOT'S SPOT

FIG. 7. KERATOMALACIA (LATE, WITH NECROSIS OF CORNEA)

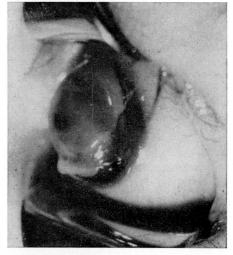

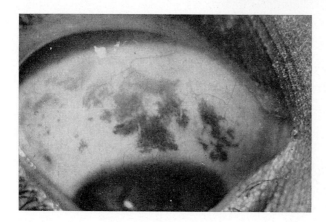

FIG. 8. SCLERAL PIG-MENTATION

Extrusion of the lens and loss of vitreous may occur; in untreated cases, panophthalmitis not infrequently supervenes.

Angular palpebritis (angular blepharitis) (Plate II B). The lesion is characterized by excoriation and fissuring of the external canthi, and it is often associated with angular stomatitis.

Group 2

Corneal vascularization (Plate II B). This represents an invasion of all quadrants or the whole of the periphery of the cornea by fine capillary blood vessels. Early changes can be defined only by biomicroscopic examination. It is due to congestion of the normal limbal plexus. It is non-specific and can occur in any inflammatory or irritative process affecting the cornea.

Conjunctival injection and circumcorneal injection. The terms are self-explanatory.

Conjunctival and scleral pigmentation (Fig. 8). The nature and location should be described. The following classification is suggested by McLaren (1963).

(*a*) Diffuse conjunctival pigmentation. A generalized brownish pigmentation of the bulbar conjunctiva, most marked in the interpalpebral fissure. The condition is common in older children and adults in dark-skinned peoples and is of no significance. In young children, however, it is abnormal if marked, and is then usually associated with xerosis conjunctivae (see above).

(*b*) Speckled areas of pigment, associated with healed Bitot's spots.

(*c*) Circumcorneal pigment ring.

(*d*) Particles of blue-black choroidal pigment visible through gaps in the sclera around the perforating branches of the anterior ciliary arteries.

Items (*c*) and (*d*) have no nutritional significance.

Corneal opacities and scars. Their nature (fine or dense, deep or superficial) and position (which quadrant of the cornea) should be noted. They may result from previous infection, including ophthalmia neonatorum, trachoma and congenital syphilis, from trauma or from malnutrition, especially from past avitaminosis A, which can leave the eye damaged with nebulae, leucomata, anterior staphylomata or phthisis bulbi (Oomen, McLaren & Escapini, 1964; McLaren, Oomen & Escapini, 1966).

Group 3

Pingueculae (Fig. 9). These are unilateral or bilateral, whitish or yellowish circumscribed thickenings of the conjunctiva. They are yellowish accumulations of fatty material, generally on the lateral side of the sclera, placed close to the corneal margin. They are more common in adults than in children, and occur both in well-nourished and in poorly-fed communities.

FIG. 9. PINGUECULA

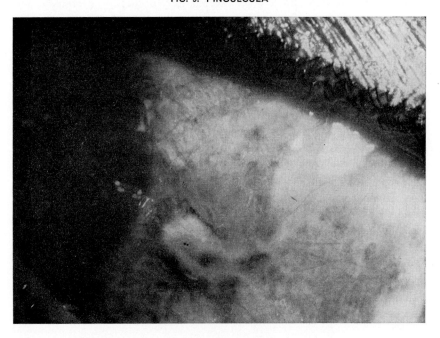

FIG. 10. PTERYGIUM

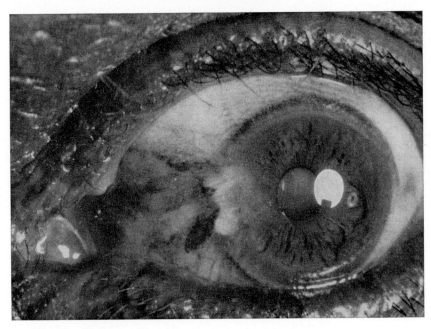

PLATE I

A. DYSSEBACEA

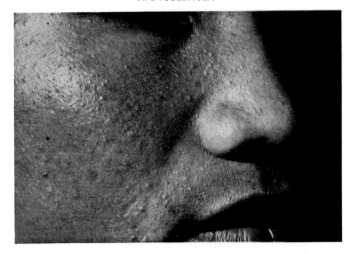

B. CONJUNCTIVAL XEROSIS

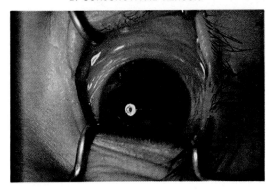

C. CORNEAL XEROSIS AND EARLY KERATOMALACIA

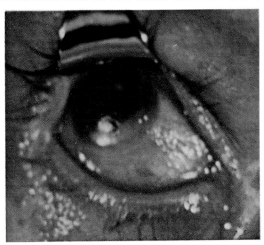

PLATE II

A. KERATOMALACIA INVOLVING WHOLE CORNEA

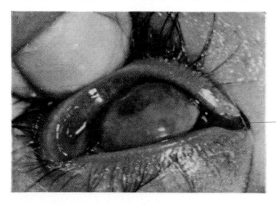

B. CORNEAL VASCULARIZATION WITH ANGULAR PALPEBRITIS

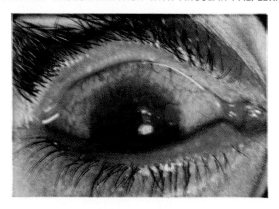

C. ANGULAR STOMATITIS

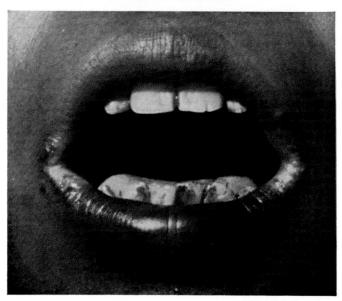

PLATE III

A. ATROPHIC PAPILLAE

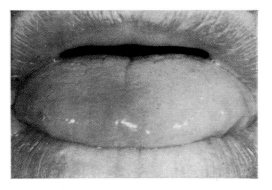

B. FISSURES OF THE TONGUE

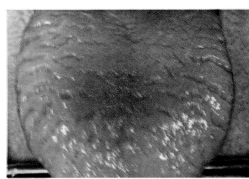

C. EARLY MOTTLING OF THE TEETH
(WHITE PATCHES)

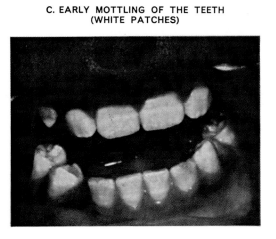

D. LATE MOTTLING OF THE UPPER INCISORS

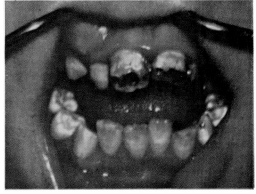

PLATE IV

A. SPONGY BLEEDING GUMS

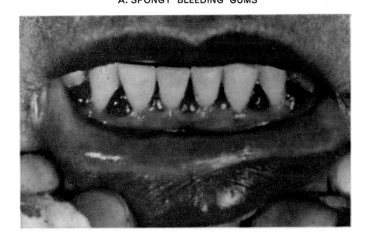

B. PYORRHOEA

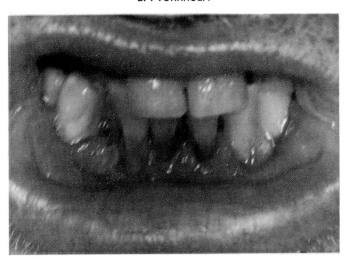

C. ACUTE PELLAGROUS DERMATOSIS ON FOREARMS AND HANDS

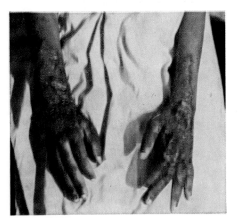

D. CHRONIC PELLAGROUS DERMATOSIS ON FOREARMS

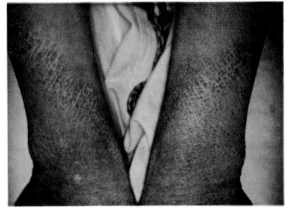

Pingueculae are intra-conjunctival, while Bitot's spots are epithelial in origin and are superficial plaques lying *on* the conjunctiva.

Pterygium (Fig. 10). This lesion, so-called because of its wing-shaped appearance, is produced by a fleshy double fold of conjunctiva, growing progressively laterally across the cornea. Its cause is unknown, but appears to be related to prolonged irritation, as from sun-glare. It has no nutritional significance.

Pannus. This is a characteristic lesion of infection of the cornea with the trachoma virus. It is due to invasion of the cornea by blood vessels and infiltration. If advanced, it has the clinical appearance of a superficial opacity of the cornea, especially in its upper part. In early cases, vessels which are always present can be seen only with a biomicroscope.

4. Lips

Group 1

Angular stomatitis (Plate II C). The term is used to describe sodden and excoriated lesions associated with fissuring at the angles of the mouth. The fissures may be shallow or deep, confined to a small area of the angles of the mouth or extending into the buccal cavity and a few millimetres onto the skin outside. Milder lesions are discerned more easily with the mouth half open. The sign should be reported as positive only if both angles of the mouth are involved.

Angular scars. Healed angular stomatitis may result in pink or blanched scars at the angles of the mouth, depending on the interval since the acute episode. In older children, the possibility of the scars being healed rhagades of congenital syphilis requires consideration.

Cheilosis (Fig. 11). This lesion is characterized by vertical fissuring, later complicated by redness, swelling and ulceration of the lips, other than the angles. The centre of the lower lip is most usually affected. Climatic factors, such as cold and wind, may sometimes be responsible.

Group 2

Chronic depigmentation of the lower lip. This is usually central and may, in some cases, represent the site of an old, healed cheilosis.

5. Tongue

Signs in the mouth affecting the tongue or gums must be considered in relation to local trauma, as from spicy foods and false teeth, as well as to nutritional deficiency.

Group 1

Oedema of tongue. This can be detected by the indentations made by pressure of teeth along the edges of the tongue.

3

FIG. 11. CHEILOSIS

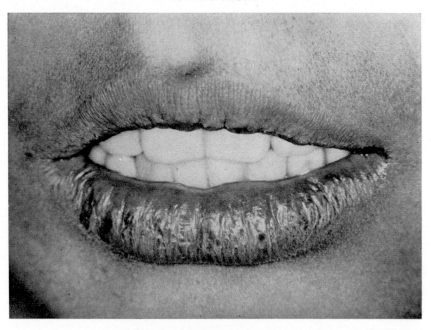

FIG. 12. HYPERTROPHIC PAPILLAE

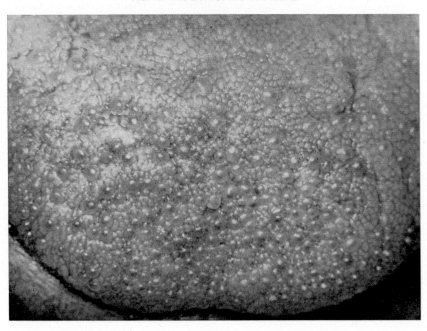

Scarlet and raw tongue. The tongue is bright red in colour, usually of normal size or slightly atrophic, denuded and very painful.

Magenta tongue. The tongue is purplish red in colour; numerous morphological changes may co-exist.

Atrophic papillae (Plate III A). The filiform papillae have disappeared, giving the tongue an extremely smooth appearance. The distribution may be central or marginal. Permanent records of the lesion can be made with " tongue prints ", although this is rarely practicable or necessary.

Group 2

Hyperaemic and hypertrophic papillae (Fig. 12). The papillae are hypertrophic and red or pink, and give the tongue a granular or pebbly appearance (red strawberry).

Fissures (Plate III B). Cracks on the surface of the tongue with no papillae on their sides or floors. These must not be confused with the congenital ridging and convoluted appearance known as " scrotal tongue ", which has no nutritional significance.

Geographic tongue. The tongue has irregularly distributed patchy areas of denudation and atrophy of epithelium. It is painless and symptomless. Its etiology is obscure and no treatment appears to be effective.

Pigmented tongue. Punctate or patchy areas of blue-black mucosal pigmentation are present, sometimes associated with similar patches on the gums. Present evidence suggests that they are of no significance (Raper, 1948).

6. Teeth [1]

Group 1

Mottled enamel (Plate III C and D; Fig. 13). The teeth are mottled with white and brownish patches, with or without erosion or pitting of the enamel, usually best seen in the upper incisors. Various other conditions, genetic and of other etiologies, can also produce mottling, and the differential diagnosis between mild fluorosis and non-fluoride opacities has been given by Russell (1961) (Table 2) and by Dean (1934, 1942).

Group 2

Caries. The presence of decayed, missing or filled teeth (DMF) is often used to record the amount of caries present in a community, although teeth may be missing for other reasons, including chronic pyorrhoea, trauma, or —in parts of rural Africa—removal because of local custom.

---

[1] Details of methods and techniques for specialist dental surveys are given in the report of the WHO Expert Committee on Dental Health (1962).

TABLE 2. DIFFERENTIAL DIAGNOSIS: MILDER FORMS OF DENTAL FLUOROSIS
(QUESTIONABLE, VERY MILD, AND MILD) AND NON-FLUORIDE
OPACITIES OF ENAMEL*

	Milder forms of fluorosis	Non-fluoride enamel opacities
Area affected	Usually seen on or near tips of cusps or incisal edges	Usually centred on smooth surface; may affect entire crown
Shape of lesion	Resembles line shading in pencil sketch; lines follow incremental lines in enamel, form irregular caps on cusps	Often round or oval
Demarcation	Shades off imperceptibly into surround-ing normal enamel	Clearly differentiated from adjacent normal enamel
Colour	Slightly more opaque than normal enamel; " paper-white." Incisal edges, tips of cusps may have frosted appear-ance. Does not show stain at time of eruption (in these milder degrees, rarely at any time)	Usually pigmented at time of erup-tion; often creamy-yellow to dark reddish-orange
Teeth affected	Most frequent on teeth that calcify slowly (cuspids, bicuspids, second and third molars). Rare on lower incisors. Usually seen on six or eight homologous teeth. Extremely rare in deciduous teeth	Any tooth may be affected. Frequent on labial surfaces of lower incisors. May occur singly. Usually one to three teeth affected. Common in deciduous teeth
Gross hypoplasia	None. Pitting of enamel does not occur in the milder forms. Enamel surface has glazed appearance, is smooth to point of explorer	Absent to severe. Enamel surface may seem etched, be rough to explorer
Detection	Often invisible under strong light; most easily detected by line of sight tangen-tial to tooth crown	Seen most easily under strong light on line of sight perpendicular to tooth surface

* Reproduced by permission from Russell (1961).

In children in most tropical areas with inadequate dental services, only the presence of decayed teeth with cavities can be recorded. The method of examination must also be noted. This will usually be by inspection alone.

The prevalence of caries is suggested by the percentage of the adult population with one or more teeth decayed or missing or filled (DMF), or, in the case of children, of those with one or more teeth decayed or filled (DF). The intensity of caries in a community is calculated by the average number of DMF teeth per person.

While malnutrition in the pregnant woman plays a part in the etiology of caries in the first dentition, caries in both deciduous and permanent teeth is more related to local effects of the foods consumed, especially to the dietary content and frequency of ingestion of sugar, over-milled flour and other highly refined carbohydrate foods.

Attrition (Fig. 14). The cutting borders of incisors and molars may be worn down and flattened. This seems related principally to the toughness

FIG. 13. LATE MOTTLING

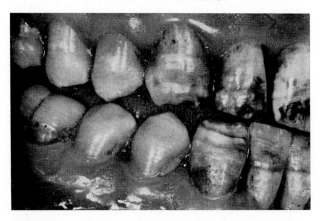

FIG. 14. DENTAL ATTRITION

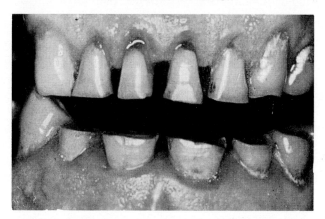

FIG. 15. ENAMEL HYPOPLASIA

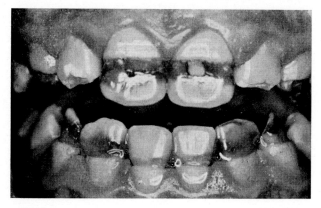

of the diet, especially its content of hard foods requiring prolonged masti-
cation.

Enamel hypoplasia (Fig. 15). Defective formation is usually generalized
over the tooth surface, especially the medial third.

Enamel erosion (Fig. 15). The term describes the sharply defined areas,
usually around the gum margin, where the tooth enamel has become eroded.

7. Gums

Group 1

Spongy, bleeding gums (Plate IV A). Purplish or red spongy swelling of
the interdental papillae and/or the gum margins, which usually bleed easily
on slight pressure.

This sign can occur with chronic intoxication with certain drugs, especially hydantoinates. It is absent even in cases of severe lack of ascorbic acid
in young children (infantile scurvy) until the teeth have erupted.

Group 2

Recession of gums. Atrophy and recession of the gums occur sometimes,
exposing the roots of the teeth. This is usually secondary to pyorrhoea.

Group 3

Pyorrhoea (Plate IV B). Suppuration of gum margins, which are red and
bleed easily with no hypertrophy.

8. Glands

Group 1

Thyroid enlargement (Fig. 16-19). The gland is visibly and palpably
enlarged. The enlargement may be diffuse or nodular. Inspection and
palpation while the subject swallows may be helpful in diagnosis.

For more specialized endemic goitre surveys, the technique and classification of Perez, Scrimshaw & Munoz (1960) should be followed. In this
classification, three grades are recognized:

(*a*) Grade 1—persons with palpable goitres. The thyroid is probably
enlarged more than four to five times, although not visible with the head in
the normal position. Most cases will be readily visible with the head thrown
back and the neck fully extended (Fig. 17). Palpation is carried out by the

FIG. 16. TECHNIQUE USED IN EXAMINATION   FIG. 17. GROUP 1 THYROID GLAND
OF THYROIDS

FIG. 18. GROUP 2 THYROID GLAND   FIG. 19. GROUP 3 THYROID GLAND

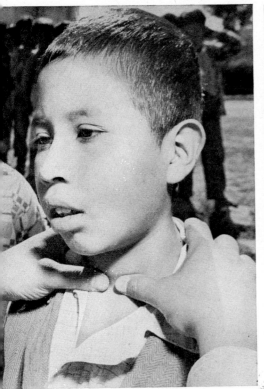

16

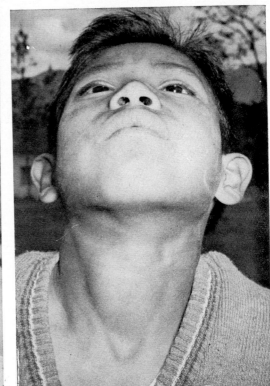

17

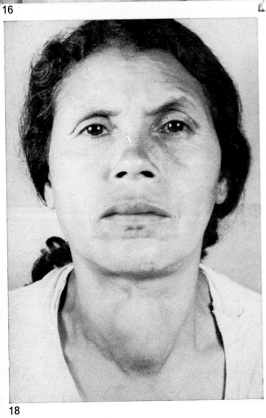

18

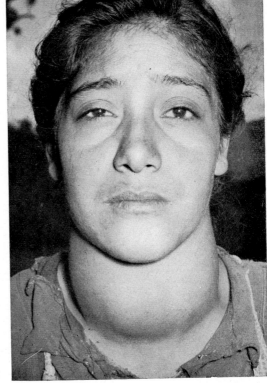

19

examiner sitting or standing facing the subject and placing his thumbs gently on either side of the thyroid area (Fig. 16).

(*b*) Grade 2—persons with visible goitres. Goitres in this category (Fig. 18) are easily visible with the head in the normal position; they are, however, smaller than those in Grade 3.

FIG. 20. PAROTID ENLARGEMENT

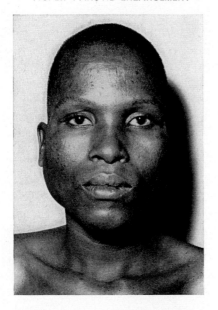

(*c*) Grade 3—persons with very large goitres. Goitres in this category can be recognized at a distance (Fig. 19). They are grossly disfiguring and may be of such a size as to cause mechanical difficulties with respiration and with the wearing of clothes.

Parotid enlargement (Fig. 20). This sign is positive if there is a chronic, visible, non-inflammatory, bilateral swelling of the parotids. The glands are firm, non-tender and painless. The overlying skin is unchanged. If the swelling is marked, the lobules of the ears are hidden when the subject is viewed from the front. It is most usually seen in schoolchildren and adults.

Parotid enlargement is usually recorded as only positive, without grading according to size. If grading is required, the technique of Shaper (personal communication, 1965) may be used (Fig. 21).

FIG. 21. MEASUREMENT OF PAROTID ENLARGEMENT
(SHAPER—PERSONAL COMMUNICATION, 1965)

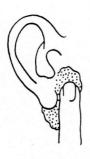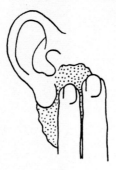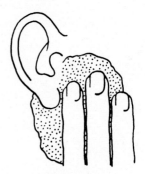

Grade 1   Grade 2   Grade 3

Group 2

Gynaecomastia. Bilateral, visible and palpable enlargement of the nipple and glandular subareolar breast tissue in males.

9. Skin

Group 1

Xerosis. Generalized dryness with branny desquamation. Factors to be considered when interpreting this and other skin signs are environmental, such as dirt, lack of washing, a dry, hot, windy climate, and the habitual use of oil on the body, and, more rarely, genetic, as in the case of the uncommon condition, congenital ichthyosis.

Follicular hyperkeratosis (Fig. 22). Two clinical types are recognized:

(*a*) Type 1, in which the lesion consists of hyperkeratosis surrounding the mouths of hair follicles and forming plaques that resemble spines. It is readily detected by the spiky feeling it gives when the palm is passed over an area of affected skin. Its characteristic distribution is frequently confined to the buttocks, thighs and especially the extensor aspects of the legs and arms, particularly the elbows and knees. The surrounding skin is dry and lacks the usual amount of moisture and oiliness. In early literature on the subject, the condition was termed " phrynoderma " (toad skin).

(*b*) Type 2, in which the lesions have a similar appearance, but the mouths of the hair follicles contain blood or pigment. The intervening skin is not unusually dry. The condition is seen mostly in adults. The distribution is usually over the abdomen and the extensor aspects of the thighs.

Petechiae. Small haemorrhagic spots in the skin or mucous membranes. Application of a blood pressure tourniquet may sometimes produce additional petechiae.

Pellagrous dermatosis (Fig. 23 (*a*) and (*b*); Plate IV C and D). Typical pellagrous skin lesions are symmetrical, clearly demarcated, hyperpigmented areas with or without exfoliation. The lesions are common in parts of the body exposed to sunlight, including the cheeks and the forearms; when they appear around the neck the condition is called " Casal's necklace ".

In acute cases, the skin is red, slightly swollen and may show vesiculation, exudation and cracking. The lesion itches and burns. In chronic cases, the dermatosis occurs as a roughening and thickening of the skin with dryness, scaling and brown pigmentation.

Flaky-paint dermatosis (Fig. 24 (*a*) and (*b*)). Extensive, often bilateral hyperpigmented patches of skin which desquamate to leave hypopigmented skin or superficial ulceration, often resembling a second-degree burn. It can occur anywhere, but characteristically on the buttocks and the back of the thighs. The lesion was once termed "crazy-pavement dermatosis".

FIG. 22. FOLLICULAR HYPERKERATOSIS

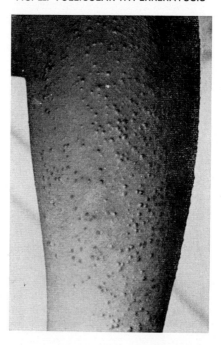

FIG. 23. PELLAGROUS DERMATOSIS

(a) Both forearms and hands   (b) Face and neck (Casal's necklace)

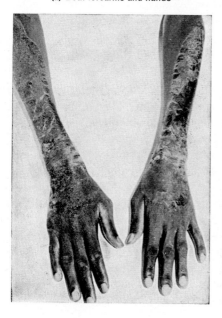
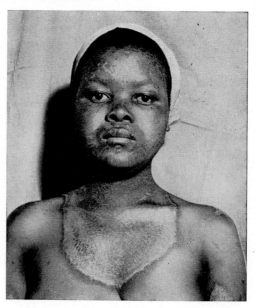

FIG. 24. FLAKY-PAINT RASH
(a) Forearms

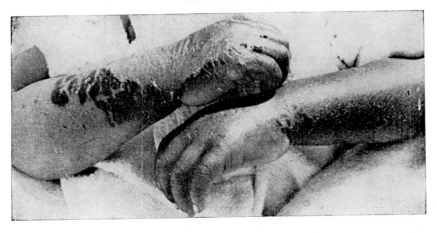

(b) Backs of legs

FIG. 25. SCROTAL DERMATOSIS

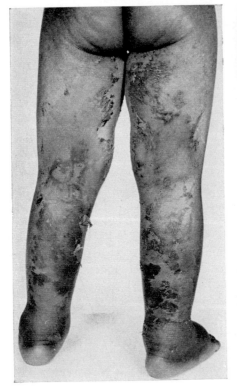

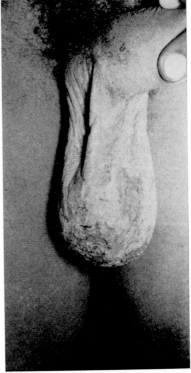

Scrotal and vulval dermatosis (Fig. 25). A desquamating lesion of the skin of the scrotum or vulva, often highly itchy. Secondary infection may supervene.

Group 2

Mosaic dermatosis. Large mosaic plaques, firmly adherent in the centre, but showing a tendency to peel at the periphery, present bilaterally on both shins.

Thickening and pigmentation of pressure points. Diffuse thickening, with pigmentation of the pressure points, such as the knees, elbows and front and back of the ankles. The knuckles may also be involved. The affected areas may be wrinkled, with or without fissuring.

Intertriginous lesions. Raw, red and macerated lesions in the skin flexures prone to constant friction, such as groins, buttocks and axillary folds, which frequently become secondarily infected.

10. Nails

Group 1

Koilonychia. Bilateral, spoon-shaped deformity of the nails in older children and adults.

Slightly spoon-shaped nails can be found commonly, affecting the toenails only, in barefooted communities; the condition appears to have no significance.

Group 2

Transverse ridging or grooving of nails.[1] This should be recorded if present in nails of more than one extremity.

11. Subcutaneous tissues

Group 1

Oedema. Usually first apparent over the ankles and feet, it may extend to other areas of the extremities. It may involve the genitals, face and hands. In early stages, it can be detected by firm pressure for three seconds with one digit on the lower portion of the medial surface of the tibia. The sign is taken as positive if there is a visible and palpable pit that persists after the pressure is removed. It is recorded only if present bilaterally.

Subcutaneous fat. An approximate estimate of any increase or decrease can be gauged by palpation of a skin-fold. If possible, detailed measurements with skin-fold calipers should also be made (see page 72).

---

[1] Other nail changes have been suggested as signs of malnutrition, including paired transverse lines (Muehrcke, 1956) and dark brown or black bands running longitudinally (Bisht & Singh, 1962). They require further investigation. A study in South Africa did not find any association between Muehrcke's lines and kwashiorkor (Catzel & Basson, 1956). Mottled nails have been described as occurring in fluorosis (Grech & Latham, 1964).

12. Muscular and skeletal systems

Group 1

Muscular wasting. This can be detected by observation and palpation of the upper arm, especially the biceps. Measurement of muscle should be carried out wherever relevant.

In children particularly, muscle wasting, accompanied by hypotonia, can result in pot-belly, lordosis and a winged appearance of the scapulae.

In severely affected children with protein-calorie malnutrition, including kwashiorkor, the degree of muscle wasting can be roughly assessed by testing the child's ability to hold up his head when pulled gently from a lying to a sitting position (Smythe, 1958).

Craniotabes. This sign consists of areas of softening of the skull, usually involving the occipital and parietal bones. Affected areas dent on pressure and spring back after the pressure is removed. The sign is positive only in infancy.

Frontal and parietal bossing. Localized thickening and heaping up of the frontal and parietal bones of the skull. Bossing may have a nutritional cause, but it can also occur in children of African ancestry with sickle-cell anaemia and appears to be recognized by some communities as a possibly familial characteristic.

Persistently open anterior fontanelle. This may be defined as an anterior fontanelle which is open on palpation after the age of eighteen months.

The sign is not specific and can be found in hydrocephalus and other conditions.

Epiphyseal enlargement (Fig. 26). Enlargement of the epiphyseal ends of long bones, particularly affecting the radius and ulna at the level of the wrist, and the tibia and fibula at the level of the ankle. In the assessment of this sign, allowance must be made for the degree of subcutaneous fat present. In wasted persons, the ends of the long bones appear unusually prominent.

Beading of the ribs (Fig. 27). A symmetrical nodular enlargement of the costo-chondral junctions, producing a " rosary " effect. It is essentially a special localized form of epiphyseal enlargement.

Knock-knees.

Bow-legs (Fig. 28).

Diffuse or local pelvic skeletal deformities.

Deformities of the thorax. The two most important are Harrison's sulcus (Fig. 29)—an indentation running laterally around both sides of the chest—and pigeon chest. However, many common thoracic deformities are unrelated to malnutrition (e.g., funnel chest, Fig. 30).

FIG. 26. EPIPHYSEAL ENLARGEMENT

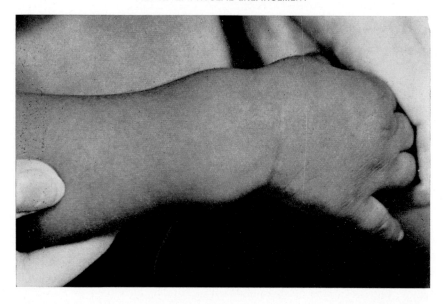

FIG. 27. RICKETY ROSARY

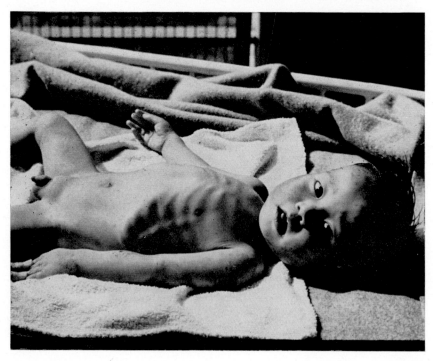

FIG. 28. BOW-LEGS   FIG. 29. HARRISON'S SULCUS

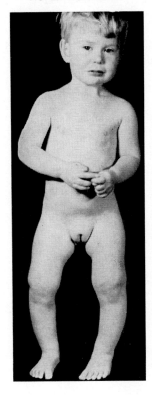 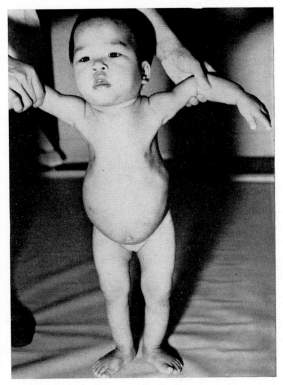

FIG. 30. FUNNEL BREAST

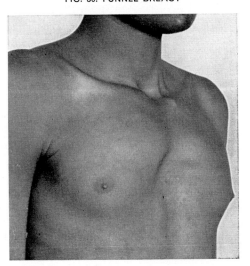

Musculo-skeletal haemorrhages. Larger haemorrhages may occur as (*a*) intramuscular haematoma, usually of the calf or thigh, (*b*) haemarthrosis, (*c*) subperiosteal haemorrhage. These may be suspected clinically, but can be confirmed only by detailed clinical examination and by special tests, such as aspiration for haemarthrosis, and radiology for subperiosteal haemorrhage.

13. Internal systems

GASTRO-INTESTINAL SYSTEM

Group 1

Hepatomegaly. The abdomen should be palpated in a standard position, that is, with the subject lying down, with the hips and knees flexed, if it is intended to measure the exact size. This can be recorded in centimetres below the costal margin.[1]

In the case of a young child, if the exact size is not to be recorded, examination can be carried out with the child reclining on the mother's lap, which reduces the likelihood of struggling. In any case, the position at examination should be noted.

Hepatomegaly in young children can occur solely as a result of a low protein, largely carbohydrate diet. It is particularly common in the West Indies. However, the enlarged palpable livers found in young children in many tropical regions appear to have mixed etiologies, including chronic malaria, malnutrition and possibly the result of the migration of helminth larvae through the liver.

NERVOUS SYSTEM

Psychomotor change. Listlessness can occur at any age, but is most strikingly seen in severe protein-calorie malnutrition of early childhood (see Fig. 49). This is especially so in kwashiorkor, when the child is apathetic, withdrawn and lacking in liveliness and interest in his surroundings. It is difficult to measure exactly, but can be crudely tested by watching the reaction to a brightly coloured object or light.

Mental confusion (Fig. 31). This may include psychosis.

Clinical tests of the central nervous system may include sensory loss, motor weakness, loss of position sense, loss of vibration sense, loss of ankle or knee jerks, and calf tenderness.

These tests are extremely difficult to carry out with any accuracy under field conditions. Even in hospital the problem of obtaining accurate, repeatable results with knee and ankle jerks is well recognized. With

---

[1] Precise studies of liver enlargement in young children can be undertaken by *averaging* the size of the liver found by palpating the abdomen in the mid-line and in the nipple-line ("average palpable liver size") (Oomen, 1957a).

apprehensive subjects hastily examined in rural survey, it is even more difficult, especially when testing for calf tenderness and vibration sense.

From the practical viewpoint, the tendon jerks should always be reinforced, tested in two positions and verified by a second examiner. Only absolute and bilateral loss should be reported (ICNND, 1961c).

If required, vibration sense can be tested with a tuning fork of 128 vibrations per minute (ICNND, 1963). Motor weakness in adults is classically judged by the "squatting" test—that is, the ability to squat and rise four times successively.

Subjective symptoms suggestive of possible neurological involvement, such as paraesthesia, are even less reliable, and, on the whole, history-taking in nutrition prevalence surveys in developing regions is of limited value, owing to the many problems of language, cultural interpretations and witness reliability.

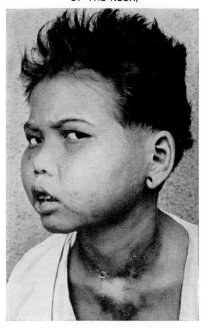

FIG. 31. MENTAL DERANGEMENT (WITH PELLAGROUS DERMATOSIS OF THE NECK)

CARDIOVASCULAR SYSTEM

Group 1

Cardiac enlargement. The simplest test of value in survey work is an examination by palpation to assess the presence of cardiac enlargement. However, with the practical exceptions of anaemia and beriberi, causes of cardiomegaly are essentially non-nutritional.

Tachycardia. The resting pulse rate may be of value in a nutritional status survey, because tachycardia can occur in anaemia, beriberi and certain probably nutritional cardiopathies. The rate must always be compared with "normal" values for the appropriate age-group. It will, of course, be very difficult to obtain a resting pulse under survey conditions. If felt to be of importance, a sample of those attending can be rested and examined, but usually this will be neither practicable nor worthwhile.

Group 2

Blood pressure. If the blood pressure is taken, the technique employed must be carefully standardized.

Interpretation of Signs in Relation to Nutrient Deficiencies

The concept of the " key sign ", introduced by Jolliffe et al. (1958), was based on the association of a certain sign with a given nutrient deficiency, such as angular stomatitis and riboflavin lack. With few exceptions—for example, thyroid enlargement and iodine deficiency—this concept is no longer regarded as valid, because of the lack of specificity of the signs recorded and because it is unusual for the diet of a community to be deficient in one nutrient only.

The fact that most clinical signs are non-specific does not preclude their use as indices of malnutrition. The frequent occurrence of one particular sign may give a lead to further investigations, while its association with other related signs at once raises its nutritional significance, both in the individual patient and in the community.

The interpretation of clinical signs can then be best made by using a " grouping of signs " which have been commonly found to form a pattern associated with the deficiency of a particular nutrient. Thus, while angular stomatitis can have various etiologies, if it is associated, in the individual or in a community, with one or more of the other signs in the " riboflavin deficiency " group, the likelihood of ariboflavinosis being present increases. The more numerous the signs present in one of the " groupings ", the more probable the diagnosis of deficiency of the particular nutrient.

However, the clinical patterns on which these " groupings of signs " are based differ, in detail or in the most prevalent combinations of signs, in various parts of the world, depending upon the quality, degree, duration and speed of onset of the malnutrition. Other factors may include the balance of other foods in the prevailing diet, genetic influences, the age and activity of the person, and the environment in which he lives, as regards both environmental hygiene and climate, and exposure to infection and parasitism (Leitch, 1963).

Age plays a particularly important part in the clinical signs produced by nutrient deficiency. The different pictures produced in young children and in adults as a result of ascorbic acid lack or protein-calorie malnutrition are clear-cut instances. Furthermore, age plays a significant, though not fully understood, part in determining the incidence and nature of the eye manifestations of vitamin-A deficiency. In particular, the signs in early childhood appear to differ from those seen in schoolchildren (McLaren, 1963.)

Patterns of clinical signs associated with specific nutrient deficiency cannot be standardized precisely for all areas of the world, although there is always a substantial agreement on the major features encountered. For example, the clinical picture of kwashiorkor, while varying in detail from one region to another, retains a core of signs found universally.

In some instances, a clinical appraisal of certain signs may be all that is required for a rapid screening survey, as in the use of the " niacin deficiency " group of signs to ascertain the prevalence of overt pellagra. More often, however, survey work based on clinical signs, even with the groupings suggested, is best supported and confirmed by (a) appropriate anthropometric measurements, (b) selected biochemical tests, and (c) investigation of the local diet, preferably by food-consumption surveys, considered in relation to local ecological circumstances. Each of these methods is imperfect and incomplete; used together, in carefully planned and locally relevant combinations, they can give the fullest information.

Guide to the Interpretation of Groupings of Clinical Signs

1. Protein-calorie malnutrition

Protein-calorie malnutrition in adults and schoolchildren

The usual signs of protein-calorie malnutrition in adults and schoolchildren are:

> diminished subcutaneous fat, and
> muscle wasting.

Other associated signs may include parotid enlargement, especially in schoolchildren (Gounelle, 1952; Raoult et al., 1957), oedema of the ankles, and gynaecomastia in males (Venkatachalam, 1962b).

Anthropometric measurements. There will be a low body weight for height, and measurements of subcutaneous fat and muscle will be considerably below the standard of reference.

Biochemical tests. Hypo-albuminaemia may be present in advanced cases.

Protein-calorie malnutrition in young children

The signs suggestive of protein-calorie malnutrition in young children are:

> oedema,
> dyspigmentation of the hair,
> easy pluckability of the hair,
> thin sparse hair,
> straight hair,
> muscle wasting,
> diffuse depigmentation of the skin,
> psychomotor change,
> moon-face,
> hepatomegaly, and
> flaky-paint dermatosis.

The clinical picture varies greatly in protein-calorie malnutrition in the early years of life, not only between the two major severe syndromes, kwashiorkor and nutritional marasmus, but with regard to the lesser and much commoner degrees of deficiency. Differentiation of the various syndromes of protein-calorie malnutrition in young children, and possible clinical, biochemical and anthropometric methods of assessment of mild and moderate degrees of involvement in the community are considered in a later section (see page 179).

Anthropometric measurements. Growth retardation, as shown by a low body weight for age and by muscle depletion are characteristic findings (see page 182).

Biochemical tests. Hypo-albuminaemia is present in advanced cases, and a low urinary creatinine excretion may be found. Poor dietary protein intake is reflected by a low excretion of urea per gram of creatinine. The serum amino-acid imbalance test and the hydroxyproline excretion test (page 86) may show abnormality (Whitehead, 1965).

Caloric overnutrition in children and adults (obesity)

The signs of caloric overnutrition are:
    increased subcutaneous fat, and
    increased abdominal girth.

Anthropometric measurements. High weight for height, excessive skin-folds and an abnormally high abdomen/chest-circumference ratio (see page 217).

2. Vitamin-A deficiency

The signs suggestive of vitamin-A deficiency are:
    Bitot's spots,
    conjunctival xerosis,
    corneal xerosis,
    keratomalacia,
    xerosis of skin, and
    follicular hyperkeratosis (type 1).

The clinical signs of avitaminosis A vary with age (McLaren, 1963). In particular, keratomalacia is principally seen in infancy and the pre-school-age group, often associated with protein-calorie malnutrition, while Bitot's spots and conjunctival xerosis are more common in schoolchildren.[1]

Recent studies have suggested that both xerosis of the skin and follicular hyperkeratosis (type 1) are more usually due not to lack of vitamin A but to other environmental and dietary factors, including a low fat diet deficient in essential unsaturated fatty acids such as linoleic acid (Hansen et al., 1962).

---

[1] Ocular xerosis may also result from scar damage to lachrymal ducts, conjunctival overexposure due to distortion of the eyelids, or dehydration (Shevalev, 1962).

Biochemical tests. Serum levels of carotene and vitamin A have been used.

Biophysical test. Classically, the dark-adaptation test has been employed for the detection of night blindness (hemeralopia), but is difficult to use in survey work, especially in young children.

3. Riboflavin deficiency

The signs suggestive of riboflavin deficiency are:
  angular stomatitis (or angular scars),
  cheilosis,
  magenta tongue,
  atrophic lingual papillae,
  dyssebacea,
  angular papebritis (angular blepharitis),
  scrotal (or vulval) dermatosis, and
  corneal vascularization.

Recent work has indicated the non-specificity of corneal vascularization and has also suggested that it is more commonly due to causes other than ariboflavinosis (McLaren, 1963).

Biochemical tests.[1] Category 1 : urinary riboflavin. Category 2: red-blood-cell riboflavin, load test.

4. Thiamine deficiency

The common suggestive signs are:
  oedema,
  loss of ankle jerks,
  loss of knee jerks,
  motor weakness (squatting test),
  calf-muscle tenderness,
  sensory loss,
  cardiac enlargement, and
  tachycardia.

Apart from oedema and signs of cardiovascular dysfunction—cardiac enlargement and tachycardia—the clinical signs associated with thiamine deficiency are all related to the central nervous system. The necessary tests are simple in theory, but extremely difficult to carry out satisfactorily in practice, especially among less sophisticated and often apprehensive rural populations during prevalence surveys. In these circumstances, subjective symptoms, such as paraesthesia, are even more unreliable. When communi-

---

[1] When appropriate, biochemical tests are given in the two categories suggested by the WHO Expert Committee on Medical Assessment of Nutritional Status (1963) (Table 7).

cation is difficult, for linguistic and cultural reasons, and time is limited, histories of such complaints are rarely worth collecting.

Thiamine deficiency in babies (infantile beriberi) has a completely different clinical picture. Usually it is one of convulsions and acute cardiac failure in the early months of life. Assessment of the incidence of this condition is difficult owing to the acuteness of the illness and because of the other diseases that produce a similar clinical picture at this age. The age-specific mortality rate between two and five months is a useful guide, while indirect evidence may be gained by estimating the thiamine content of breast milk (Simpson & Chow, 1956).

Biochemical tests. Category 1: urinary thiamine. Category 2: load test, blood pyruvate, blood lactate, red-cell haemolysate transketolase.

5. Niacin deficiency

The signs suggestive of niacin deficiency are:

> pellagrous dermatosis,
> scarlet and raw tongue,
> atrophic lingual papillae,
> tongue fissuring, and
> malar and supraorbital pigmentation.

Biochemical tests. Category 1: urinary methyl-nicotinamide. Category 2: load test, urinary pyridone.

6. Vitamin-C deficiency

The signs suggestive of vitamin-C deficiency are:

> spongy and bleeding gums,
> petechiae,
> ecchymoses,
> follicular hyperkeratosis (type 2),
> intramuscular or subperiosteal haematoma, and
> epiphyseal enlargement (painful).

The clinical picture varies greatly with age. Infantile scurvy is characterized more by lassitude, anaemia, haematoma formation, especially subperiosteally, and painful epiphyseal enlargement, particularly at the costochondral junctions. Spongy, bleeding gums do not occur in the absence of teeth.

When teeth are present, the commonest cause of bleeding gums, in the absence of hypertrophy, is a varying degree of marginal gingivitis or pyorrhoea.

Biochemical tests. Category 1: Serum ascorbic acid. Category 2: White-blood-cell ascorbic acid, urinary ascorbic acid, load test.

7. Vitamin-D deficiency

Active rickets (in young children) is typically suggested by:
    epiphyseal enlargement (painless) (over 6 months of age),
    beading of ribs,
    persistently open anterior fontanelle (after 18 months of age),
    craniotabes (under 1 year of age), and
    muscular hypotonia.
Healed rickets (in older children or adults) is suggested by:
    frontal or parietal bossing,
    knock-knees or bow-legs, and
    deformities of the thorax (Harrison's sulcus, pigeon chest).

Osteomalacia (in adults) may give rise to local or generalized skeletal deformities, especially of the pelvis, with tender bones.

The lack of specificity of these signs, including bow-legs, Harrison's sulcus and craniotabes, has suggested that a minimum of *three* signs are needed for diagnosis, preferably backed by biochemical and radiographic evidence.

Biochemical tests. Serum alkaline phosphatase level.

Radiographic examination. Changes in the ends of long bones, especially at the wrist.

8. Iron deficiency

Iron deficiency is suggested by:
    pale conjunctiva,
    koilonychia (in older children and adults), and
    atrophic lingual papillae.

Biochemical and haematological tests. Category 1: haemoglobin, thin blood film and haematocrit. Category 2: serum iron, bone-marrow iron and percentage saturation of transferrin.

Additional investigations. These may be necessary to exclude other nutritional causes of anaemia (e.g., folic acid or vitamin-B_{12} deficiency), and to assess possible contributory causes of the anaemia. They may include a stool examination for hookworm ova and occult blood, a thick blood film for malarial parasites and, in populations of African descent, a sickling preparation and electrophoresis for abnormal haemoglobins.

9. Folic acid or vitamin-B_{12} deficiency [1]

This condition is usually accompanied by pale conjunctiva due to anaemia.

---

[1] Hyperpigmented extremities have been described in vitamin-B_{12} deficiency in Indian infants (Jadhav et al., 1962).

Biochemical and haematological tests. Category 1: haemoglobin, thin blood film. Category 2: serum concentrations of folic acid and vitamin B_{12}.

10. Iodine deficiency

A deficiency of iodine produces enlargement of the thyroid.[1]

Biochemical tests. No simple tests are available, nor are they required for standard goitre surveys. For research purposes and if elaborate equipment is available, the urinary iodine can be assessed and various tests for thyroid function undertaken.

11. Excess of fluorine (fluorosis)

An excess of fluorine is suggested by mottled dental enamel.

This sign, however, has to be distinguished in its early stages from enamel hypoplasia and from various congenital conditions (Russell, 1961). According to Grech & Latham (1964), mottling of the finger nails may also be found.

Radiographic examination. Although rarely of practical importance in a prevalence survey, in chronic advanced cases radiographic examination of the spine will show increased density of the bones, with calcification of ligaments.

Chemical test. If possible, analysis of representative water samples should be made. More than 2 ppm of fluoride is a positive result.

Therapeutic Trials

Therapeutic trials can be a useful extension of clinical assessment where the need is to establish the identity of a deficiency syndrome or to differentiate between two conditions with similar clinical manifestations. They can, for example, be of value in defining the nutritional etiology of anaemia, when effectiveness will be assessed by haematological response, as judged by a rise in the reticulocyte count and haemoglobin level (Stott, 1960).

This type of investigation will generally be carried out at the end of a survey or as part of a follow-up on a limited number of affected persons. The trial will also be guided by biochemical and dietary findings.

Therapeutically effective doses of the single nutrient being investigated are given to the selected persons for what is judged to be a sufficient time to produce results. If the nutrient is not given parenterally, biochemical tests to ensure that absorption has occurred are desirable.

At the same time, a control group of people with the same clinical features should be given a placebo in order to eliminate changes that could

---

[1] Size assessed by the technique of Perez, Scrimshaw & Munoz (1960).

occur spontaneously, such as those due to seasonal factors. The trial should be a " double-blind " test in that the clinical observer should not be able to differentiate between nutrient and placebo until after the trial is completed.

Clinical change must be critically evaluated, preferably quantitatively, as by measurement of the size of a lesion, or by before-and-after photographs, preferably in colour.

Rapid Clinical Surveys

These are designed to detect the most characteristic signs of one or several nutritional deficiencies. They are of most value when the plane of community nutrition is low. They can be carried out by medical staff or by paramedical personnel who have been specially selected and trained and are working under the supervision of a competent nutritionist. The data collected should be recorded on a special record form, which lists the signs that are considered to be both particularly characteristic and easily identifiable during a field survey.

Experience has shown that if these rapid surveys are to be of real value, they must be carried out on samples that are sufficiently large, when judged by standard statistical considerations.

A simple schedule will be employed, which may include some or all of the following signs:

Hair :
  dyspigmentation
  easy pluckability
  sparseness

Face :
  moon-face

Eyes :
  Bitot's spots
  conjunctival xerosis
  pale conjunctiva

Mouth :
  angular stomatitis
  cheilosis
  glossitis
  swollen, bleeding gums

Thyroid gland :
  goitre

Skin :
  oedema (bilateral)
  follicular hyperkeratosis (type 1)
  pellagrous dermatosis

Skeleton :
  epiphyseal enlargement (wrist)
  rickety rosary
  persistently open anterior fontanelle
  Harrison's sulcus
  bossing of skull
  knock-knees
  bow-legs

Rapid surveys of this type are usually mainly clinical, but may include limited anthropometry, especially weight measurements. They have limited objectives and are often concerned with a specific problem, such as goitre or protein-calorie malnutrition. They are inexpensive, speedy and require only limited staff. However, they are at best screening procedures that indicate whether more detailed surveys are desirable.

Occasionally, rapid screening surveys may be based solely on a laboratory test, such as the haemoglobin estimation for anaemia or the urinary thiamine test for deficiency of this vitamin.

NUTRITIONAL ANTHROPOMETRY[1]

Nutritional anthropometry is concerned with the measurement of the variations of the physical dimensions and the gross composition of the human body at different age levels and degrees of nutrition.

In its modern scientific form, it is a comparatively recent development requiring well-organized research centres, elaborate equipment and highly sophisticated mathematical knowledge. Its newer techniques have been used to a limited extent in the developing regions of the world, especially in young children. The interpretation of findings anywhere is always complex and often controversial, even to leading authorities. The normal healthy well-fed human body can vary so much that interpretation of the nutritional significance of variations in physical dimensions is peculiarly difficult.

The present account, together with subsequent sections dealing with the interpretation of results and with special problems in different age-groups, is not concerned with the nutritional assessment of the individual, but rather suggests simple methods that will supply useful, if approximate, information concerning the nutritional profile of the community and be of value in guiding public health programmes.

The methods suggested here can be carried out with a small staff and little equipment. At the same time, they must be regarded as to some extent of an interim nature, in so far as they require much additional large-scale evaluation in the field and may be superseded by newer procedures.

Growth is influenced by biological determinants, including sex, intra-uterine environment, birth order, birth-weight in single and multiple pregnancies, parental size and genetic constitution, and by environmental factors, including climate, season and socio-economic level. In the final analysis the environment seems to produce its effect mostly by the presence (or absence) of infective, parasitic and psychological illnesses (Patton, Gardner & Richmond, 1963) and, above all, by the plane of nutrition.

In general, recent work tends to suggest that environmental influences, especially nutrition, are of greater importance than genetic background or other biological factors. Certainly the physical dimensions of the body are much influenced by nutrition, particularly in the rapidly growing period of early childhood. Selected body measurements can therefore give valuable information concerning certain types of malnutrition in which body size and gross body composition are affected.

---

[1] A valuable guide to nutritional anthropometry has recently been prepared in Spanish by Ramos-Galvan (1965).

Dramatic historical examples of the effect of nutrition on anthropometric measurements are demonstrated in the lower weights and heights of European schoolchildren in Paris (Gounelle, Vallette & Moine, 1942; Laporte, 1946) following prolonged and severe war-time dietary restrictions. Conversely, and probably mainly because of improving nutrition, the stature and weight of children and adults have increased progressively over the past hundred years in both North America (Meredith, 1941) and Europe (Clements, 1953), and more recently in Japan (Mitchell, 1962) and Jamaica (Ashcroft & Lovell, 1965).

Growth and physique can also be affected by bacterial, viral and parasitic infections. These factors require differentiation, but, under practical circumstances in many developing tropical regions, they may together form part of a person's total disease burden, and have secondary nutritional consequences. It is difficult, if not impossible, to disentangle these secondary effects underlying primarily dietetic malnutrition. This is especially so in kwashiorkor—one of the two principal forms of severe protein-calorie malnutrition of early childhood. This condition is almost never exclusively dietary in origin, but rather the result of other cumulative stresses as well, including the nutritional ill-effects of intestinal helminths, bacterial and viral infections (such as tuberculosis, whooping cough and measles), persistent malaria, and psychological trauma associated with weaning (Patton, Gardner & Richmond, 1963).

The methods and the measurements employed in anthropometry can vary greatly in number and complexity. Obviously those chosen will depend on the purpose and objectives of the particular survey or study. Detailed, elaborate and time-consuming techniques and analyses, such as refined scientific procedures for estimating body composition, can usually be carried out only by the laboratory research worker.

For the practical nutritionist in the field, the problem is:

(a) to select the minimum number of relatively simple methods that can give useful, if approximate, practical information on a community basis;

(b) to understand thoroughly the practical techniques involved; and

(c) to interpret the results and express them in a way that is understandable to workers anywhere in the world.

Much of the world literature on nutritional anthropometry is concerned with adults, especially in well-fed communities where obesity is a health problem, so that the estimation of body fat in relation to weight and height figures prominently. Similarly, investigations of children have also been concerned mainly with the evolution of " standards ", and with problems of growth and development among children in North America and Europe.

For the field worker in a developing tropical country, nutritional anthropometry appears to be of greatest value in the assessment of growth failure and undernutrition, principally from lack of protein and calories. In particular, the often numerous less advanced states of protein-calorie malnutrition in early childhood can probably be best detected objectively by deviations from the usual rapid growth pattern characteristic of this age-group, as shown especially by a low body weight and by depletion of protein stores, as indicated by a subnormal muscle mass.

Standardization of Techniques

Methods

The apparent simplicity of making measurements is deceptive (Brozek, 1956), and yet in a survey such measurements as weighing may be delegated to the most junior, least well trained member of the team, who is commonly left to work without adequate supervision and without regular checking of his apparatus. The effects are particularly unfortunate, since the inaccurate results obtained are expressed numerically and too often viewed as scientifically precise and objective data.

The time spent in obtaining a measurement is only a small fraction of the time required for subsequent calculations and interpretation, and effort as well as time are wasted if the original measurement is inaccurate.

The techniques employed, including such apparently simple and common-place procedures as weighing, must be carefully carried out, standardized, thoroughly understood by all team members, and given adequate preliminary practical testing to ensure uniformity of results. Details of standardized techniques for the most useful procedures are set out in a subsequent section. Particular accuracy of both technique and equipment is needed with small children, especially when growth is being assessed by the measurement of small increments.

If many people are to be examined, sufficient personnel should be available to permit of rest periods. Otherwise the repetition, monotony and physical strain of making large numbers of precise measurements, especially on uncooperative young children, lead to fatigue, boredom and inevitable error. Lastly, the average time required to carry out procedures must be known, in order to determine how many subjects can be dealt with at each session.

Instruments

The selection of suitable instruments is extremely important. They must be sufficiently accurate for the particular study, simple to use, inexpensive and " readily portable and rugged enough to withstand severe handling " (Pett & Ogilvie, 1956). They require careful pre-testing and frequent checking and calibration. Details of appropriate instruments for various practical procedures are given later.

Description of methods

In all published results, the fullest details of methods used must be clearly stated. For example, the precise technique used for weighing (e.g., the scales used, whether clothes worn or nude) must be set down.

If possible the investigator should dictate each measurement to a recorder, who repeats aloud the figure as it is given to him. This method speeds up the procedure and reduces clerical error.

Standards of Reference

Community standards for anthropometric measurements are difficult to define.[1] What is usually meant are values that can be employed as a " frame of reference ".

Standards for a community are usually obtained by measuring a statistically adequate sample of a healthy, well-fed segment of the population whose ages are known with certainty. For all age-groups, measurements made cross-sectionally will suffice.

For children, however, values should, if possible, also be obtained by more time-consuming longitudinal methods—that is by serial measurements of a sample of children over some years—in order to determine the pattern of growth for the particular population in relation to known episodes in the children's lives.

As a compromise between these two methods, the accelerated longitudinal method of Bell (1964) or the mixed longitudinal method (Harrison et al., 1964) may be employed.

From this type of data, the range of distribution of values for these normals can be determined and the results expressed as the average or mean value plus or minus *twice* the standard deviation (mean $\pm$ 2 S.D.) (Falkner, 1962a).[2] The most useful and practical ways of expressing results below these standards are considered in a later section.

However, it must again be stressed that the most desirable, or optimal, anthropometric values or standards are not known with certainty for any community. There has been a constant secular trend in the past century towards heavier and taller populations in the western world (Meredith, 1941) that has made previous "standards" progressively out-of-date.[3]

---

[1] The desired end-product of optimal nutrition at present lacks definition, and Barness & György (1962) stress the uncertainty of whether the goal is " to produce muscle-men, geniuses, giants, dwarfs or Methuselahs".

[2] Twice the standard deviation ($\pm$ 2 S.D.) covers 95% of the distribution and permits percentiles to be calculated later, if required.

[3] According to Norwegian records, this secular trend commenced in the 1830s, and in Western Europe as a whole there has been a consistent increase in adult height by about 1 cm per decade over the past century (Harrison et al., 1964). The possibility that this trend has ceased in the USA is suggested by recent measurements of private-school children (Bakwin & McLaughlin, 1964).

That a secular trend of this type can be downwards is suggested by the smaller sizes of preserved skeletons in mediaeval Iceland, when adverse climatic conditions developed (Harrison et al., 1964), and by the inferior stature of the modern Peruvian peasants compared with their pre-Conquistador ancestors, which Graham (1966) suggests may be due to dietary change and, in particular, the abandonment of high-protein quinoa (*Chenopodium chinoa*) as the main staple.

That this runs parallel with an improvement in nutrition and other environmental influences, such as disease control, seems certain. At the same time, there may well be developing an undesirable relation between larger, early-maturing, possibly overfed populations and a subsequent disease pattern in adulthood that includes, among other things, an increasing incidence of atherosclerosis and obesity.

Optimum growth levels can be evaluated logically only in relation to present and future health. Evaluation of this kind is difficult to do in a long-lived species such as man, but it is the basis for the " desirable " standards of weight for adults laid down by the Society of Actuaries (1959), which are related to cardiovascular disease and longevity.

Local standards of reference. It should be the ultimate aim of nutritionists to prepare and use local standards for different ethnic groups with potentially different patterns of growth. To cite an extreme instance, height standards for the pygmies of Rwanda are obviously inappropriate for their extremely tall nilo-hamitic neighbours, the Tutsi.

Body proportions appear to vary in different groups of peoples. This is partly genetic, possibly being related in some instances to climatic adaptation, as exemplified by the contrasting shape and size of the Arctic-dwelling Eskimo and the tall, slender Dinka of equatorial Africa.

However, physique is also related to nutrition, as has been demonstrated by the increase in height as well as weight of second- and third-generation Japanese Americans in California compared with their ancestral stock in Japan (Greulich, 1957).

Difficulties in preparing local standards are great. Large numbers of careful measurements have to be made among the healthy, well-fed section of the community whose ages are known. This is a major undertaking, but, when staff and other priorities permit, a carefully planned accumulation of these important base-line data should be carried out, using standardized techniques, fully detailed in the recording of the results.

It is particularly desirable to collect reliable present-day local standards for young children, but this is often especially difficult (Dean, 1965). In some cases, only a small proportion of children may be well fed, healthy and with their ages known exactly, owing to inadequate birth registration. If practicable, measurements should be made of singleton children of the educated, prosperous élite section of the community, if such exist in sufficient numbers, excluding those with serious illness or congenital abnormalities. In all instances, the group measured should be ethnically homogeneous, fully described and statistically adequate numerically.

Many so-called " standards " that have been compiled for pre-school children in developing tropical countries are based on measurements of children from lower socio-economic groups, who are, in fact, usually under-nourished from six months of age onwards and continuously exposed to a succession of infective and parasitic diseases (Dean & Jelliffe, 1960). Optimum data from the offspring of the truly well-fed, medically and socially protected élite are much needed and should be the aim when local standards are being constructed.

Ideally, both cross-sectional and longitudinal serial measurements are needed for children, but the latter take years of patient supervision and careful collection of data, to ensure the accurate recordings of small increments. Longitudinal measurements offer the advantages of permitting accurate knowledge of age, ensuring genetic homogeneity and enabling growth to be correlated with each child's history and background, including diet, minor illnesses and socio-economic circumstances. They give information on possible variations in patterns of growth and developmental phases, such as adolescence, but may be already out-of-date by the time they are ready for use. More often only cross-sectional measurements are practicable. They are more quickly obtained and give information on current conditions.

For convenience, measurements have often been made in easily accessible groups, such as schoolchildren and adults, especially in the police or armed forces. However, because of the age distribution of protein-calorie malnutrition, it is most important to have standards of growth for the first five years of life.

To prepare local growth standards by cross-sectional methods to cover the vulnerable first five years of life, it is necessary to measure at least 30 children of each three-month period and to calculate the means (averages) plus or minus *twice* the standard deviation ($\pm$ 2 S.D.). Results may sometimes be more vividly portrayed as a graph. Separate results can be collected for each sex, but, for practical nutritional anthropometry in the community, standards for boys and girls may be considered together in these early years. Apart from the measurement of subcutaneous-fat thickness, there is not much difference in the commonly employed measurements.

In later childhood and for adults, separate standards are required for the sexes, and must be based on the examination of statistically adequate groups.

The need for different standards of weight and height (and other linear measurements) for different age-groups is obvious. In addition, however, consideration has to be given to *relative* rates of growth and of maturation of different tissues at various ages, and to the possible effects of malnutrition at different periods of life.

Normal growth is an uninterrupted process, although the rate is uneven, with recognized periods of rapid increase, particularly the first six months of life and the puberty " spurt ". In protein-calorie malnutrition, however, it is slowed or even halted. Suggested average expected weight gains at different periods of childhood are given in a later section (Table 19, page 196).

Differences of body proportion at various stages of human development are also well recognized—for example, the relatively large head of the new-born compared with that of the adult. Of particular interest in nutritional anthropometry is the variation of subcutaneous fat and muscle at different ages. The thicker layer and different distribution of fat in healthy babies make different standards necessary for this age and for the normally leaner pre-school-age child.

A local anthropometric standard will often have a usefulness extending beyond the actual group for whom it was originally prepared. It may be appropriate to use the same standards for groups of similar genetic stock, although it will always be difficult to know how far afield the same values may be employed with exactness. For example, growth standards compiled for Baganda children could be used among the Basoga, another genetically similar Bantu community in Uganda. In some parts of the world, as in the West Indies, where people of different ethnic groups often intermarry, it may be difficult to decide on precise local standards that cover all genetic possibilities.

General standards of reference

As noted, carefully compiled local standards, based on statistically adequate samples, are difficult to prepare. Many workers have noted that really well-fed people of various ethnic groups tend to approximate to standards, especially weight levels, similar to those found in well-nourished Caucasians in Europe and the USA.[1] This secular trend has already been noted for Japanese Americans (Greulich, 1957), and for Japanese children of the upper socio-economic group in the homeland in the last decade (Mitchell, 1962).

Furthermore, Ford (1964) has collected evidence that well-nourished infants and pre-school children of various genetic backgrounds attain weight levels so near to those obtained in the Harvard Longitudinal Studies [2] (Stuart & Stevenson, 1959) that these values may be used for assessing malnutrition. Similar findings have been reported for Central American pre-school children (Hurtado, J. J.—personal communication, 1962), and for West Indian schoolchildren in Haiti (King et al., 1963) and Jamaica (Ashcroft & Lovell, 1964; Ashcroft et al., 1965).

It follows that the use of such general standards of reference appears to be of value as a public health approximation (Woodruff, 1966), with the proviso that, wherever feasible, control measurements should also be made locally from children of the well-fed élite. Obviously, the genetic extremes among the sub-groups of mankind, such as the pygmies, cannot be included.

Other indirect evidence supporting the feasibility of using general standards of reference includes the increased birth-weight in well-nourished

---

[1] This may take two well-nourished generations, as a small malnourished mother will give birth to a low-birth-weight neonate.

[2] These measurements are referred to as " the Harvard Standards " throughout this monograph.

sections of tropical communities, and the excellent weight gain of most babies in developing regions while on the abundant, protein-rich diet furnished by on-demand breast feeding in the early months of life. Conversely, following the years of war-time nutritional deprivation, the weights and heights of some groups of European children fell to levels comparable to those " normally " found in some developing countries (Laporte, 1946).

In any case, it is often necessary, because of a lack of local measurements, to use a (possibly) genetically less appropriate but widely available general standard. Several of these are available, but it is suggested that the Harvard Standards should be used for weight and height measurements in young children. These data, although derived from the growth of Caucasian children in Boston from 1930 to 1956, offer the advantages of having been carefully compiled longitudinally on a large series, of being widely available in Nelson's *Textbook of Pediatrics,* and of being used already by paediatricians in many countries. For schoolchildren where weight-for-height-for-age data are required, the Baldwin-Wood Standards should be used (Baldwin & Wood, 1923; Baldwin, 1925). The Harvard data have not been analysed in this way, but can be used for weight-for-height standards where the age is not known.

Sources of general standards of reference for other measurements (e.g., triceps skin-fold, arm circumference etc.) are given in Annex 1.

For adults, the weight-for-height tables suggested are derived by ICNND (1963) from the figures compiled by the Society of Actuaries (1959) [1] and considered to be " desirable ".

Sources of other general standards suggested for older children and adults are given in Annex 1.

Despite the practical usefulness of the general standards of reference given, their arbitrariness must also be noted, because the figures for different age-groups and measurements have been collected by various investigators using varying techniques in non-identical populations in different, recent decades.

Conclusion

Local anthropometric standards should be prepared and used wherever possible, because they may often be considered a more realistic goal. They are, however, very difficult to collect.

In addition, general standards of reference should be employed, for, although they may be genetically unsuitable, they supply a yardstick with which results from surveys at different times and places can be compared. While they may be locally relevant as a goal, they are more usually of value as a standard of reference.

Where available, results should be expressed in terms of *both* standards. In all cases, precise details of the standards employed must be known

---

[1] These measurements are referred to as the " Actuaries Standards " throughout this monograph.

(e.g., techniques, groups, age assessment, etc.) and must be clearly stated in the published results.

Age Assessment

Many persons living in the developing regions of the tropics are ignorant of their exact age, or occasionally may employ a system of age classification different from the western method. This is understandable since precise age has little significance unless it has a recognized social value, e.g., in relation to legal responsibility, admission to school, pension rights, etc. Among some peoples, functional or physiological age-groups are recognized—e.g., " big enough to be able to herd goats ", or " capable of carrying a younger sibling ", or " marriageable ".

Often transitions from one group to another are recognized by special ceremonies and by the wearing of different clothes, decorations or hair style thereafter. These include initiation rites in some communities, e.g., the elaborate ceremony and short hair-cut carried out before a girl can enter the marriageable group among the San Blas Indians of Panama (Jelliffe et al., 1961b).

For adults, all that may be possible is to consider the two sexes in broad age-groups—young adults, adults, old adults. However, differentiation may sometimes be difficult in groups where the scalp hair is shaved, where there is no " middle-aged " obesity, and where facial wrinkles are less prominent against a darker complexion, or, conversely, where women age rapidly with continuous child bearing and too much work. A long-term local calendar of important events may have to be constructed.

More-exact age-assessment is desirable in the anthropometry of young children, when protein-calorie malnutrition has its main incidence. When dealing with infants and pre-school children, ages should, if possible, be known to the month. For schoolchildren, assessment of ages to the nearest three months should be attempted.

In field-survey circumstances, age assessment in young children may be attempted in various ways. Documentary evidence may, though rarely, be forthcoming, including birth certificates, horoscopes and baptismal certificates. Careful prior enquiries must always be made and, wherever possible, the parents must be encouraged to bring these vital papers.

Sometimes, the mother may not know the child's age, but may be able to recite the month of birth, and occasionally the day as well. If this is so, the mother will often recall details of the youngest child only, not those of the older siblings. If dates are known, they should be recorded as given and the ages calculated later.

In some communities, the period of the year in which the child was born can be recognized by the name given, e.g., " born during millet harvesting ", or as belonging to a certain ritual age-set; or there may be a local lunar calendar, as among the San Blas Indians of Panama, e.g., iguana egg-laying moon, corn-sprouting moon, etc. (Jelliffe et al., 1961b). It may be possible to obtain information in relation to Muslim lunar months.

Often the only practicable method may be to construct a locally relevant calendar (Tukei, 1963) based on events in the preceding years, including agricultural, climatic and political occurrences, as well as natural or man-made disasters (Table 3). However, such a calendar takes weeks to prepare and pre-test in the field, while its use in survey circumstances is laborious, time-consuming, and least satisfactory with the unsophisticated communities for which it is intended. Calendars will plainly have to be specific for different communities.

As approximate supporting evidence, the young child's deciduous dental eruption should be noted on the survey form, the standard visual coding shown in Fig. 32 being used. It has been shown that the time-range of eruption in inadequately nourished children of lower socio-economic groups in Peru (Graham & Morales, 1963), in various parts of Africa (Welbourn, 1956; Sénécal, Masse & Moreigne, 1959), and in the New Guinea Highlands (Voors & Metselaar, 1958; Bailey, 1963a) is similar to that found among children in Europe and North America, although Puyet, Downs & Budeir (1963) found some delay in Arab children.

FIG. 32. STANDARD VISUAL CODING OF DECIDUOUS DENTITION

(Right upper jaw) E D C B A	A B C D E (Left upper jaw)
(Right lower jaw) E D C B Ⓐ	Ⓐ B C D E (Left lower jaw)

Code: A = central incisor; B = lateral incisor; C = cuspid; D = first molar; E = second molar.

Example shows both lower central incisors erupted.

However, times of dental eruption can vary greatly in normal children, and further work is needed to establish local standards, because some presumed genetic differences in tooth-eruption timing have been noted in different parts of the world (Garn, Lewis & Kerensky, 1964). Strangely little precise information appears to be available on the effect of kwashiorkor on the appearance time of deciduous teeth, although the clinical impression is that it is little affected, if at all. Trowell, Davis & Dean (1954) remark on " the incongruous sight of the tiny child with his mouth crowded with teeth ".

Evidence concerning the time of dental eruption in children suffering from nutritional marasmus is incomplete. In experimentally severely under-nourished piglets, dental eruption is not delayed (McCance, 1964), although

TABLE 3. CALENDAR FOR THE ASSESSMENT OF THE AGE OF YOUNG BAGANDA CHILDREN *

Main events of the year	Rainy seasons	Month	Recalled seasonal or special events	Age on 31.12.1962	
				years	months
1959		January	Beginning of New Year Picking and selling of cotton crop	4	
Year of trade boycott (*okubaliga ya Kamya*)		February	Children go back to school End of cotton picking; selling continues Queen Mother visited Uganda	3	11
Queen Mother visited Uganda	*Togo*	March	Muslim Fast, ending with Id celebration (*okusiiba bya abasiramu*)	3	10
	Rains	April	Easter (*paska*) celebrated White ants fly	3	9
		May	Early cotton planting	3	8
		June	Main cotton planting Weeding early cotton	3	7
		July	Main cotton weeding	3	6
		August	Main groundnut harvest	3	5
	Dumbi	September	Coffee picking	3	4
		October		3	3
	Rains	November	Kabaka's birthday	3	2
		December	Christmas (*Noeli*) End of year	3	1
1960 Year following the trade boycott		January	Beginning of New Year Picking and selling of cotton crop	3	
		February	Children go back to school End of cotton picking; selling continues	2	11
	Togo	March	Muslim Fast, ending with Id celebration (*okusiiba bya abasiramu*)	2	10
	Rains	April	Easter (*paska*) celebrated White ants fly	2	9
		May	Early cotton planting	2	8
		June	Main cotton planting Weeding early cotton	2	7
		July	Main cotton weeding	2	6
		August	Main groundnut harvest	2	5
	Dumbi	September	Coffee picking	2	4
		October		2	3
	Rains	November	Kabaka's birthday	2	2
		December	Christmas (*Noeli*) End of year	2	1
1961 Year when Buganda declared Independence		January	Beginning of New Year Picking and selling of cotton crop Buganda declares Independence (*Okuwofeguwa Baganda*)	2	

* Reproduced by permission from Tukei (1963).

TABLE 3. CALENDAR FOR THE ASSESSMENT OF THE AGE OF YOUNG BAGANDA CHILDREN
(*continued*)

Main events of the year	Rainy seasons	Month	Recalled seasonal or special events	Age on 31.12.1962	
1961 Year when feasting for Kabaka's return from London Conference		February	Children go back to school End of cotton picking; selling continues	1	11
Year of initial Congo refugees	*Togo*	March	Muslim Fast, ending with Id celebration (*okusiiba bya abasiramu*) Democratic Party win general elections, boycotted by Buganda	1	10
Year which ended with bad floods closing many roads	Rains	April	Easter (*paska*) celebrated White ants fly	1	9
		May	Early cotton planting	1	8
		June	Main cotton planting Weeding early cotton	1	7
		July	Main cotton weeding	1	6
		August	Main groundnut harvest	1	5
	Dumb	September	Coffee picking Very heavy rains and flooding of roads	1	4
	Rains	October	Kabaka went to first London Conference	1	3
		November	Kabaka's birthday General feasting for Kabaka's return from Conference	1	2
		December	Tanganyika became independent Christmas (*Noeli*) End of year	1	1
1962		January	Beginning of New Year Picking and selling of cotton crop	1	
The year Uganda became independent	*Togo*	February	Children go back to school End of cotton picking; selling continues		11
	Rains	March	Muslim Fast, ending with Id celebration (*okusiiba bya abasiramu*) Kabaka-Yekka won the Lukiiko elections		10
		April	Uganda People's Congress-Kabaka-Yekka won National Assembly elections Easter (*paska*) celebrated White ants fly		9
		May	Mr Obote succeeded Mr Kiwanuka as Prime Minister Early cotton planting		8
		June	Main cotton planting Weeding early cotton		7
		July	Main cotton weeding		5-6
		August	Main groundnut harvest		5-6
	Dumbi	September	Coffee picking		4
	Rains	October	Uganda became independent		3
		November	Kabaka's birthday		2
		December	Christmas (*Noeli*) End of year		1-0

McLaren, Ammoun & Houri (1964) have shown that deciduous teeth erupt later in marasmic infants.

A method of assessing approximately the age-range from dental eruption is suggested in Table 4 as judged by average eruption times. Bailey (1963a) has suggested that, as an approximation, the simple addition of 6 to the number of teeth erupted—that is, with the crown of the tooth visible through the gum—gives the rough age in months, and this proposal has the advantage of requiring no memorizing or consulting of tables.

TABLE 4.   AVERAGE ERUPTION TIME OF DECIDUOUS
TEETH *

Tooth	Lower jaw	Upper jaw
Central incisor [a]	6 months	7 ½ months
Lateral incisor [a]	7 months	9 months
Cuspid	16 months	18 months
First molar [b]	12 months	14 months
Second molar [b]	20 months	24 months

* From Massler & Schour (1944). Copyright by the American Dental Association. Reprinted by permission.
[a] Incisors: range ± 2 months
[b] Molars: range ± 4 months

The stage of dental eruption can be combined with a careful measurement of head circumference as a method that may narrow the range. It is obvious that although, at best, these methods can act only as guides, they can certainly suggest the *lower* age limit. Other physiological yardsticks, such as bone age and sexual maturation, are also variable, and anyhow not relevant or practicable in cross-sectional prevalence-survey work.

The stage of neuromuscular development is usually of only slight value, as it is very variable in the healthy, and particularly difficult to test in anxious children in the field. The picture may also be obscured by the muscle wasting and weakness characteristic of protein-calorie malnutrition.

The presence of older or younger siblings, or a pregnant mother, may provide further useful information in guiding age-assessment of the individual child, although in some groups it is difficult for the observer in a prevalence survey to discover whether the children do in fact belong to the particular women. For example, among the Baganda, the sending of young children to stay with relatives is widely practised and, by local convention, the woman with whom they are staying will not like to say that a particular child is not her own. A knowledge of children's ages is one of the advantages of long-term longitudinal studies.

Age-assessment can sometimes be best attempted by a *combination* of dental eruption, head circumference, local calendar and presence of siblings. However, as age is still often difficult to evaluate, attention is given later to methods that can be used to assess growth-failure where the age is not known (Table 22, page 200).

For schoolchildren, attempts should be made to assess the age to within three months. Parents or teachers may supply information or documentary evidence. A local calendar covering an adequate time-range can be constructed for use with parents. The eruption of the permanent dentition can be noted (Table 5), but the significance must be interpreted cautiously, in view of individual variation and evidence that genetic factors may influence the time of eruption (Chagula, 1960).

TABLE 5. AVERAGE ERUPTION TIME OF PERMANENT TEETH *

Tooth	Lower jaw (years)	Upper jaw (years)
Central incisors	6-7	7-8
Lateral incisors	7-8	8-9
Cuspids	9-10	11-12
First bicuspid	10-12	10-11
Second bicuspid	11-12	10-12
First molar	6-7	6-7
Second molar	11-13	12-13
Third molar	17-21	17-21

* From Massler & Schour (1944). Copyright by the American Dental Association. Reprinted by permission.

Measurement Techniques [1]

Of the almost unlimited number of possible body measurements, those selected should be the simplest and quickest to take and the easiest to reproduce that will give the maximum information concerning the particular nutritional problem under investigation. In the developing regions of the world, this will almost always be the problem of protein-calorie malnutrition, both in adults, schoolchildren and, especially, pre-school-age children—in direct contradistinction to many studies carried out in both America and Europe, where the treatment of the problem has often centred on obesity and excessive weight.

---

[1] The techniques suggested are based on those described by the Committee on Nutritional Anthropometry (1956), Falkner (1960, 1962b), and Prinsloo (1964).

The most usual measurements are those made to assess (*a*) body mass, as judged by weight; (*b*) linear dimensions, especially height; and (*c*) body composition and reserves of calories and protein, as judged by the principal superficial soft tissues—subcutaneous fat and muscle.[1]

Measurements should be made and recorded in the metric system.

However, in areas where the only available weighing machines record in pounds and ounces, measurements may be taken in these units and later converted into metric units prior to comparison with standards of reference (Annex 1).

1. Weight

Weight is the anthropometric measurement most in use. Its potential value, especially for children, is appreciated not only by health personnel, but often by less educated parents, for whom it is useful as a source of health education.

In developing regions, the prevalence of protein-calorie malnutrition appears to be best indicated by weight deficiency in all age-groups and by growth failure in children. Weighing is the key anthropometric measurement.

Weight estimations can be made on isolated occasions, as in many surveys, or repeated at intervals under special conditions, as at child-welfare clinics, schools, prenatal clinics, or in longitudinal studies. These serial measurements give a better index of actual growth or growth failure, but attention should be paid to possible difficulties of identification that may arise if the particular population is mobile and if name-changing is a common practice culturally.

The evaluation of the significance of weight measurements must take into account length, frame size, proportions of fat, muscle and bone, and the presence of pathological weight due, for example, to oedema or spleno-megaly. Accordingly, weight measurements should be combined with other appropriate measurements and with clinical examination.

Equipment. The choice of suitable scales is a difficult matter. They must be sturdy, inexpensive, easily transportable, and accurate to within the limits required (e.g., 0.1 kg). They must be checked frequently through the complete range of weights envisaged, at least twice daily during a survey,

---

[1] Photography can be a valuable tool for the assessment of nutritional status in the laboratory, as well as under field conditions, but is too expensive and time-consuming to be commonly used, except in a general way.

To be of value, anthropometric photography requires adequate standardization of procedure, i.e., posture, avoidance of distortion, uniform lighting, etc. The scale used should always be included in the photograph, and should be located in the same plane as the subject. Proper identification is essential.

Measurements from photographs require uniform positioning which is almost impossible to obtain in mass surveys of young children. In older children and adults, valuable anthropometric and clinical information can be obtained. With suitable arrangements, photography can substantially reduce the time required for field measurements. The great advantage of photographs is that one can always return to the original records for checks on doubtful data at a more leisurely pace than is possible under field survey conditions.

Selected photographs can be of considerable value in illustrating nutritional aspects and various features in the local ecology. They are particularly needed to illustrate subjective judgements of health and nutritional status.

by the use of objects of known weight supplied for this purpose. The scales should be corrected in the light of the tests, or—less satisfactorily—allowance made in the results.

Weighing machines based on two different principles are available: beam balance scales and spring scales. The latter should not be used because they easily become stretched and inaccurate from frequent use or with the expansion of the spring that occurs in unduly hot weather.

Beam, or lever, balance scales (Fig. 33) are preferable, as they are less likely to be inaccurate if carefully looked after. Their accuracy depends, however, on the integrity of their knife-edge balancing part or fulcrum. Beam balance scales are usually of the familiar type supplied by UNICEF for young children, measuring up to 16 kg (35 lb) with increments of 100 g (3½ oz) or the platform type for adults or older children. Both are rather heavy to transport and can become mechanically inaccurate after jolting on a rough road journey. The use of a locking device or wedging the moving

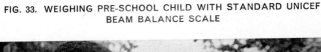

FIG. 33. WEIGHING PRE-SCHOOL CHILD WITH STANDARD UNICEF BEAM BALANCE SCALE

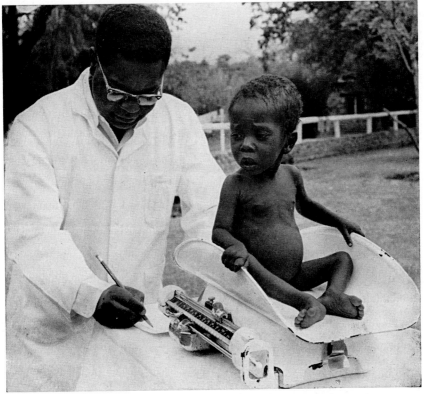

FIG. 34. WEIGHING PRE-SCHOOL CHILD WITH MODIFIED STEELYARD

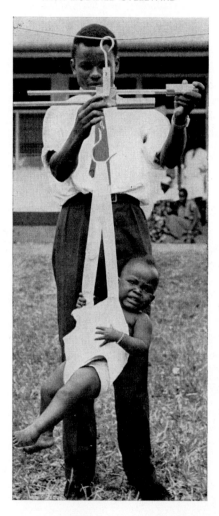

parts before journeys is advisable. They must be used on a firm, non-tilted surface, and checked before use.

Another type of scale, employing the beam-balance principle, is the butcher's steelyard (Fig. 34), which is an ancient, simple and inexpensive weighing apparatus. It is compact and can be easily transported, usually weighing up to 20 kg (44 lb) with an accuracy of up to 0.1 kg. It has to be suspended from the branch of a tree or roof beam, but can be read accurately as there is little oscillation (Welbourn, 1956).

Technique. Young children should be weighed nude. If bells or heavy charms are worn, as in some rural African communities, they should be removed, if permissible and practicable. Otherwise, due allowance should be made for their weight. Scales capable of making small measurements with accuracy are needed for young children, especially for serial measurements.

With due attention to technique, relatively passive infants can be weighed on most of the scales mentioned. The problem is more difficult with larger, more active pre-school-age children. As elsewhere in the world, and especially with apprehensive children in rural tropical surroundings, it is often best to use an adult platform beam balance scale to weigh the mother alone, and then weigh her carrying her child. The advantage of this method is that the child is calmed by the mother, so that time is saved and accurate recordings can be made. The disadvantage is that two weights have to be recorded and the risk of clerical error is doubled. The subtraction required to obtain the child's weight should not be carried out in the field, but on return to base. However, occasional calculations at the time may serve as a check on the clerical recording of figures.

For schoolchildren and adults, the platform beam balance is most usually employed. Weighing should not be done after a full meal. Theoretically, the bladder should be emptied prior to measurement. In fact, this is rarely done and has little practical significance.

The subjects should stand on the centre of the platform without touching anything else. Shoes should be removed and the minimum clothing worn. For schoolchildren, if the sexes are weighed separately, it is possible for clothing to consist of a pair of drawers or shorts. For adults, especially in field circumstances, weighing usually has to be carried out while they are wearing ordinary clothing. In these circumstances, the average weight of the clothing customarily worn must be determined and due allowance made in the results. Details of this kind must always be recorded in the written reports of surveys.

Standards of reference. As noted earlier, body-weight measurements found in a community can best be compared with locally prepared standards, if such exist, and also with suggested general standards of reference (e.g., the modified Harvard Standards for young children (Annex 1, Tables (1)-(4), (10) and (11)), the Baldwin-Wood Standards for schoolchildren (Annex 1, Tables (8) and (9), and the modified Actuaries Standards for adults (Annex 1, Tables (15) and (16)).

Results. Weight assessment in community investigations in most developing countries is concerned with determining degrees of underweight, principally resulting from varying levels of protein-calorie malnutrition. It is not usually concerned with the detection of obesity.

Body weight is mainly made up of muscle, fat, bone and internal organs, with the addition, in pathological circumstances, of oedema, ascites, massive organ enlargement (e.g., splenomegaly) and even the helminth burden in severe ascariasis.

The interpretation of weights below the standard has to take account of these various components, and it can be critically analysed only if a simultaneous estimation of some of these tissues is also carried out at selected sites, especially subcutaneous fat and muscle mass.

Because of differences in growth at various stages of life, weight levels or changes in weight over a period of time have to be interpreted differently in various age-groups. These are considered in a later section for young children, schoolchildren, pregnant women, and adults.

2. Linear measurements

Two types of linear measurement are commonly employed: (*a*) height (or length) of the whole body and (*b*) certain circumferences, particularly of the head and the chest.

Height (or length)

The height of an individual is made up of the sum of four components: legs, pelvis, spine and skull. While, for detailed studies of body proportions, all of these measurements are required, in field nutritional anthropometry usually only the total height (or length) is measured.

Equipment and technique. For older children and adults, a vertical measuring rod or a scale fixed to a wall can be employed (Fig. 35). After removing the shoes, the subject should stand on a flat floor by the scale with feet parallel and with heels, buttocks, shoulders and back of head touching the upright. The head should be held comfortably erect, with the lower border of the orbit in the same horizontal plane as the external auditory meatus. The arms should be hanging at the sides in a natural manner. The headpiece, which can be a metal bar or a wooden block, is gently lowered, crushing the hair, and making contact with the top of the head. The presence of unusually thick hair requires to be taken into account. The measuring scale should be 2 m (78³/₄ in.) high and capable of measuring to an accuracy of 0.5 cm (¹/₅ in.).

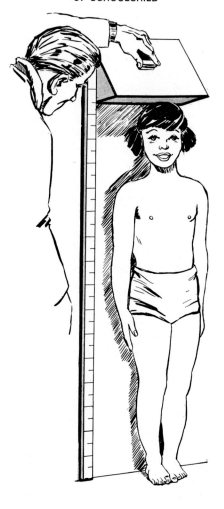

FIG. 35. HEIGHT MEASUREMENT OF SCHOOLCHILD

For infants and pre-school children, recumbent length (crown-heel length) has to be employed, as the measurement of standing height is either impossible or very inaccurate with an uncooperative child. This is usually carried out with a wooden length-board (Fig. 36).

The infant is laid on the board which is itself on a flat surface. The head is positioned firmly against the fixed headboard, with the eyes looking vertically. The knees are extended, usually by firm pressure applied by an assistant, and the feet are flexed at right angles to the lower legs. The upright sliding foot-piece is moved to obtain firm contact with the heels and the length read to the nearest 0.1 cm.

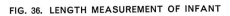

FIG. 36. LENGTH MEASUREMENT OF INFANT

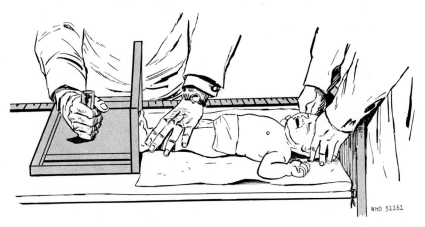

WHO 51161

The difficulties of using a length-board for measuring terrified, struggling young children in rural surveys are considerable. Much practice and the assistance of two, or preferably three, people are required to make adequately accurate readings.

Standards of reference. Results should be compared with local standards, if such exist, and with general standards of reference (Annex 1, Table (2)).

The usefulness and the interpretation of this measurement in various age-groups are given in other sections.

Head circumference

The measurement of head circumference is a standard procedure in paediatric practice, usually to detect pathological conditions accompanied by a large head or one of increasing size, as, for example, with hydrocephalus, or too small a skull, as with microcephaly.

Head circumference is related mainly to brain size and—to a small extent—to the thickness of the scalp tissues and the skull. Brain-size increases rapidly during the first year, when head circumference normally reflects age rather than health or nutrition. However, brain-size and both the thickness of scalp soft tissues and the skull can vary with nutritional status, so that head circumference is slightly affected in the second year of life in protein-calorie malnutrition (Robinow & Jelliffe—in preparation), although much less so than chest circumference.

In nutritional anthropometry, the chest/head circumference ratio is of value in detecting protein-calorie malnutrition in early childhood (see page 196). The head circumference may also be used as a rough additional guide in age assessment.

Equipment and technique (Fig. 37). Measurements should be made with a narrow (less than 1 cm wide), flexible, non-stretch tape, made of steel or

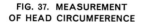

FIG. 37. MEASUREMENT
OF HEAD CIRCUMFERENCE

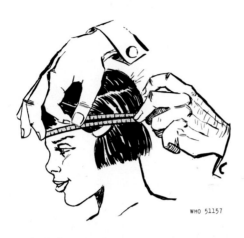

WHO 51157

preferably fibre-glass. Cloth tapes should be avoided as they tend to stretch in use. If they have to be used, they should be checked frequently.

The child's head should be steadied and the greatest circumference measured, by placing the tape firmly round the frontal bones just superior to the supra-orbital ridges, passing it round the head at the same level on each side, and laying it over the maximum occipital prominence at the back. Measurements should be made to the nearest 0.1 cm.

Standards of reference. Little work appears to have been done in this field among children in different parts of the world. Variations in skull appearance occur in different ethnic groups, presumably on a genetic basis, although the possibility of other factors playing a part in these differences cannot be overlooked.[1] These may include cultural practices in infancy —seen in an extreme form in the head-binding of certain South American Indians, in the large skulls sometimes found in rickets, or in such pathological conditions as sickle-cell anaemia.

Local standards require to be constructed. In the meantime, figures given by Watson & Lowrey (1958) can be used for reference purposes.

Chest circumference

Again, the main practical field use of this measurement will be in the second, and perhaps third, years of life. This is because the circumference of the head and the chest are about the same at six months of age. After this, the skull grows slowly and the chest more rapidly (Table 6). Therefore, between the ages of six months and five years, a chest/head circumference ratio of less than one may be due to failure to develop, or to wasting of the muscle and fat of the chest wall, and can be used as community indicator of protein-calorie malnutrition of early childhood. It also has the advantage of not requiring even a tape measure, as the two circumferences can be compared with a piece of string (Dean, 1965).

Equipment and technique. A narrow, flexible non-stretch steel or fibre-glass tape should be used, and measurement made at the nipple line, prefer-

---

[1] Variations in skull shape may be recognized—for example, among the Baganda, who have different words for bossing in different places (e.g., *mpumi* for frontal bossing, *masiga* for parietal bossing, and *nkona* for occipital bossing).

TABLE 6. HEAD AND CHEST CIRCUMFERENCE
MEASUREMENTS IN FIRST FIVE YEARS OF LIFE *

Age (months)	Head (cm)	Chest (cm)
Birth	35.0	35
3	40.4	40
6	43.4	44
12	46.0	47
18	47.4	48
24	49.0	50
36	50.0	52
48	50.5	53
60	50.8	55

* From *Growth and development of children*, 4th ed., by
E. H. Watson and G. H. Lowrey. Copyright © 1962, Year Book
Medical Publishers, Inc. Reproduced by permission of Year
Book Medical Publishers.

ably in mid-inspiration (Fig. 38). Practical problems may be considerable, as it is difficult to obtain accurate readings if the child is screaming or breathing irregularly. Consequently, this procedure is best carried out with the child sitting on its mother's lap. Measurement should be made to the nearest 0.1 cm.

3. Soft tissues

The brain, liver, heart, kidneys and other internal organs together make up an appreciable part of the body weight, but are *relatively* unchanged by weight in malnutrition. Muscle and fat constitute the soft tissues that vary most with a deficiency of protein and calories. Tissue anthropometry can be carried out on both of these in the assessment of the nutritional status of a community.

FIG. 38. MEASUREMENT
OF CHEST CIRCUMFERENCE

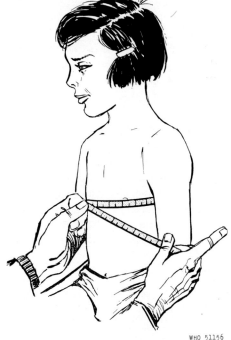

WHO 51156

Subcutaneous fat

Body composition studies, including information concerning the amount and distribution of human subcutaneous fat, and hence of calorie reserves, can be carried out by various methods,[1] including the following:

physical and chemical analysis (by whole-body analysis at autopsy)

ultrasonics

densitometry (by water displacement in a densitometer, or underwater weighing)

gaseous uptake of fat-soluble gases

radiological anthropometry (using soft-tissue exposures) [2]

physical anthropometry (using skin-fold calipers).

Equipment. While all the techniques listed above can be important tools in detailed nutritional investigation in well-equipped research centres, only physical anthropometry using skin-fold calipers is practicable in field circumstances and, even then, great care has to be taken with the technique employed and with the interpretation of results. It may be noted, however, that the correlation between caliper measurements, radiological findings and direct measurements at surgical operations is good (Tanner, 1959; Garn, 1962).

Various skin-fold calipers have been devised, but experience has shown that the instrument used should have a standard contact surface or " pinch " area (20-40 mm^2), should read to 0.1 mm accuracy and exert a constant pressure (10 g/mm^2) through the whole range of skin-fold thicknesses at all distances of separation of the jaws.

In practice, three instruments at present seem to be most often used: the Harpenden calipers (Edwards et al., 1955) (Fig. 39), the Lange calipers (Lange & Brozek, 1961) (Fig. 40), and the USAMRNL calipers [3] (Best, 1953, 1954; Consolazio, Johnson & Pecora, 1963). Where possible, the dial must be carefully reset to zero before each day's work, if practicable, or due allowance made for zero error.

Technique. The skin-folds measured consist of a *double* layer of skin and subcutaneous fat. The most appropriate " pinch " sites depend on the purpose of the study, the age of the population examined (fat distribution varies with age, even in childhood), sex, precision in locating the particular site, the relative homogeneity of the thickness of the layer of fat and skin in a given region, and the ease or otherwise of accessibility when problems of undressing and modesty exist (Garn, 1957; Lewis, Masterton & Ferres, 1958). The left side of the body should be used for this and all other measurements (Falkner, 1960).

---

[1] Full documentation on the latest scientific advances in this field are given by Forbes (1962) and by the Annals of the New York Academy of Sciences (1963), Vol. 110 (2 parts).

[2] Garn (1962) has pointed out that this supplies a permanent record. It is possible that radiological films taken for orthopaedic reasons in developing regions or elsewhere might be analysed.

[3] US Army Medical Research Nutrition Laboratory, Chicago, Ill., USA.

FIG. 39. HARPENDEN SKIN-FOLD CALIPERS

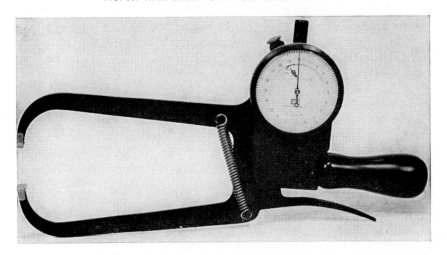

FIG. 40. LANGE SKIN-FOLD CALIPERS

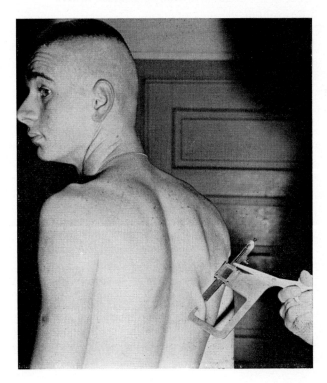

In most large-scale surveys, in both adults and children, major emphasis has usually been on obesity due to caloric overnutrition. With this in mind, workers, including Hammond (1955b), have suggested that *total* body subcutaneous fat can be calculated from measurements made at several places, such as the triceps, the abdomen, and subscapular and subcostal sites.

Similar methods can be employed in communities in developing regions, but large numbers of measurements will not usually be indicated or feasible. Despite the fact that increase or depletion of subcutaneous fat stores is not uniform all over the body, the essence of the problem is to select one or two easily accessible sites that may be expected to give an approximate practical indication of calorie reserves. For this purpose, both with poor calorie stores and in obesity, the triceps skin-fold is the most practical measurement for all age-groups.

Furthermore, in young children, the triceps skin-fold is not only useful as an index of calorie reserves but enables the underlying mid-upper arm muscle circumference to be calculated (see Fig. 44).

At all sites, a lengthwise skin-fold is firmly grasped and slightly lifted up between finger and thumb of the left hand, care being taken not to include underlying muscle. The calipers are applied about 1 cm below the operator's fingers at a depth about equal to the skin-fold, while the skin-fold is still gently held throughout the measurement. Three measurements should be made and the results averaged. Difficulties in obtaining accurate results can occur because of increased compressibility in frank, or even subclinical, oedema, and possibly because of the normal occurrence of softer fat in infants than in adults.

The technique is by no means easy and requires prolonged supervised practice and repetition to obtain reliable and reproducible results.

Triceps skin-fold (upper arm, dorsal arm, arm skin-fold). As the fat in this region is not uniform in thickness, the site is carefully selected, halfway down the arm, between the tip of the acromion process of the scapula and the olecranon process of the ulna (Fig. 41). The measurement is made with the arm hanging relaxed at the side. The skin-fold parallel to the long axis is picked up between the thumb and forefinger of the left hand, clean away from the underlying muscle, and measured at this point (Fig. 42) (Committee on Nutritional Anthropometry, 1956).

Subscapular skin-fold (infrascapular, back skin-fold). The subscapular skin-fold is measured just below and laterally to the angle of the left scapula. The fold should be in a line running at approximately 45° to the spine, in the natural line of skin cleavage. It is often used as a secondary site for adults. It has the advantage of providing a uniform layer of subcutaneous fat, not requiring precise localization. It has the disadvantage of inaccessibility.

Standards. With the considerable variation in fat distribution with age, both in early childhood and in later life, separate standards are needed for different age-groups. Likewise, sex differences occur throughout life, with skin-folds greater in females from birth onwards. Also, limb skin-folds, including the triceps measurement, can yield falsely low results if the skin and subcutaneous fat are stretched by considerable underlying muscle hypertrophy.

Appropriate standards for use in communities in developing tropical regions are difficult to lay down with certainty. It is possible that a lesser insulating layer may be usual in warmer climates, and also that figures obtained so far from Europe and North America are too high, reflecting a too-generous calorie intake, which may well not be optimal. Also, a variation in fat composition may occur with different diets and environmental temperatures, possibly associated with atypical physical properties, such as compressibility (MacDonald, 1961; McLaren & Read, 1962), while a genetic difference in subcutaneous-fat distribution has been suggested (Robson, 1964b).

It is therefore desirable that local standards should be prepared and compared with those already available from well-fed Caucasian populations. In the meantime, general standards of reference are given in Annex 1, Tables (5), (12) and (17).

Muscle

Poor muscle development or muscle wasting are cardinal features of all forms of protein-calorie mal-

FIG. 41. ASSESSING MIDPOINT OF UPPER ARM (HALFWAY BETWEEN THE ACROMIAL PROCESS OF THE SCAPULA AND THE OLECRANON PROCESS OF THE ULNA)

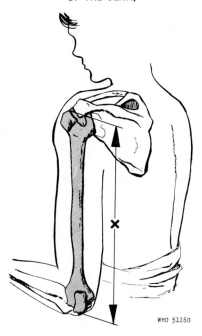

WHO 51160

FIG. 42. MEASUREMENT OF TRICEPS SKIN-FOLD WITH HARPENDEN CALIPERS

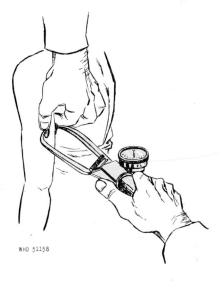

WHO 51158

nutrition, especially those of early childhood. In older children and adults, muscle mass is also related to general exercise and to special increased use of certain muscle groups.

Muscle mass [1] may be assessed in various ways (Standard, Wills & Waterlow, 1959):

(a) Total: body analysis (at autopsy) (Garrow, Fletcher & Halliday, 1965)

     body radio-active potassium (as a measure of cellular mass, of which muscle is the principal component)

     chemical urine analysis (for muscle breakdown products, e.g., creatinine excretion)

(b) Localized: soft tissue radiology (of leg or arm)

     physical anthropometry (by measurement of a limb).

For practical purposes, with the possible exception of urine samples for creatinine excretion, the only practical field method is by direct physical anthropometry of a limb.

Technique. In practice, two limbs have been used—the mid-calf and the mid-upper arm. Both are roughly circular and heavily muscled.

Measurements of the mid-upper arm appear to be most useful in practice. This region is easily accessible, even with a young child sitting in front of the examiner on his mother's lap. Also, in kwashiorkor the upper arm is not usually clinically oedematous, while it has been shown that the mid-upper arm is markedly wasted in this condition.

The arm circumference is measured to the nearest 0.1 cm with a flexible steel or fibre-glass tape, which must be placed gently, but firmly, round the limb to avoid compression of the soft tissues (Fig. 43). In young infants, it is difficult to measure the small circumference of the arm with a steel tape, and it is necessary to use a glass-fibre one.

The left arm is measured, while hanging freely, at its mid-point, which is selected in the same way as for the triceps skin-fold. Secondly, the over-lying subcutaneous fat is measured in the triceps region with skin-fold calipers as described earlier (p. 74).

From these two measurements, it is possible to calculate the inner circle, which is composed principally of muscle, with a small central core of bone. It is usually assumed that the bone is relatively constant in size, and the calculated value is termed the " mid-arm-muscle circumference ".[2] Alternatively, it is possible to make allowance for the humerus by subtracting an approximate standard value according to the age of the subject, but usually this is not done. A formula for the calculation of the mid-arm-muscle

---

[1] Measurement of muscular strength by dynamometry is not usually practicable in survey work, as it is time-consuming, influenced by psychological factors, and impossible to use in young children. It may sometimes be of value for adults and schoolchildren.

[2] Alternatively, the I.A.D. (" inner arm diameter "), composed principally of muscle and bone, has been calculated as a gauge of muscularity (McFie & Welbourn, 1962).

FIG. 43. MEASUREMENT OF MID-UPPER-ARM CIRCUMFERENCE

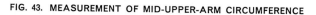

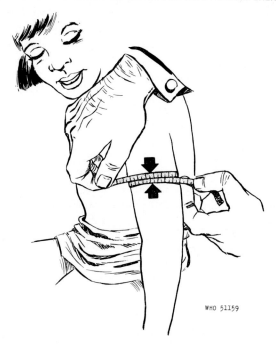

WHO 51159

circumference is given in the caption of Fig. 44 (based on Jelliffe & Jelliffe, 1960).

An apparent disadvantage of this type of measurement is that it is a linear expression of a three-dimensional tissue, which should, ideally, be given by weight or volume. However, this single measurement cor-

FIG. 44. CALCULATION OF MID-UPPER-ARM-MUSCLE CIRCUMFERENCE

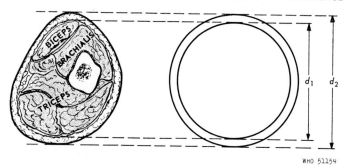

WHO 51154

Measurements are made of arm circumference C_1 and triceps skin-fold S. Let d_1 = arm diameter and d_2 = muscle diameter. Then skin-fold $S = 2 \times$ subcutaneous fat = $d_1 - d_2$, and arm circumference $C_1 = \pi d_1$. Now, muscle circumference $C_2 = \pi d_2 = \pi [d_1 - (d_1 - d_2)] = \pi d_1 - \pi(d_1 - d_2)$. Hence, $C_2 = C_1 - \pi S$.

relates well with more general manifestations of protein-calorie malnutrition. Also, it is an attempt to assess a body-wide tissue, which may be affected unequally in different muscle groups, by a measurement at a single site. Nevertheless, the arm-muscle circumference does represent a practical, if approximate, gauge of muscle tissue, and one that can be easily obtained.

An even simpler measurement, that of the arm circumference, may be used by itself, because it has been shown to correlate well with the calculated muscle circumference (Robinow & Jelliffe—in preparation) and to be much reduced in all severer forms of protein-calorie malnutrition of early childhood (see page 196).

Standards. Values for arm-muscle circumference are not easily available for well-nourished communities. Approximate general standards of reference are given later for this calculated measurement and also for arm circumference for different ages and both sexes (Annex 1).

Recommended basic measurements for surveys

The following basic measurements should be made on all age-groups: weight, height (or length), triceps skin-fold, and arm circumference.

In young children, these should be supplemented by measurements of the head circumference and of the chest circumference.

BIOCHEMICAL TESTS[1]

Although biochemical estimations of nutritional significance can be carried out on a variety of body tissues, including liver, muscle (Waterlow & Mendes, 1957) and bone, in practice, in field surveys, tests are confined to two fairly easily obtainable body fluids: blood and urine.

The range of biochemical tests that can be employed for assessing malnutrition is considerable. However, in rural field conditions, this will be limited by many factors, including the need for single-specimen samples, rather than the collection of "timed" samples or the use of loading tests; the age-groups concerned (and the difficulty in securing large samples of venous blood from young children); and the limitation of laboratory facilities, especially of skilled laboratory staff.

Defining ideal criteria for biochemical tests suitable for field work, Whitehead (1965) stresses that these should be easily collectable (this implies a finger-prick sample of blood or a random specimen of urine), stable during transport (preferably not requiring refrigeration), not affected by a recent meal or by water load, and capable of giving information not already available by non-biochemical techniques, so that they can be used either for objective quantitative assessment or as a screening procedure.

---

[1] This section has been based largely on the report of the WHO Expert Committee on Medical Assessment of Nutritional Status (1963), on the work of Goldsmith (1959) and Wilson et al. (1964), and on the manual prepared by the ICNND (1963). These publications should be consulted for additional technical details, including laboratory control, reproducibility, etc.

Generally, intricate biochemical tests are costly and time-consuming to carry out. In all surveys, the expected value of results to be obtained by particular methods in the assessment of nutritional status must be weighed against the problems of collection, transport, laboratory analysis and interpretation. In addition, while some tests are of considerable assistance, many have as yet uncertain " standards " for less advanced forms of malnutrition, especially in young children. In fact, valuable nutritional surveys of limited scope can be undertaken with a small team by means of clinical assessment, anthropometry, dietary inquiry, and with no laboratory investigation other than haemoglobin estimation.

Appropriate biochemical tests will have to be selected for the particular survey contemplated. The range to be employed may embrace some, or all, of the tests listed in category 1 (Table 7), or may be much more restricted. For a nutrition survey to produce useful information, it is not always necessary to have the large number of personnel and the quantities of equipment required for a wide range of biochemical tests.

Sometimes laboratory investigations may be practicable on a limited sample of those covered by the survey, particularly if specimens can be air-freighted to a regional centre. Selection, again, may be by subsampling, or by choosing subjects considered, on clinical evidence, as likely to be deficient. Thus, more detailed haematological tests may be carried out on only a small percentage of those found to be definitely anaemic by clinical assessment or by haemoglobin level. Also, vitamin " loading " tests with riboflavin may be feasible in a sample of persons with angular cheilosis and other suggestive signs of ariboflavinosis.

As with all methods of assessment, the nutritional significance of the results of biochemical tests in a community has to be correlated with all the other findings—clinical, anthropometric, dietary and ecological.

Collection of samples

Numbers. When the appropriate biochemical tests for the particular survey have been chosen, a decision must be made on the number of specimens that can be collected and processed, since this will determine the required amount of collecting equipment. The number of specimens will depend on statistical considerations in relation to the total number of persons examined clinically in the field and on the limitations imposed by facilities for transport, storage and actual analysis. A sub-sampling technique will normally be required.

Blood samples. Plasma is required for examinations for albumin, vitamin A, carotene, ascorbic acid and alkaline phosphatase, and will have to be prepared from oxalated whole blood by centrifugation. Fresh whole blood or blood preserved with sequestrene is used for the determination of haemoglobin and haematocrit, and for the preparation of thin and thick blood films, if these are to be included.

TABLE 7. BIOCHEMICAL TESTS APPLICABLE TO NUTRITION SURVEYS *

Nutritional deficiency	First category [a]	Second category
(1) Protein	Amino acid imbalance test Hydroxyproline excretion test (F) Serum albumin Urinary urea (F) [b] Urinary creatinine per unit of time (T)	Serum protein fractions by electrophoresis
(2) Vitamin A	Serum vitamin A Serum carotene	
(3) Vitamin D	Serum alkaline phosphatase (in young children)	Serum inorganic phosphorus
(4) Ascorbic acid	Serum ascorbic acid	White blood cell ascorbic acid Urinary ascorbic acid Load test
(5) Thiamine	Urinary thiamine (F) [b]	Load test Blood pyruvate Blood lactate Red blood cell haemolysate transketolase
(6) Riboflavin	Urinary riboflavin (F) [b]	Red blood cell riboflavin Load test
(7) Niacin	Urinary N-methylnicotinamide (F) [b]	Load test Urinary pyridone (n-methyl-2-pyridone-5-carbonamide)
(8) Iron	Haemoglobin Haematocrit Thin blood film	Serum iron Percentage saturation of transferrin
(9) Folic acid Vitamin B_{12}	Haemoglobin Thin blood film	Serum folate (*L. casei*) Serum B_{12} (*E. gracilis*)
(10) Iodine		Urinary iodine (F) Tests for thyroid function

* Adapted from WHO Expert Committee on Medical Assessment of Nutritional Status (1963)
[a] Urinary creatinine used as reference for expressing other urine measurements in first category.
[b] Expressed per gram of creatinine.
(F) In a single urine specimen, preferably fasting.
(T) In timed urine specimens.

Blood tests are often carried out with macro-methods, although the relatively large quantities required can be obtained in field circumstances only from adults or school-age children. Venous samples are preferably taken by vacuum tube (such as the Vacutainer), or with disposable needles attached to plastic tubing, to avoid contamination and the need for cleaning and sterilizing syringes in the field. The latter is the easiest and cheapest method of obtaining blood samples, especially if used with a sphygmomanometer rather than a tourniquet, and it also permits several samples of blood to be taken into different containers during one venepuncture, if required.

Equipment for washing out and unplugging syringes and needles must be immediately at hand when samples are taken. Needles must be sharpened as necessary. The technique for drawing blood must be thoroughly known and practised.

Blood samples are collected into stoppered or screw-capped glass vials, containing an anticoagulant, such as dried oxalate or heparin lithium. Each container should have a previously affixed blank label.

Some of the biochemical tests used for nutritional appraisal can be carried out by micro-methods. These methods are particularly important where young children are concerned. Blood obtained by finger-prick can be collected in heparinized capillary tubes, and sealed by heating in a flame or by using commercial clay, specially prepared for this purpose.

All blood samples must be kept chilled until tested. In the field, this is achieved in thermos flasks, in plastic cooling bags (with tins of freezing mixture) or, rarely, in mobile refrigerators. In the laboratory, the specimens are kept in an ordinary household refrigerator.

Urine samples. Difficulties in collection from adults are largely related to modesty. For young children, only boys can have this undertaken easily by fixing a test-tube (preferably of plastic) to the penis, although a relatively expensive plastic disposable collecting device, which sticks to the perineum, can be used for little girls. Sometimes, however, it may suffice for plastic jars to be given to mothers for them to " catch " a specimen during the survey period.

For the commoner urinary analyses (e.g., urea, thiamine, riboflavin, N-methyl-nicotinamide), fasting samples passed in a definite time-period are ideal, but not usually practicable under field conditions, especially with children. Single random specimens must often suffice. However, when used as a measure of body-muscle mass, urine for creatinine estimation has to be collected over a timed period—minimally 3 hours, and preferably 24 hours.

Urine should be collected in sturdy screw-capped glass or, preferably, plastic bottles containing hydrochloric acid as a preservative and as an inhibitor of bacterial growth. The amount of hydrochloric acid should be such as not to dilute the sample greatly: one drop of concentrated hydrochloric acid should be enough for about 25 ml of urine. The specimen can then be kept at room temperature or stored in a refrigerator.

Laboratory considerations

Site. The various laboratory tests differ in complexity in respect of the staff and facilities required, and the time within which they have to be performed once the sample has been taken.

One, or all, of three laboratory sites have to be considered:

(*a*) survey site facilities for taking, lableling, packaging and refrigerating samples;

(b) a field laboratory adjacent to, or not far distant from, the survey site. Adequate bench or table space should be available, as well as a water supply, a refrigerator, cylinders of gas and, if possible, electricity;

(c) a base laboratory, often situated in a central institution, such as a medical school or an agricultural research station.

The most suitable arrangement for a given survey depends upon the tests envisaged, the availability and location of existing laboratories, the distances and communications involved, and the funds available. In some surveys, it may be possible to build up a new laboratory, or to help one develop or expand.

In most developing countries, laboratory services are limited outside main centres, and plans must be made to take most of the samples back at the end of a survey, or to send them at intervals during the field work, depending on local circumstances. The necessary funds for staff, including drivers, and for equipment, including refrigeration, must be budgeted for in whatever scheme is considered to be appropriate.

In many shorter surveys, it is easier and more economical to make it a rule that, whenever possible, specimens should be collected in the field, preserved or refrigerated suitably, and ultimately taken back to the base laboratory at the end of the survey.

Equipment. Initial and recurrent equipment needed must be calculated as far as possible on an estimate of the numbers of samples likely to be collected and their possible storage and transport. A 20% excess is desirable for field work to cover breakage, loss and any initial underestimate of attendance.

Supplies should be standardized, as far as possible. Containers should be labelled prior to the field work and held ready for use (e.g., with anticoagulants already in them). They should be as strong as possible and of suitable shape to facilitate packing and minimize breakage (e.g., sturdy, flat-bottomed, thick-glass or plastic, screw-capped vials).

Techniques. Laboratory techniques must be selected for their accuracy, sensitivity, reproducibility, and practicability within the technical resources available. Methods commonly used and of proved value are suggested in subsequent sections dealing with individual nutrients. In all cases, the method employed must be described in reports, and, if it is a modification of a standard procedure or a new technique, details must be given.

Details must also be given of procedures used in the collection, transport and storage of specimens, including, if relevant to the particular tests, the time when taken, possible exposure to sun, heat and air, and the period between collection and testing.

Interpretation of biochemical tests

The significance and accuracy of results of biochemical tests are related to standards of collection, methods of transport and storage, including possible exposure to ultraviolet light, heat and shaking, and the actual technique used including laboratory control using control sera (Sinclair, 1964).

The interpretation of results varies with knowledge of the unique metabolism of each particular nutrient, including its storage in the body, the possibility of synthesis and the mode of excretion. The tests employed usually assess one of two aspects of nutritional inadequacy, although their specificity may be less than is at present appreciated.

First, a biochemical investigation may give information on the nutrient supply to the body, as reflected by levels in a particular tissue, most often the serum, e.g., ascorbic acid. However, the concentration of an essential nutrient in a body fluid may be reduced as a result of dietary deficiency, poor absorption, impaired transport (as can result from the decreased plasma proteins in protein-calorie malnutrition), abnormal utilization, or a combination of these. The presence of haemoconcentration, as in dehydration, or of haemodilution, as in pregnancy, requires consideration. While the measurement of nutrient concentration is helpful in suggesting the possibility of malnutrition, it does not indicate the presence, or define the degree, of nutritional disease.

Secondly, some biochemical tests can be undertaken that reveal metabolic changes resulting from tissue malnutrition due to inadequate levels of essential nutrients, often of long duration. The detection of such metabolic changes aids in the assessment of nutritional status and, in many instances, indicates a state of deficiency with greater certainty than does a mere lowering of tissue concentration of essential nutrients. Furthermore, these changes sometimes precede the appearance of clinical manifestations of malnutrition. However, in some instances, biochemical tests relate to both the causes mentioned.

In addition to interpretation in relation to biochemical significance, levels of nutrients in the body have to be compared with the standards of reference, if possible, appropriate for the age and sex. Often these will have been constructed from results from the normal range found in well-fed healthy groups and from results from patients obviously clinically ill with the particular form of malnutrition. In such circumstances, it may be possible to sort out the findings into various highly tentative groups, with descriptive labels, such as " deficient ", " low ", etc. (Tables 8 and 9).

Often, however, standard values are not known, especially for children. The results then are necessarily expressed in relation to whatever data are available, even though the age-group is inappropriate.

Whether there is sufficient information to sort into specific " labelled " groups or not, it is always necessary in addition to report results mathematically, including the number examined and the results expressed as means (averages), standard deviations, and in numbers and percentages in convenient groups.

TABLE 8. SUGGESTED GUIDE TO INTERPRETATION
OF URINARY VITAMIN EXCRETION DATA,
YOUNG ADULT MALES *

	" Low "	" Deficient "
N¹-Methylnicotinamide:		
mg/6 hours	0.2-0.59	<0.2
mg/gm creatinine	0.5-1.59	<0.5
Riboflavin:		
mcg/6 hours	10-29	<10
mcg/gm creatinine	27-79	<27
Thiamine:		
mcg/6 hours	10-24	<10
mcg/gm creatinine	27-65	<27

* The urinary values indicated are based on an average creatinine coefficient of 23 and on an expected excretion of 1.5 g/day of creatinine by a 65-kg man.
Reproduced by permission from ICNND (1963).

TABLE 9. SUGGESTED GUIDE TO INTERPRETATION
OF BLOOD DATA, YOUNG ADULT MALES *

	" Low "	" Deficient "
Serum albumin:		
g/100 ml	2.80-3.51	<2.80
Serum ascorbic acid:		
mg/100 ml	0.10-0.19	<0.1
Serum vitamin A:		
mcg/100 ml	10-19	<10
Serum carotene:		
mcg/100 ml	20-39	<20

* Reproduced by permission from ICNND (1963).

Tests for specific nutrients

Although it may sometimes be difficult to find a biochemical test that will determine the presence of one specific nutrient, certain tests can be regarded as having some degree of specificity or, rather, indicativeness. From the practical point of view, these tests may be divided into two categories (Table 7):

First category. Those which have been most extensively used in past nutrition surveys and have a demonstrated usefulness. The necessary samples are relatively simple to collect, and the tests are easy to carry out in general nutrition laboratories. The urine tests included can be carried out on a single specimen.

Samples of blood and urine are preferably collected from subjects in the fasting state, but as this is not usually practicable, the investigator may have to resort to random specimens.

Second category. Methods of performing the tests in this category are complicated and are based on samples that are difficult to collect. In addition, the methods used are designed, in most instances, to gain more accurate and specific knowledge of particular nutritional inadequacies suggested by first-category tests, as well as by other survey data. They will be employed only in research investigations. They are set out in Annex 2.

The following sections are concerned with the commoner biochemical methods of assessing nutrient intake and nutritional status that have proved to be most applicable to nutrition prevalence surveys. References to commonly used biochemical procedures are also given in the text.

1. Proteins

Biochemical tests may be employed to test three aspects of protein nutrition:

(*a*) the relative adequacy of dietary intake;

(*b*) metabolic changes due to tissue malnutrition; and

(*c*) depletion of body stores of protein.

Dietary adequacy

The urea-nitrogen/creatinine-nitrogen excretion ratio is an approximate index of dietary protein related to muscle protein stores, although the result is affected by the preceding water load (Arroyave, Jansen & Torrico—in preparation). Although a 24-hour collection period probably gives more reliable results, a 3-4-hour period has been suggested (Powell, Plough & Baker, 1961). Once again, the collection of samples may present difficulties in the field (Luyken & Luyken-Koning, 1960). Recently, Dugdale & Edkins (1964) have suggested that an index of 30 or lower in a random sample is indicative of malnutrition.

The estimation itself is simple to carry out using an adaptation of the picrate method of Folin & Wu (1919) given by Consolazio, Johnson & Marck (1951), or by micro-methods (Toal & Daniel, 1950). Urea can be estimated in many ways; the method of Archibald (1945) is often used.

Metabolic changes

Alterations in amino acid metabolism have been demonstrated in kwashiorkor. They are probably due both to widespread metabolic changes, possibly caused by enzyme defects, and to immediate inadequacy of dietary protein. Thus, Holt et al. (1963) have shown that " plasma aminograms " from hospitalized cases of kwashiorkor in many parts of the world showed a similar pattern—namely, a reduction in most of the essential amino acids and certain inessential amino acids, and unaffected, or even high, values for most of the inessential group.

Recently, a new abbreviated test for imbalance of amino acids in the serum has been introduced that promises to be of value in survey work (Whitehead, 1964, 1965; Whitehead & Dean, 1964; McLaren, Kamel & Ayyoub, 1965). It consists in separating and assessing quantitatively four " indispensable " amino acids (leucine, isoleucine, valine, methionine) and four " dispensable " amino acids (glycine, serine, glutamine, taurine), by one-dimensional paper chromatography.

This test has the advantage that it is carried out on a capillary tube of blood obtained from a finger-prick, which has to be centrifuged immediately, but is stable for some days at room temperature thereafter, although preferably kept cool at icebox temperature (5°C) (Whitehead, 1965). It must not be frozen or haemolysis will occur. The test has the added merit of being independent of age.

Disadvantages include the need for chromatographic apparatus, although this can be quite easily used by specially trained junior laboratory technicians, and the fact that the test is normal in children in the marasmus " line of development ". Also, the test is invalidated by a recent high-protein meal, but this effect can be minimized by taking the specimen after a wait of four hours at the collecting point. Such a meal is in any event unlikely in the case of pre-school children in developing regions.

The result is expressed as a ratio of dispensable to indispensable amino acids which is high (5-10) in kwashiorkor and low (less than 2) in well-fed, healthy pre-school children. Initial studies also suggest that the ratio increases between these two levels with the degree of protein-calorie malnutrition in less affected children in the kwashiorkor " line of development ", and in particular it correlates with the only simple objective criteria—weight for age. Recent studies by Whitehead (1965) have suggested the following levels: below 2, " ideal "; 2-3, " doubtful "; above 3, " abnormal ". This test plainly merits further field trial; so far, it seems to be of value only in the kwashiorkor line of development (see Fig. 53).

More recently, Whitehead (1965) has introduced another test for marginal malnutrition based on the urinary excretion of hydroxyproline, which is low in malnourished children, being a product of collagen metabolism. In field surveys, random samples of urine are collected, and the hydroxyproline excretion is correlated to creatinine content per kilogram of body weight. Indices for normal children range between 2.0 and 5.0 (mean 3.0), and there is little variation between 3 months and 7 years of age. Clinically malnourished children have indices between 0.5 and 1.5 (mean 1.0), and in marginally malnourished children the values range between 1.0 and 2.0. Abnormal values are found in children deficient in both protein and total calories (nutritional marasmus), so that Whitehead (1965) has suggested that the measurement of both the amino-acid ratio and the hydroxyproline index may be of value in determining the diet of communities of marginally malnourished children.

A similar approach has been suggested independently by Picou et al. (1965).

Depletion of body stores

The plasma proteins, especially albumin, are much reduced in kwashiorkor. However, it is generally agreed that the body's ability to synthesize serum albumin is affected relatively late, and that the primary effect of protein lack is depletion of muscle tissue. Levels of total plasma protein are even more difficult to evaluate, as raised globulin levels, due to infections, including chronic malaria, are likely to influence the results.

It is usually believed that the level of serum albumin falls significantly only in severe protein depletion, thus serving " only as a confirmation of a condition already clinically evident " (Arroyave, 1961), and that it is not of value for detecting " marginal " mild-moderate cases (Waterlow, 1963).

Nevertheless, it must be admitted that investigations among children with protein-calorie malnutrition have mostly been concerned with total plasma proteins in hospitalized children. It does seem justifiable to reinvestigate the usefulness of serum albumin levels in community studies (Schendel, Hansen & Brock, 1960; Woodruff & Pettit, 1965), although it cannot be considered an established procedure in general surveys.

Further comparative studies between plasma albumin and other parameters of protein-calorie malnutrition disease are needed, based on field work, when results should be reported in various levels in grams per 100 ml (e.g., up to 2 g, 2.1 to 3 g, 3.1 to 4 g, 4.1 to 5 g, and over 5 g).

This test has the advantage of simplicity. Total protein can be carried out on a small quantity of serum by a modified Biuret method (ICNND, 1963), and the serum albumin estimated afterwards by paper electrophoresis.

Urinary excretion of creatinine during a timed period—as a minimum, 3 hours, but preferably 24 hours—is considered to be roughly proportional to the body's muscle mass in man (Stearns et al., 1958) and in sheep (Van Niekerk et al., 1963), although unexplained variations in excretion can occur from time to time (Forbes, 1962). Moreover, the intake of flesh foods can affect results, but this will have little significance in most tropical communities, especially in children. This technique has been used from the converse point of view—that is, for the assessment of obesity in adults (Garn & Clark, 1955) and schoolchildren (Talbot, 1938).

According to Clark et al. (1951), the creatinine coefficient (mg of creatinine excreted per 24 hours per kg body weight) is 22.0 (range 14.2-32.0) from birth to 24 months of age, and 25.0 (range 16.3-36.2) in subjects aged between 2 and 18 years. Oomen (personal communication, 1965), however, found lower figures for young healthy adults in the Netherlands—males and females, 19 mg—and for " normal " young adult sweet-potato eaters in New Guinea—males, 17 mg; females, 14 mg.

The expression of results as " mg of creatinine in 24 hours per cm of body height " is to be preferred to " per kg of body weight ", since variations in fat deposits affect the latter (Arroyave & Wilson, 1961).

Further research tests are given in Annex 2.

2. Vitamin A

Vitamin A is stored in the liver, and a direct assessment of body reserves can be made on liver biopsy material, but this is not practicable under field conditions.

The most useful biochemical test for survey work is the actual estimation of serum vitamin A, especially in young age-groups. However, because of hepatic storage of this vitamin, a low serum level reflects not only an inadequate recent intake, but also exhaustion of liver reserves. It is therefore related to prolonged severe dietary deficiency—probably of up to one year in adults and of up to four months in young children.

It has been shown that low levels of serum vitamin A are found in acute infections (McLaren, 1966) and in kwashiorkor; these low levels are probably due in part to liver dysfunction and in part to impairment of blood transport of the vitamin (Arroyave et al., 1965). Caution may therefore also be required in interpreting results in populations among whom lesser degrees of protein-calorie malnutrition are common (Leonard—personal communication, 1964). In addition, high levels of beta-carotenoids interfere technically with the estimation of serum vitamin A.

In young adult males, the following levels of serum vitamin A have been suggested: " low ", 10-19 mcg; " deficient ", < 10 mcg (ICNND, 1963). Similar standards may be used arbitrarily for all age-groups, although more data are required for pre-school children. In all investigations due attention must also be given to correlation with food-consumption studies, with clinical signs suggestive of avitaminosis A, and, in older children and adults, with results of dark-adaptation tests, if practicable. It seems probable that low serum-vitamin-A levels and abnormal dark-adaptation tests usually antedate the appearance of clinical signs as community indicators of inadequate vitamin-A nutrition.

Serum-carotene estimations are of less value as they merely reflect levels of dietary intake of carotene-containing foods and their digestion and absorption by the body. They are not indicative of vitamin-A nutrition as such, particularly as some are not utilizable by the body (McLaren, 1966). At best, low levels are related to a low intake of carotene-containing foods, which is often important in tropical populations whose diet is deficient in pre-formed vitamin A.

Again, for young adult males, serum-carotene levels can be tentatively classified as " low " if they are less than 40 mcg per 100 ml and acceptable if they are above this figure (ICNND, 1963).

Estimations are made by spectrophotometry, using either macro- or micro-methods (Consolazio, Johnson & Marck, 1951; ICNND, 1963).

3. Vitamin D

Adequacy of vitamin-D nutrition is not related to dietary intake alone, because body synthesis can produce part or all for the daily needs, provided that the skin is exposed to sufficient sunlight.

In severe shortage of vitamin D—manifested as rickets in young children and as osteomalacia in adult women—an excessive, though incomplete, bone development is associated with a rise in alkaline phosphatase enzyme in the serum.

In young children, the normal serum alkaline phosphatase ranges between 5 and 15 Bodansky units per 100 ml, and in clinical rickets it usually rises to above 20 units. Similarly, in osteomalacia in adult women, the serum alkaline phosphatase is above the usual adult level of 3 to 5 Bodansky units.[1]

The serum-alkaline-phosphatase level in groups of children is not a generally accepted criterion for the detection of subclinical deficiency of vitamin D, as it is too unreliable in the early stages. Caution in interpreting findings is also necessary because this enzyme has been shown to be reduced in kwashiorkor (Dean & Schwartz, 1953) and appears to be affected in lesser degrees of protein-calorie malnutrition (Mannheimer, 1966).

Surveys of young children principally concerned with vitamin-D deficiency should be based on a combination of clinical signs, serum-alkaline-phosphatase levels, and radiological examinations.

4. Ascorbic acid [2]

The simplest biochemical test for inadequate vitamin-C nutrition is the serum-ascorbic-acid level. Unfortunately, this reflects only the recent

---

[1] Usual upper limits in King-Armstrong units are 20 units for children and 13 units for adults.

[2] A lingual screening test for tissue ascorbic acid, using sodium dichloroindophenol solution, has been introduced by Cheraskin, Ringsdorf & El-Ashiry (1964) and may be useful for survey work.

dietary intake. Even an absence of serum ascorbic acid is not diagnostic of scurvy, as volunteers on a vitamin-C-free diet had an absence of serum ascorbic acid for some three months prior to developing clinically evident disease (Grandon, Lund & Dill, 1940). For young adults, 0.10-0.19 mg per 100 ml is regarded as " low " (ICNND, 1963).

The ascorbic acid can be estimated by the dinitrophenylhydrazine method (ICNND, 1963), or by the micro-methods either of Lowry, Lopez & Bessey (1945) or of Raoul (1947). Further research tests are given in Annex 2.

5. Thiamine

Thiamine concentrations in the plasma, red blood cells and white blood cells cannot be determined with small samples, because available methods are not sufficiently sensitive (Burch et al., 1952). However, estimations of urinary excretion of thiamine have been undertaken widely and reflect the intake of this nutrient. The 24-hour output, the one-hour excretion on fasting, or the thiamine content of a random sample per gram of creatinine can be used. Tentative guide figures for thiamine excretion for adults and children are given in Tables 8 and 10.

Urinary thiamine is estimated fluorometrically (Mickelson & Yamamoto, 1958; ICNND, 1963). Further research tests are set out in Annex 2.

TABLE 10. TENTATIVE GUIDE FOR THE INTERPRETATION OF THIAMINE EXCRETION IN CHILDREN *

Age (years)	" Low " thiamine excretion (mcg/g creatinine)	" Deficient " thiamine excretion (mcg/g creatinine)
1-3	120-175	<120
4-6	85-120	<85
7-9	70-180	<70
10-12	60-180	<60
13-15	50-150	<50

* Adapted by permission from Pearson (1962).

6. Riboflavin

In field surveys, riboflavin may be determined in a single random urine specimen, preferably collected from a fasting subject. The following standards for young adult males have been suggested (ICNND, 1963):

riboflavin per 6 hours: " low " 10-29 mcg, " deficient " <10 mcg

riboflavin per gram creatinine: " low " 27-29 mcg, " deficient " <27 mcg.

Normal values for young children are uncertain, although it is stated that excretion is 2-3 times as great as in adults when expressed per gram of creatinine (Table 11).

Urinary riboflavin can be estimated by the method of Morell & Slater (1946). Further research tests are set out in Annex 2.

TABLE 11. TENTATIVE GUIDE FOR THE INTERPRETATION OF RIBOFLAVIN EXCRETION IN CHILDREN *

Age group (years)	" Low " riboflavin excretion (mcg/g creatinine)	" Deficient " riboflavin excretion (mcg/g creatinine)
1-3	150-499	<150
4-6	100-299	<100
7-9	85-269	<85
10-15	70-199	<70

* Adapted by permission from Pearson (1962).

7. Niacin

This water-soluble vitamin differs from others of the B complex because an amino acid, tryptophan, serves as its precursor in man, and because it is not secreted in the urine as such, but is metabolized to at least two derivatives, N'-methylnicotinamide and N'-methylpyridone.

In field surveys, excretion of these niacin metabolites in the urine over a timed interval—e.g., 6 hours, or, more usually, in a single random (preferably fasting) urine sample, expressed per gram of creatinine, provides information concerning the dietary intake of niacin and tryptophan.

As about equal quantities of the two metabolites are excreted, an assay of N'-methylnicotinamide is recommended, as this is technically less time-consuming than an assay of N'-methylpyridone. The suggested levels of urinary excretion for young adult males are:

N'-methylnicotinamide per 6 hours: " low " 0.2-0.59 mcg, " deficient " < 0.2 mcg

N'-methylnicotinamide per gram creatinine: " low " 0.5-1.59 mcg, " deficient " < 0.5 mcg.

Assessment is made photocolorimetrically by the method of Carpenter & Kodicek (1950). Further research tests are set out in Annex 2.

8 and 9. Iron, Folic Acid and Vitamin B₁₂

Anaemia can occur from deficiency of various nutrients (Wadsworth, 1959). The principal ones are iron, folic acid and vitamin B_{12}.

Iron deficiency may exist in the body as a result of inadequate dietary intake, poor absorption or excessive loss (especially as a result of severe hookworm infection), or a combination of these. This is especially likely to happen in early childhood, when the iron needs are high and the foods eaten tend to be poor sources of this metal.

Possible early effects of iron lack upon the body's enzyme systems and myoglobin synthesis are not at present measurable, so that the detection of an iron-deficiency anaemia is the only practical method of assessing an iron lack.

In field surveys, this can be best undertaken by haemoglobin estimations,[1] associated with the examination of thin blood films and haematocrit estimations, if practicable.

The haemoglobin can be estimated in various ways, using, for example, the grey wedge photometer, the Spenser haemoglobinometer, or the battery-operated haemoscope (Lewis & Carne, 1965). These three methods are especially indicated if the estimations have to be carried out in the field. The Talquist and Sahli methods are too inaccurate to be recommended, and the results expressed in figures give a false impression of scientific precision.

The cyanmethaemoglobin method is often suitable (Cannon, 1958). In this method, 0.02 ml of fresh or oxalated blood, obtained by finger- or heel-prick without squeezing, is added to 4 ml of Drabkin's cyanide-ferricyanide solution, which acts as a preservative, if protected from the sunlight, and which also allows the resulting cyanmethaemoglobin to be estimated colorimetrically with an electrical photometer at leisure on return to base, or even days later. If kept over a week, however, flocculation or fungus infection can occur. The photometer requires careful testing and calibration. It can be worked off a car battery.

A field modification of this test has been suggested by workers in Thailand in which the blood (0.02 ml) is run on to a strip of Whatman filter paper (2 cm $\times$ 4 cm) and allowed to dry. Specimens can be transported in small individual envelopes, and ultimately dissolved for 30 minutes in the Drabkin's solution and estimated in the usual way. In the climatic conditions of Bangkok, filter paper specimens can be used up to 10 days after collection (Sundharagiati & Harinasuta, 1964).

Standards of haemoglobin suitable for the particular age-groups will have to be applied, while adjustment may be required for altitude. Suggested levels are shown in Table 12.

Haemoglobin levels are independent of climate, but attention may have to be paid to the effects of high altitude, as well as to other possible causes of anaemia, such as malaria, sickle-cell disease and folic-acid deficiency.

---

[1] The International Committee for Standardization in Haematology recommends that only methods based on estimation of cyanmethaemoglobin or oxyhaemoglobin should be used (*British Medical Journal*, 1965).

TABLE 12. HAEMOGLOBIN LEVELS BELOW WHICH ANAEMIA
CAN BE SAID TO EXIST, AND ASSOCIATED PACKED CELL
VOLUMES (PCV %) FOUND IN IRON DEFICIENCY *

Age (years)	Sex	Hb (g/100 ml)	PCV %
0.5-4		10.8 ⎫	32
5-9		11.5 ⎬ 11.5	33
10-14		12.5 ⎭	37
Adults	Male	14	42
	Female	12	36
	Pregnant female	10	30

* Reproduced from WHO Study Group on Iron Deficiency Anaemia
(1959).

The thin blood film, stained with Wright's stain, can be examined for
cell morphology, especially for the presence of characteristic microcytes,
hypochromia, anisocytosis and poikilocytosis.

Megaloblastic anaemias, due to folic-acid or vitamin-B_{12} deficiency,
are suggested by a low haemoglobin, associated with a thin film showing
macrocytes, hypersegmented (5-7 lobed) neutrophil polymorphs and
reduced numbers of platelets.

Haematocrit estimations are practicable in some surveys, especially if
micro-methods are used (Guest & Siler, 1934). A capillary tube of blood is
centrifuged at 3000 r.p.m. on an electrical micro-haematocrit which can,
if required, be run off a car battery. With young children, when fresh blood
is used from a finger-prick, this has to be done as soon as possible, so that
a separate " station " with one or two persons will be required to carry out
the centrifuging and to measure the results. Packed-cell-volume readings
suggestive of iron-deficiency anaemia are given in Table 12.

Results of community surveys should be expressed in relation both to
" anaemia levels " (Table 12) and to spaced levels of haemoglobin—
for example: up to 4 g/100 ml; 4.1-7 g/100 ml; 7.1-10 g/100 ml; 10.1-12
g/100 ml; over 12 g/100 ml. At times it may also be useful and practicable to
classify different levels of haemoglobin " functionally "—that is, in relation
to the type of management required—e.g., hospitalization, various types of
therapy, close observation, etc.

If community anaemia surveys are to be carried out in a more complete
manner, in many tropical regions the following range of tests will be required,
especially in children : haemoglobin, thin blood film, micro-haematocrit,
thick blood film (stained with Giemsa to show intensity of infection with
malarial parasites), a second thin blood film (stained with cresyl blue for

reticulocytes,) a stool sample (taken from young children with a glass anal tube, stored in 10% formol saline as a preservative and later examined for occult blood, for the ova of hookworm, and for a rough gauge of approximate worm burden). In African populations, a test for sickling should be included. This may be done by the standard method of a coverslip ringed with vaseline and examined 24 hours later in the field, and by micro-electrophoresis of the packed cells remaining in the capillary tube after micro-haematocrit estimations have been made.

Community anaemia surveys may often best be based on widespread haemoglobin estimations and thin blood film examinations, with sub-sampling for more complex tests, and with appropriate therapeutic trials, both on severely affected individuals and in the community itself (Stott, 1960).

Further research tests are given in Annex 2.

10. Iodine

A decreased availability of iodine to the thyroid may be the result of an inadequate intake, or possibly of goitrogenic factors in the food.

Field surveys are usually based entirely on the detection of the principal physical sign of iodine lack—thyroid enlargement, especially in accessible age-groups likely to be affected, e.g., schoolchildren, pregnant women.

Further research tests are given in Annex 2.

BIOPHYSICAL METHODS

Radiographic Examination [1]

While routine radiographic studies of population groups are rarely possible, or indeed required, it is sometimes valuable to carry out these investigations on a sample of a population if the physical signs and other circumstances suggest that rickets, osteomalacia, fluorosis or beriberi may be present. This type of survey may also sometimes be of value in the retrospective assessment of malnutrition, as with rickets and possibly protein-calorie malnutrition in early childhood.[2] In such circumstances, the following are the principal signs sought:

Rickets

(*a*) Active: widened concave (cupped), rarefied, frayed distal ends of long bones, usually the radius and ulna;

---

[1] This section is based largely on WHO Expert Committee on Medical Assessment of Nutritional Status (1963), p. 26.

[2] Recent evidence suggests that transverse trabeculation at the growing ends of long bones in young children may be a result of protein-calorie malnutrition (Platt & Stewart, 1962; Stewart, 1965). Garn and his associates have stressed the *measurable degrees* of osteoporosis and reduction of compact bone (Garn, 1966).

(*b*) Healed: concave line of increased density at distal ends of the long bones, usually the radius and ulna.

Osteomalacia

Deformity and loss of density of bones, especially the pelvis.

Infantile scurvy

(*a*) Loss of density, ground-glass appearance of long bones;

(*b*) Line of increased density, sometimes with lateral spur formation due to increased calcification of metaphysis, with underlying zone of rarefaction, usually best seen at the knee.

Beriberi

Increased cardiac size.

Advanced fluorosis

Increased density of bones, with coarse trabeculation and thickening of the cortex; calcification of ligaments; osteophytic outgrowths at tendinous insertions, and marginal lipping of vertebrae. Changes most marked in the spine (Grech & Latham, 1964).

Tests of Physical Function [1]

The main purpose of biophysical tests is to assess alterations in function associated with inadequate nutrition. Many tests have been devised to determine deviations in visual acuity, dark-adaptation of the eye, capillary fragility, nerve accommodation, physical performance (dynamometry, etc.), muscle co-ordination, and so on, in different deficiency states. Their nutritional significance has been critically discussed by Sinclair (1948), who points out that most of them have an uncertain value. They are not usually of practical importance in survey work, although dynamometry was used in the classical study of Orr & Gilks (1931).

Of these tests, dark-adaptation is the most widely used. Although this measurement can be valuable in the objective evaluation of the complaint of night-blindness, one of the causes of which is vitamin-A deficiency, it has several limitations (Kinney & Follis, 1958). The main drawbacks are: (*a*) tests of dark-adaptation are not a specific measure of vitamin-A deficiency and other factors responsible for its impairment are difficult to eliminate; (*b*) it is not easy to conduct them in certain age and population groups; and (*c*) responses to the tests are not entirely free from subjectivity. In spite of all these difficulties, dark-adaptation measurements are of value in special circumstances—for example, in epidemics of night-blindness where the authenticity of the complaint itself needs to be established.

[1] This section is based largely on WHO Expert Committee on Medical Assessment of Nutritional Status (1963), p. 27.

Cytological Test

The examination of stained epithelial smears obtained from the buccal mucosa has been suggested by Squires (1965). Results in malnourished children and experimental animals suggest that the percentage of cornified cells increases with the degree of protein-calorie malnutrition present. Cornified and non-cornified cells can be differentiated by the colour reaction to Schorr's stain (Schorr, 1941).

Buccal smears from healthy children show 60-70% non-cornified cells, while in protein-calorie deficiency this proportion drops to about 20% or less (Squires, 1965).

Further field testing is required. If of confirmed value, the test may be important because it is independent of age. Present evidence suggests that the test may not be positive in marasmus. The effect of other conditions likely to produce changes in the buccal mucosa requires investigation, including febrile illnesses, dehydration and vitamin-A deficiency.

3 Indirect Nutritional Assessment of Human Groups

Vital Statistics

Malnutrition influences morbidity rates for various diseases (such as tuberculosis), maternal and perinatal mortality rates, life expectancy and other health statistics. A variety of vital statistics may therefore be considered as indirect indicators of the nutritional status of the community.

Difficulties in using data of this sort as indirect public health indicators of malnutrition are, first, the usual problems of collecting accurate information in the cross-cultural circumstances found in developing regions of the world. Before interpretation, it is necessary to ascertain not only the availability of local statistics, but their probable reliability, which will be related to the method of collection and its acceptability by the public, the percentage of deaths certified by doctors, occurring in hospital or autopsied, etc. The situation varies greatly from one country to another, and in some areas the numbers of deaths are recorded with comparative reliability, although the stated causes of death may be quite unreliable.

Secondly, problems of interpretation are considerable in relation to many other concurrent factors, such as a high incidence of infectious disease, overwork, poor housing and other socio-economic conditions.

This type of data, analysed where possible according to region, season, sex and age-group, should, then, be considered as important and suggestive, but not specifically indicative of the plane of nutrition of the community.

As far as morbidity and mortality are concerned, widespread malnutrition has its most marked general ill-effect among young children and pregnant women, and statistics relating to these groups are considered in detail both at this point and in subsequent sections.

Age-Specific Mortality Rates

Some types of malnutrition have a particularly high incidence at certain ages, so that the mortality rates at these specific age-periods have been suggested as indicators of the incidence of certain types of malnutrition.

2-5-month mortality rate

In areas where thiamine deficiency is a potential danger, it has been shown that there is a relatively high mortality rate due to infantile beriberi between 2 and 5 months of age, compared with similar areas where dietary lack of thiamine is uncommon (Aykroyd & Krishnan, 1941).

In view of the difficulty of assessing the incidence of infantile beriberi by other means, the 2-5-month mortality rate may be a valuable public health index. It will, of course, be imprecise, because other diseases, including pneumonia and diarrhoea, can be important causes of death in this age-range, although mortality is usually relatively low at this time in fully breast-fed babies in traditional tropical circumstances, except where the mothers are thiamine-deficient.

1-4-year mortality rate [1]

While the infant mortality rate has long been used as an indicator of the health of a community, it is now realized that, while the IMR in developing regions of the world may be 10 times as high as in industrialized countries in Europe and North America, the 1-4-year mortality rate may be 30 to 50 times as great (Table 13).

TABLE 13.   MORTALITY RATES PER 1000 CHILDREN
1-4 YEARS OF AGE IN SELECTED COUNTRIES *

Country	Mortality rate in 1-4-year-olds per 1000
United States of America	1.1
Denmark	1.1
Colombia	18.6
Mexico	19.3
El Salvador	26.6
Ecuador	28.5
Federation of Malaya	45.1
Guatemala	46.6
Guinea	54.8

* Reproduced by permission from Scrimshaw (1964).

This is because the so-called pre-school-age period, especially its earlier part, is a time of combined nutritional, infective and psychological stress, and the high 1-4-year mortality rate is due to an accumulation of infections,

---

[1] The 1-4-year period includes children from 12 to 59 months (i.e., below their fifth birthday).

parasitism and malnutrition during this vulnerable period, which is normally characterized by rapid growth and high nutritional needs. The precise details of the responsible conditions will vary from one area of the world to another, but in most developing regions the principal factor is protein-calorie malnutrition of early childhood. The use of the 1-4-year mortality rate as a public health index of malnutrition has been particularly suggested in the West Indies (Wills & Waterlow, 1958; Harney, 1958; Uttley, 1963).

Estimation

In common with the collection of any statistics, there will be great difficulty in assessing the 1-4-year mortality rates in most developing countries. However, an estimate may be attempted in the following ways:

(*a*) *Analysis of birth and death records.* Records of births and deaths should be consulted, if available. These may be kept by a local authority, such as a chief or mayor, or by a religious leader, such as the priest or a missionary. If these are complete and accurately kept, which is unusual, it may be possible to calculate the infant mortality rate and the 1-4-year mortality rate, and to enumerate the commoner causes of death in various age-groups. However, with precise ages not known, with no cultural incentive to register births and deaths, and with little likelihood of medical certification of the cause of death, it is unusual to obtain much useful information. Nevertheless, it is worth while examining available records. Sometimes, at least, it may be possible to note which causes of death are notified, although these may be diagnosed only symptomatically or by means of the vernacular name.

(*b*) *Calculation from census figures.* This will be practicable only if a careful census has been repeated at intervals in the area (Rao et al., 1959).

(*c*) *Questionnaire at village level.* A sample of mothers may be questioned carefully, by someone speaking the vernacular and preferably from the local community, on the number of children they have had, the number that have died, and the approximate ages at death, which may have to be expressed in general terms in descriptive age-groups, such as " still on breast ", " able to walk ", " circumcised ", etc. The cause of death may also be sought and may be expressed symptomatically, e.g., " diarrhoea ", " convulsions ", " voiceless crying " (infantile beriberi), or as a syndrome recognized in the local culture, e.g., *obwosi*—one of the terms used for kwashiorkor by the Baganda people.

However, this type of inquiry is laborious and time-consuming, and may prove inaccurate. Where the birth-rates are high and many children die, mothers often do not remember details exactly. Also, there may be local concepts that confuse such data as are obtained. Thus, an abortion or the placenta may be classified by local custom as a separate " child ", or it may be considered inauspicious to enumerate children, whether alive or dead.

Further attempts to obtain figures concerning family structure and particularly child mortality may be carried out by questionnaire and by observation in the course of rapid ecological visits. The same difficulties arise as those connected with the questioning of mothers at the survey site. Moreover, in large extended polygamous families, or those with closely-knit clan ties, it may be extremely difficult to sort out the relationships of children and adults, especially if it is customary for children to stay for prolonged periods with relatives. Also, in some groups, it may be considered incorrect behaviour for a woman not to acknowledge all the young children in her house as her own. Nevertheless, useful information has been obtained through this type of approach, as in Kenya, where Grounds (1964) calculated the infant and total child wastage rates, expressed per 1000 live births for different regions of the country.

Expression of results

Mortality in early childhood can be expressed in various ways:

(*a*) *Percentage of deaths of children below 5 years in relation to total deaths at all ages.* This can be calculated either from birth and death records or from census data. Figures in Western Europe and North America are below 10%, while in some developing regions they may exceed 50% (Table 14). However, it is difficult to compare figures from developing and developed countries owing to the different population structures (Bengoa—personal communication, 1965).

(*b*) *Annual 1-4-year deaths per 1000 of the 1-4-year population.* This method has the disadvantage that it is necessary not only to have a good registration of deaths but to know the size of the 1-4-year population in the area, which is difficult to estimate. Rates of 10 : 1000 or over indicate a high mortality in this group, suggestive of widespread protein-calorie malnutrition (Bengoa, Jelliffe & Perez, 1959). In some developing regions, this figure may reach 20 to 200 : 1000, whereas in Europe and North America the corresponding figures are usually 1 to 2 : 1000.

(*c*) *Percentage of childhood deaths occurring in the 1-4-year period.* This information, with all the inaccuracies implicit in the method, can sometimes be sought by questioning the mothers.

(*d*) *Ratio of 1-4-year mortality rate to that of infants aged 1-12 months.* This method of expressing the 1-4-year mortality rate was suggested by Wills & Waterlow (1958), based on experience in Jamaica, as an index of protein-calorie malnutrition of early childhood in the community. However, this depends on the assumption that complicating factors, such as infections and incomplete birth registration, are common to both age-groups, and that malnutrition affects mainly the 1-4-year-old children.

This is not always the case. In some areas, nutritional marasmus is the most common form of protein-calorie malnutrition of early childhood and

TABLE 14. INFANT AND CHILD MORTALITY IN COUNTRIES WHERE PROTEIN-CALORIE MALNUTRITION IS UNKNOWN OR EXTREMELY RARE, AND WHERE IT HAS BEEN FREQUENTLY ENCOUNTERED *

Country	Infant mortality per 1000 live births	Proportion of mortality, all ages (%)
Protein-calorie malnutrition unknown or rare		
Canada	28.4	10.8
Czechoslovakia	25.7	5.0
England and Wales	22.2	3.7
Japan	33.7	9.2
USA	26.4	7.8
Protein-calorie malnutrition frequent		
Chile (1958)	127.7	41.6
Mexico	74.4	46.3
Ceylon	57.5	39.1
India (1956)	101.8	38.4
Philippines (1958)	109.2	49.9

* The figures given in the table are for 1959 and 1960, unless otherwise stated, and are taken from *Annual Epidemiological and Vital Statistics* 1959 and 1960, published by the World Health Organization.

occurs mainly in the first year of life, as in Chile. In some more urbanized regions, the age-incidence of kwashiorkor itself has fallen with the decline in breast feeding, as, for example in Trinidad, where the peak incidence (86%) is in the first year of life (Jelliffe, Symonds & Jelliffe, 1960). In either of these circumstances, protein-calorie malnutrition will be related more to the infant mortality rate.

Furthermore the 1-4-year period often has a much higher incidence of certain parasitic infestations, such as malaria and hookworm, and of infectious diseases—e.g. tuberculosis and measles—than occurs in infancy, which is often relatively protected by close contact with the mother and by some persistence of transplacentally acquired antibodies.

A further problem is that children in the early pre-school-age group in some parts of the world—e.g., in Gambia (McGregor, Billewicz & Thomson, 1961)—can have a high mortality even where severe primary, dietary malnutrition appears to be uncommon, but where infections such as malaria are widespread.

It may be concluded that at the present time in many developing countries the 1-4-year mortality is much influenced by malnutrition—the influence being greater than during infancy—and that this can be a useful index of malnutrition. However, in whatever way the mortality rate is expressed, to be of value it must be interpreted in the light of the knowledge of the local disease-pattern in early childhood, and particularly of the age distribution of the different forms of protein-calorie deficiency disease, and of bacterial and parasitic infections in infancy and the 1-4-year period, and of an analysis of the ecological factors responsible for malnutrition in the particular region.

As a refinement of this concept, mortality rates in early childhood need to be analysed by one-year age-groups, so covering periods more specific to the peak-age occurrence of malnutrition in the particular region (Aykroyd, 1965). These would vary in different parts of the world, depending upon such factors as the age of " weaning " and other infant-feeding practices. As a generalization, the 13-24-month (or " second year ") death rate would yield useful information in many countries, as this is the classical age-group principally affected by kwashiorkor, when the child is experiencing the " transitional " dietary period, when the main foods are likely to be largely carbohydrate pastes and gruels, and when the child is between the breast-fed sufficiency of early infancy and the omnivorousness of later childhood.

Morbidity and Cause-Specific Mortality

Information concerning the incidence and mortality of certain forms of malnutrition may be available, if looked for, while data concerning the commonness and mortality rates of certain " nutritionally relevant " diseases also require to be collected, if practicable.

Malnutrition

Once again, information specifically concerning protein-calorie malnutrition should be sought.

Surveys. The prevalence of the major, clinically identifiable syndromes, such as kwashiorkor, nutritional marasmus, pellagra, keratomalacia, etc., can be noted in the course of a community-wide nutritional survey, and will provide useful information on prevalence provided that note is also made at the same time of cases admitted from the same area to adjacent hospitals, and care is taken to ensure that affected persons are not being hidden.

Health centres. Useful, though biased, information concerning geographical distribution and seasonal incidence can be obtained by training staff, including paramedical personnel, to recognize kwashiorkor and nutritional marasmus at health centres and to record cases attending with these conditions (Gongora and McFie, 1961; Burgess and Dean, 1962). Diagnostic signs should be simple, clearly understood and taught to personnel by means of practical demonstrations and photographs. Kwashiorkor should be recorded for every young child with oedema, poor growth (low weight) and wasted muscles, and nutritional marasmus diagnosed by very low weight with marked wasting of muscles and subcutaneous fat, with no oedema. Results can be expressed as percentages of children under 5 years of age attending the centre.

In well-organized young children's clinics, the percentage attending with " inadequate weight gains " (see Table 19) can be determined.

Hospitals. Lastly, hospital statistics can be of some value, although they do not reflect the actual community conditions. Difficulties of interpretation arise from the inadequacy of local transport and communications, the available bed-space, the admission policy and the attitudes of indigenous people to the hospital and to the causation of malnutrition and its therapy. At present, hospital data often fail to furnish as full information as they could do, because protein-calorie malnutrition of early childhood is not identifiable in the disease classification used. In addition, confusion may occur with regard to the diagnostic labelling of malnourished children who are also suffering from multiple infections.

It is suggested that *all* cases of kwashiorkor and marasmus, as defined later, should be recorded at hospitals, and that secondary conditioning factors should also be noted, especially associated infections. Annual figures can best be reported as percentages of the total number of patients under 5 years of age admitted to the wards. Similar records should be kept for out-patients. Care must be taken to avoid duplication of reporting if children with malnutrition are first seen in the out-patients' department and subsequently admitted. Figures should be broken down in relation to infants and 1-4-year-old children, and, if age assessment has been sufficiently accurate, figures for the latter should be analysed in yearly age-intervals.

Hospital admissions with kwashiorkor and nutritional marasmus can also be used to supply information on the seasonal incidence and the geographical distribution of these conditions in the surrounding area. The plotting of home sites of affected children on superimposed transparent nylon-acetate maps may permit correlation with local ecological factors, including population distribution, urbanization and staple food crop.

Children admitted to hospital with severe forms of protein-calorie malnutrition or keratomalacia can yield valuable information on important local conditioning factors in the etiology of these conditions (Oomen, McLaren & Escapini, 1964). For this, detailed clinical histories concerning feeding practices, method of " weaning " from the breast and antecedent infections, as well as laboratory and other investigations, including a tuberculin test, a stool examination for helminth ova, a thick blood film for malarial parasites, etc. will have to be carried out.

Lethality figures for various hospitalized forms of malnutrition, such as beriberi or kwashiorkor, should be available, but, of course, these give no indication of mortality from these causes in the community. They are biased by the various factors common to all hospital data, and, in the case of kwashiorkor, by the associated conditioning infections common in the particular region and by the effectiveness of the treatment employed.

In relation to the assessment of the prevalence of avitaminosis A, Oomen, McLaren & Escapini (1964) have suggested that the age-specific blindness rate can be related to past keratomalacia, in that blindness occurs between 1 and 4 years of age, and is suggested by the presence of leucomata, staphylomata or phtisis bulbi in older children or adults, dating from the preschool period.

Finally, where autopsies are obtainable, post-mortem evidence of protein-calorie malnutrition and causative conditioning diseases may be available.

Cause-of-death records. Where official records are reasonably accurate, the specific death rates due to malnutrition in 1-4-year-old children can be very useful, as has been shown in Venezuela (Bengoa, 1940, and personal communication, 1965). Results are best expressed per 100 000 population in this age-group.

However, official notification of deaths in many countries gives very distorted figures of the real problem, as a great proportion of deaths in children below five years is attributed to either diarrhoeal diseases, parasitism, respiratory conditions or some infectious diseases, particularly measles and whooping cough.

All this information is of value but requires careful interpretation.

In the absence of death certification by medically trained personnel, the percentage of deaths due to malnutrition in different age-groups may be impossible to determine. Sometimes a simple " clinical feature description " may facilitate a workable cause-of-death classification and may give information of nutritional relevance—e.g., young children dying with swelling of the legs may in some circumstances in developing regions be equated with kwashiorkor. Alternatively, there may be vernacular names for syndromes or signs of malnutrition—e.g., *obwosi* and *omusana* for kwashiorkor among the Baganda, or *sisikan* (" fish's scales ") for Bitot's spots in Indonesia (Oomen, McLaren & Escapini, 1964), and, if these are recorded, analysis may yield useful information.

Where there is no adequate coverage by medical services and the population has no inducement to report births and deaths, incidence rates and mortality rates for malnutrition in a community can be discovered accurately only in special circumstances, i.e., when circumscribed areas are under continuous direct observation. This can take place in a special long-term study in a defined area adjacent to a model health centre from which home-visiting activities are carried out, or in a small community under close continuous observation by interested people, not necessarily with specific medical training, such as anthropologists or missionaries.

Nutritionally relevant diseases

Malnutrition is an important contributory cause of morbidity and mortality in such diseases as tropical ulcer, diarrhoeas of infectious origin, tuberculosis and measles, and death certificates should include mention of severe malnutrition whenever it occurs concurrently with the principal cause of death or primary disease.

Diarrhoea is one of the principal causes of death among young children in developing regions of the world. Its etiology is often complicated and varies from region to region, but alimentary bacterial infection and protein-calorie malnutrition are probably the two main causes. They often occur together and each can influence the other adversely (" weaning diarrhoea ") (Gordon, Chitkara & Wyon, 1963). It seems probable, however, that protein-calorie malnutrition of early childhood can, in isolation, result in loose stools.

Therefore, in view of the relation between diarrhoea and malnutrition, and between these and the methods of infant feeding employed, statistics concerning the morbidity and mortality attributable to diarrhoea of early childhood may be valuable indirect evidence of malnutrition.

Measles is a world-wide disease. The attack rate remains unchanged even in countries where mortality due to the condition is now very low. As there is apparently no evidence of variation in the virulence of the measles virus, the infection represents a uniform stress all over the world.

Under this uniform stress, mortality rates and the severity of the disease seem to be in considerable measure related to the nutritional state of the group involved, although late attendance for treatment, availability of health services and their quality, associated parasitic infestations, and a younger age incidence must also be taken into account. In a careful field study carried out over a four-year period in rural Guatemala, the mortality was found to be 11.5% and 8.5% in the first and second years of life respectively (Gordon, Jansen & Ascoli, 1964), while in El Salvador in 1959, the mortality rate was 105 times as high as in the USA (Scrimshaw, 1964).

In some regions, measles is well recognized as a common precipitating factor in the etiology of kwashiorkor. Thus, in Western Nigeria, the hospital lethality rate was 25%, and 13% developed kwashiorkor (Morley, 1962).

Measles is an easily recognizable condition, well known to lay people and often with a specific local name, so that information can often be obtained readily by field workers. Attempts can therefore be made to collect data concerning mortality from measles in the community as a whole and in children admitted to hospital, for such data will provide approximate indices of the nutritional status of the child population.

8

4 Assessment of Ecological Factors

Human malnutrition is always an ecological problem in that it is the end-result of multiple overlapping and interacting factors in the community's physical, biological and cultural environments (Bengoa, 1940).

Thus, the amount of various foods and nutrients available to persons of different age-groups will depend upon such environmental conditions as climate, soil, irrigation, storage, transport and economic level of the population, as well as on such cultural influences as local cooking practices and food classifications, especially in relation to the distribution or restriction of foods for vulnerable age-groups.

Similarly, the importance of non-nutritional conditioning diseases in the production of malnutrition has become increasingly realized in recent years; in particular, the synergistic influence of bacterial, viral and parasitic infections and psychological trauma is now recognized, especially in relation to protein-calorie malnutrition of early childhood.

It is therefore necessary to make an ecological diagnosis of the various causative or co-existing factors responsible for malnutrition in a community before it is possible to elaborate a locally appropriate preventive programme that can be " aimed at the vulnerable links in the chain of multiple causation " (Scrimshaw, 1964).

Preventive programmes aimed at eradicating kwashiorkor have to suit the particular area or community. Dietetically, the lack of protein in the children's diet may be due to parental poverty, to lack of availability, to inadequate knowledge of nutritional needs, to customs that prevent young children from receiving available protein foods, or to any combination of these factors. Furthermore, kwashiorkor is almost never exclusively of dietary etiology, but is precipitated by one or more infections, such as whooping cough, measles or diarrhoea, or parasitic infestations, such as hookworm disease or malaria, or the psychological trauma of abrupt weaning, or a combination of these.

A rational preventive programme should be directed at *all* the factors considered of public health significance in the particular area, so that, apart from other considerations, an immunization programme or malaria chemoprophylaxis for pre-school-age children may be planned, quite logically, for nutritional reasons.[1]

---

[1] This broad approach to the age-group is the basis of the "Pre-school Protection Programme (P.P.P.)" (*Journal of Tropical Pediatrics*, 1963).

Ecological factors related to the etiology and prevention of malnutrition are considered in this chapter under the following six artificially separated headings: (*a*) conditioning infections; (*b*) food consumption; (*c*) cultural influences; (*d*) socio-economic factors; (*e*) food production; (*f*) medical and educational services. In fact, all these aspects of the ecology are intimately related to one another, as stressed by Scrimshaw (1964).

Methods of Obtaining Information

Information of varying degrees of usefulness and accuracy concerning ecological factors can be obtained in various ways, some of which may be more or less feasible in different circumstances.

Background data

Background data should be sought early on, prior to the preliminary visit or field reconnaissance to the survey area. Library research, using books, journals and other publications in medical, nutritional, anthropological, agricultural and other relevant fields, will be required, if available.

Inquiries should be made from the various government departments whose officials and archives may be able to supply information—census figures, statistics, maps, national and regional food production, etc. The relevant departments will have various functions in the particular country, but the ministries concerned with health, agriculture, economic development, population studies, fisheries and community development should always be approached.

Discussion should be sought with those who have had general or professional experience in the area to be surveyed. This may include both foreigners—doctors, social anthropologists and missionaries—and educated indigenous people. In all cases, the possible bias of the informant must be considered.

Further information and clarification of background data will often result from the field reconnaissance.

General survey data

Limited, but valuable information on the ecological background can be gathered in the field during, and as a part of, the actual general nutrition survey.

(*a*) *Survey site.* Observations, based largely on impressions, can be made at the actual survey site when people have been assembled for examination. Staff should be encouraged to jot points down as noted, and notebooks should be available for this purpose. Co-ordination of these impressions can often best be carried out by a team discussion each evening, and may suggest special features to be watched for in subsequent days.

Questionnaires concerning various types of information can be used on a subsample of those attending. However, other activities at the survey site may make this difficult, if not impossible. This method can, for example, be employed to obtain approximate qualitative information on the dietary pattern, especially of young children. If possible, advice on sampling should be obtained from a statistician beforehand.

(b) *Rapid ecological visits* (Fig. 45). As part of the survey, rapid ecological visits should be paid to a number of houses, cultivation sites, markets, local shops and other places associated with food production, e.g., fishing grounds, animal herds, etc. The type of information obtained, by means of observation, discussion and inquiry, is often mainly qualitative, but can be made more exact by the use of a suitable form or schedule, listing the facts to be noted on each visit. Again, a statistician should be consulted regarding the number of households, etc. to be visited.

Information obtained in the course of these rapid ecological visits is of great importance in throwing light on home life and its problems. It is so frequently neglected that, if staff resources permit, one small mobile team might with advantage be made responsible for these activities.

As a minimum, the team must include a senior person, usually either a doctor or a non-medical nutritionist, together with a respected member of the local community.

At the same time, it is desirable for *all* senior members of the survey team to take part in some visits, as personal observation of the ecological background is vital both to the subsequent interpretation of the survey findings and to the eventual planning of preventive measures.

Home visits should always be carried out in a friendly, diplomatic fashion, and with a minimum disruption of domestic privacy. The correct amount of time should be spent on greetings, which must be learnt, and local etiquette should be carefully followed. It is sound policy, as well as humane, to be willing, in the course of the visit, to treat or advise anyone who is really sick.

It is often unwise or impossible during these rapid visits to fill out a form within a household, since such action is often viewed suspiciously as being related to increased taxation. The practical extent of information to be gathered from such home visits depends on circumstances. Sometimes male visitors are debarred by custom, or the use of a questionnaire may be associated with potential witchcraft. Procedures must therefore be flexible to suit the actual on-the-spot reaction. Minimally, only observation may be possible. If completing questionnaires in households is not acceptable, a small pocket notebook may be carried, and facts obtained entered briefly between visits to houses. To facilitate this, the pages of the notebook can be prepared beforehand.

FIG. 45. ECOLOGICAL FACTORS
(a) Market sale of food, Indonesia

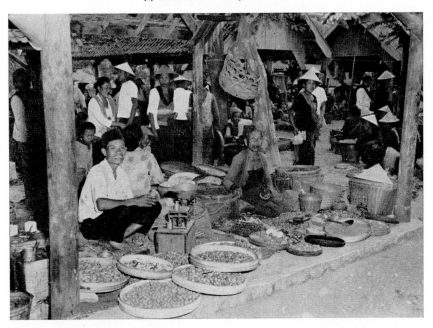

(b) Kitchen, showing food preparation, method of cooking and level of hygiene, Nile delta, rural Egypt

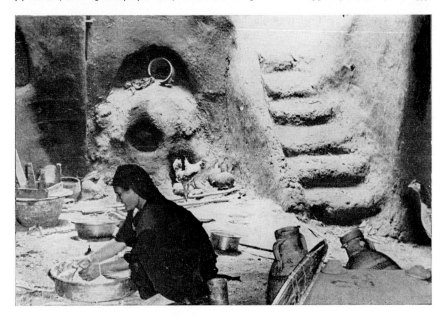

FIG. 45. ECOLOGICAL FACTORS (*continued*)

(*c*) Intra-familial food distribution at joint meal among Canadian Eskimos

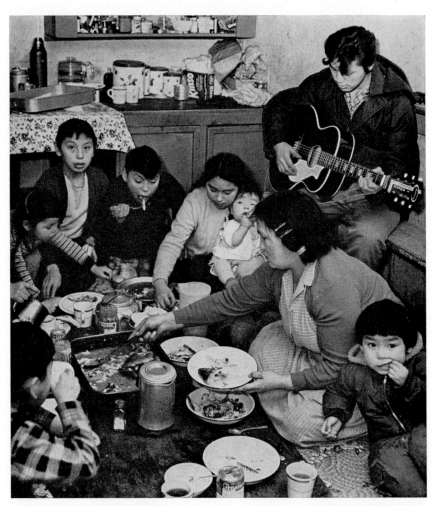

The data so obtained should be transferred to the appropriate survey forms each evening, while the day's visits are still fresh in the observer's memory.

The ecological data to be collected at the survey sites and during rapid ecological visits are considered in the present section under six artificially separated headings. In practice, a composite form will be required and should, if possible, be planned with statistical guidance. Points to be noted are suggested later (see Table 16, page 131).

FIG. 45. ECOLOGICAL FACTORS (*continued*)

(*d*) Method of infant feeding, including newly introduced bottle feeding, Sarawak

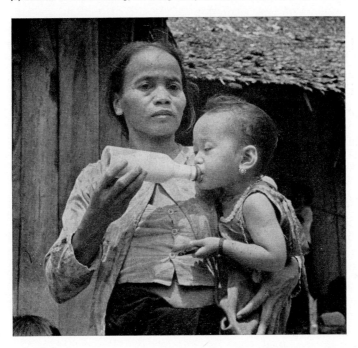

Data from case analysis

As noted earlier, clues to possible ecological factors responsible for malnutrition in the community can sometimes be obtained by investigating the detailed etiological findings of malnourished persons admitted to adjacent hospitals, including the social, nutritional and clinical history, and laboratory investigations for conditioning infections. Often, however, this will not be possible because of shortage of staff, and because the notes on cases of malnutrition admitted to the wards contain inadequate information.

Special survey data

The gathering of accurate and detailed ecological information requires highly trained specialist personnel, such as social anthropologists, who may often employ special techniques and usually need to spend long periods in the field.

Conclusion

All these four methods of obtaining data may be practicable in some community assessments of nutritional status. If so, the most valuable combinations will have to be decided upon in the light of the particular circumstances.

However, with the exception of food-consumption studies, which should, if possible, be carried out at least on a small sample, detailed special studies in depth will not usually be practicable in the course of prevalence surveys, so that approximate information on the local ecological scene will often have to be based on background data, and especially on the information obtained at the survey site and through rapid ecological visits.

In collecting data concerning ecological factors it is necessary to consider ways of recording information quantitatively and in a form capable of expressing degrees or types of information in a numerical code—e.g., type of housing, degree of literacy, etc.

Conditioning Infections

The association between bacterial, virus and parasitic infections, and malnutrition has been fully documented and critically reviewed recently by Scrimshaw, Taylor & Gordon (1959; in press). They stress that in human populations there is a synergistic interaction between nutrition and infection, and also that infections have an adverse influence on nutritional status, and may precipitate frank malnutrition.

Numerous pathological mechanisms may be responsible, either singly or together, including:

decreased intake, from poor appetite, diminished absorption or customs restricting food intake in illness;

increased loss from diarrhoea, vomiting or long-continued micro-haemorrhage;

increased needs, both for the human host and for the responsible organisms or parasites.

Nutritionally relevant infections

Bacterial, viral and parasitic infections considered most likely to be nutritionally relevant in the survey area will have to be decided upon. The list will probably be based on those of world-wide significance in this regard and on probabilities suggested by such background data as may be available.

The list of infections may include the following: *bacterial*—tuberculosis, whooping cough (Morley, Woodland & Martin, 1966) diarrhoeal disease, including "weanling diarrhoea", bacillary dysentery, amoebiasis; *viral*—measles; *parasitic*—malaria (Platt, Miller & Payne, 1961), intestinal helminths (ancylostomiasis, ascariasis).

Collection of information

Background data

Information may be available from the local health services, including hospitals and health centres, on the incidence (including epidemics) of some of these conditions. Although a biased sample, they should always be sought by means of visits to hospitals, etc., when attendances and admissions with malnutrition can also be noted. The age-incidence of the possible conditioning infections should be noted, particularly in relation to diarrhoea in young children in order to see if " weaning diarrhoea "[1] is an important local entity (Gordon, Chitkara & Wyon, 1963).

General survey data

At the actual survey site, two approaches are possible. First, a questionnaire can be used to try to determine the commonness of various infections in the community. This is rarely advantageous, as the collection of this type of retrospective medical information is both time-consuming and unreliable. Secondly, certain infections of a more chronic nature may be tested for, and may include:

(a) *Intestinal helminths*—by the testing of stool samples taken in the field (by the anal tube technique for young children) and kept in preservative (e.g., 10% formol saline, merthiolate-iodine-formaldehyde, etc.), which can be examined later, on return to base, or in camp with a standard microscope or a battery-operated portable model (McArthur, 1958);

(b) *Malaria*—by clinical examination for an enlarged spleen and by a thick blood film, stained with Giemsa or Field, etc., for malarial parasites;

(c) *Tuberculosis*—by carrying out a tuberculin test with a Heaf gun. The main difficulty here is the need to read the result of the test at a subsequent attendance 2-3 days later, which is always difficult, and may be impossible, to organize. Furthermore, tuberculin sensitivity may be influenced by protein-calorie malnutrition (Harland & Brown, in preparation).

An obvious drawback is that, unless an epidemic is occurring at the time of the survey, short-term, periodic or seasonal infections of nutritional consequence, such as measles, whooping cough and infective diarrhoea, cannot be assessed in prevalence studies, and it will be difficult to determine the importance of these illnesses as conditioning infections, except by investigating the etiology of malnutrition in adjacent hospitals. The ability to document the occurrence of such illnesses is among the advantages of longitudinal studies.

---

[1] " Weanling diarrhoea " is not a specific clinical or etiological entity, but a variable syndrome, usually due to combined intestinal infection and malnutrition at the time when other foods, likely to be both low in protein, bacteriologically contaminated and indigestible, are given to the child in addition to breast milk. Its age-incidence varies with local infant feeding practices but is often between 6 and 18 months (Gordon, Chitkara & Wyon, 1963).

Food Consumption

It is obviously important to have as much detailed knowledge as possible of the foods actually eaten in the community, both for assessing nutritional status and for discovering the dietary etiological factors that may be amenable to correction.

Collection of information

Background data

Gross food-consumption figures and food balance sheets may be available at the national or regional levels, and should be studied. Their value in the assessment of the nutritional status of a community is limited by the fact that they supply approximate information on deficiencies or otherwise for the country or region as a whole, and not for different communities, socio-economic levels, occupations or physiological groups at special risk, particularly young children and pregnant women.

Even qualitative data are, however, useful. Thus, the widespread use of low-protein high-starch staple means that protein-calorie malnutrition of early childhood is likely to occur, while data on crops, seasonal availability and methods of food storage may indicate the likelihood of a hungry season.

Unless previous dietary studies have been carried out in the region, the relevant literature is likely to give no more than outline information, mainly useful as a guide for subsequent inquiries during the survey.

General survey data

As noted earlier, it is sometimes practicable to arrange for a subsample of the persons examined to be questioned about their current diet. This should be carried out by someone speaking the local language, preferably belonging to the same community. The interview should, if possible, be held in private. The questionnaire should be simple and easy to fill up by marking written alternatives (e.g., cow's milk: yes/no—daily: $1/4$; $1/2$; $3/4$; 1 litre, etc.) and be based on indigenous foods and dishes given in their vernacular names, and on local domestic measures of weight and volume— all of which will be known from the background data, and as a result of the preliminary visit or field reconnaissance. Quantities can be described more accurately if the interviewer has with him the various locally used measures—e.g., bottles, gourds, spoons, etc.

The information thus gathered will be approximate, extremely crude and unproven. Much will depend upon the skill of the interviewer and the accuracy of the person questioned, which may be affected by exaggeration, understatement or poor memory, and upon the difficulty of assessing the foods taken outside the house, e.g., wild fruits, insects, etc. This technique is probably of more use for young children with their individualized food intakes within the family group.

Rapid ecological visits are especially important in connexion with dietary inquiries, because although quantitative data are not obtainable, an outline of the general feeding pattern will emerge, and some idea can be formed on the probable degree of reliability of the information supplied in a simple questionnaire.

The kitchen is of particular importance during home visiting. The stove or other cooking device (e.g., fire, oven, pit), the type of fuel and its apparent availability; the number, size and types of pots; the methods of cooking (e.g., boiling, steaming in leaf packets, barbecuing, roasting), the sources of water; the storage and preservation of uncooked foods and prepared dishes; and the local weights and measures, which are usually related to domestic items—spoons, bottles, gourds, coconut shells, etc.— should be noted. The preparation and cooking of food are the subject of a valuable observation, together with the inspecting and tasting of the meal when completed.

Inquiry should also be made concerning the local meal pattern, including the number of meals daily, their composition and the intrafamilial order of feeding. Special attention should be paid to the foods given to young children, e.g., how the adult dietary is fed to them, whether specially prepared dishes are made for them or not.

Special survey data[1]

For accurate dietary data most helpful in the nutritional assessment of the community, some type of family food-consumption study is indicated. Among urbanized, literate peoples, who purchase most of their food, this study can sometimes be based on results of food accounts filled in by housewives, concerning foods bought, eaten and left over at the end of the investigation period. For various reasons, including illiteracy and the common use of home-grown foods, this technique is not usually practicable in developing regions.

Household food-consumption surveys

The principles and practice of household food-consumption surveys have been very fully covered by Hollingsworth (1961), Flores (1962) and various publications of the Food and Agriculture Organization (Norris, 1949; Reh, 1962; Food and Agriculture Organization, 1964a, 1964b).

The present account is confined to a brief consideration of certain important aspects and is based largely on the above-mentioned FAO

---

[1] The dietary intake of special groups living in institutions, such as boarding schools or military forces, may be required and can be obtained fairly easily. Techniques for food-consumption studies of troops are given in ICNND (1963) and Wilson et al. (1964).

Techniques of collecting information on family food consumption include (*a*) interviewing with recall list; (*b*) food accounts, and (*c*) actual measurement of food (Food and Agriculture Organization, 1964a). Sometimes a combination may be the most suitable.

publications, which should be consulted in the planning of a family food-consumption study. Family food-consumption studies are conducted in the following successive stages (Reh, 1962):

(*a*) *Assessment of food consumption.* This is carried out by dietary survey teams that visit households and record the quantities of all foods eaten during a set period, often of seven days' duration, by weighing and measuring them in the raw state, and also, if methods of cooking are fairly standard, by weighing cooked food portions. At the same time, details of the family composition are collected.

Certain difficulties, inherent in this type of survey, comprise human problems, including establishing friendly rapport, and ensuring that the diet is typical and unmodified during the survey period, practical problems, such as the estimation of wastage and refuse, alteration of foods produced by cooking, use of local domestic units of weight and volume, the need to record some foods descriptively rather than by weight, assessment of food eaten away from home, and statistical problems, especially in relation to combining scientific sampling with practical realities, such as the lack of a local census, or the inaccessibility or hostility of certain households.

However, these intensive periods of home-visiting also permit much other valuable information to be gathered, partly by questioning and partly by observation. Food preparation (including methods of cooking, storage, the number of meals daily and the common dishes that are taken), food purchasing, local household economics, agricultural practices and social patterns can be observed and discussed.

Information can be collected by the home-visiting team on specially prepared forms (Reh, 1962). In most agricultural communities, consumption studies may require repetition to cover seasonal variations in availability of food. The home-visiting should cover a period of not less than three, and preferably of seven, days. Where relevant, a complete " eating cycle " should be covered—in many cases, of one week. Often, however, a shorter period of observation may be sufficient in developing regions where the diet tends to be limited in range and monotonous.

(*b*) *Calculation of nutritive value of food.* Initially the data collected on food consumption have to be converted into uniform terms of weight and cost, and then their nutritive values calculated, by means of appropriate food-composition tables containing references to local foods (Chatfield, 1954; Platt, 1962).

Difficulties in the use of food-composition tables arise from variations in techniques of food analysis, regional differences in composition of foods (including moisture content and methods of preparation) (Asenjo, 1962), and the fact that foods of local importance may not be included. Ultimately, tables will have to be prepared for individual regions. Some are already available and a list of these has been compiled recently. These should show values for foods AP (" as purchased ") or EP (" edible portion ") (Food and Agriculture Organization, 1964a).

Exceptionally, analysis of foods may be practicable on samples chemically preserved and brought back to the base laboratory (Wilson et al., 1964).

Food consumption should then be calculated *per capita* per day. This requires the collection of social details of the families, e.g., number of members, relationships, sex, ages, physical conditioning factors, such as pregnancy or illness, etc. Unless cooked servings are weighed, it is impossible to gauge the distribution within the family, including the amounts reaching young children.

(*c*) *Comparison with nutritional requirements.* The last stage of the analysis of food-consumption data is a comparison of the nutritive values of the diets with standard nutritional allowances, corrected, where necessary, for sex, age, body weight, environmental temperature and physiological state, especially pregnancy and lactation. Allowances suggested for calorie requirements are those laid down by the FAO Committee on Calorie Requirements (1957), and for other nutrients by the United States National Research Council (1964), although it must be realized that these are probably too generous, and that no allowance is made for possible special regional needs and adaptations. Requirements of thiamine and niacin are calculated in relation to the calorie intake.

Consumption can then be expressed as a percentage of the requirements with respect to calories, protein (total proteins and the proportions from animal and vegetable sources) and other nutrients. If practicable, an analysis of the amino acid patterns should be made, expressed as a percentage of the recommended pattern (FAO Committee on Protein Requirements, 1957). Results can also be further analysed to show the proportion of families in the survey sample whose diets reach stated levels of adequacy, or to show differences between given economic, social and cultural groups. The effect of certain non-dietary influences on intake may require consideration, e.g., iron from cooking pots and calcium from the water supply.

In presenting survey data concerning food consumption, the nutritional allowances used as standards of comparison must be clearly defined. If the food consumption of the group falls below the estimated requirements or recommended allowances for one or more nutrients, this finding should not be expressed in terms of degrees of " undernutrition " or " malnutrition ". The report should simply state the difference between the observed consumption and the allowances as a percentage of the latter (Reh, 1962).

Conclusion. Household food-consumption surveys are difficult to carry out and time-consuming; they call for carefully trained personnel capable of undertaking the meticulous work required, often under arduous field conditions. Apart from the problem of obtaining accurate data, analysis and interpretation are not easy, owing to the possible incompleteness and inconsistencies of food-composition tables (Harris, 1960) and the scientific uncertainty regarding optimum nutrient needs.

Nevertheless, the results of household food-consumption surveys greatly assist the over-all assessment of the nutritional status of the community, if read in conjunction with complementary information obtainable by clinical, anthropometric, biochemical and other methods. They serve as a basis for nutrition education, which must be based on existing practices. Every effort should be made to include at least a small subsample of household food-consumption studies in the survey.

Special problems of early childhood

Despite the frequent occurrence of malnutrition in the vulnerable period of early childhood, knowledge of food intakes in this age-group is especially scanty. Reasonably precise data are difficult to collect—more so even than with dietary studies in adults. In particular, it is difficult to assess the exact situation with regard to breast feeding, especially in late lactation. The quantity of breast-milk taken by the child varies with the output of the particular mother at that time, the daily number of feeds, the activity of the " let-down " reflex, and the time spent actively suckling the breast. Similarly, quantitative information with regard to the small, though increasing, amounts of food given to young children is not easy to obtain, especially in poorer homes in developing countries.

Basically, most accounts are qualitative, consisting of a combination of careful questioning of mothers, field observation of feeding practices (often including a note on whether the mother breast-feeds the child at the investigator's suggestion), and inspection of the local scene in the course of rapid ecological visits to homes, kitchens, gardens, markets, etc. Outline information of this type has been collected in South India (Rao et al., 1959) and in the course of East African community child health surveys— for example, among the Lugbara people of Uganda (Jelliffe et al., 1962a). It is useful to obtain an approximate outline of practices in the early years, including the number of daily meals and the preparation, or lack of preparation, of special protein-rich dishes for young children, especially for use during the dangerous, protein-deficient transitional period.

Local household utensils of known size should be used as adjuncts to the questionnaire when mothers are interviewed, in order to assess approximate quantities.

The questionnaire can be used on a sample of mothers attending, and it should aim at ascertaining only the foods taken *currently* (that is— yesterday and today), with no attempt at retrospective assessment. Its construction will be guided by background data and by information gained during field reconnaissance. Neutral, non-leading questions are preferable.

A simplified, rapid technique for use in a dietary inquiry has been suggested by Blankhart (1965) for most field work, both at the survey site and in home visits. In this, the mother is first asked to say spontaneously what the child was eating at the time. Following this, she is questioned as to how many times a day each item is being eaten. The information obtained is recorded as given by the mother, e.g., rice, twice a day, etc.

When the mother has given her spontaneous answers, questions are put systematically on the use of other foods, and, in the event of an affirmative answer, on the number of times daily.

This questioning is done quickly, as, according to Blankhart (1965), too much interrogation and cross-checking defeat their purpose and leave both the mother and the interviewer confused.

The information may be entered on double foolscap lined sheets, on which columns are ruled for each of the local foods likely to be used for young children. The frequency of use of different foods can be calculated and expressed as the number of times they have been eaten per week per child (Table 15).

TABLE 15. FEEDING OF YOUNG CHILDREN
IN A SIERRA LEONE VILLAGE *

Type of meal	Average number of times different foods taken per week at following ages (and number of children studied):		
	7-12 months (12 children)	13-18 months (15 children)	19-24 months (11 children)
Breast-milk	21	10	2
Rice	6	13	14
Cassava and *foo-foo* pap	6	3	1
Sweet potato		⅓	½
Custard or cornflour	4	2	
Leafy vegetables	1 [a]	12	10
Bananas		2	1 ½
Oranges		1	1 ½
Tomatoes			
Milk	13	1 ½	½
Egg	½ [a]		
Fresh fish			
Dried fish		5	5
Oil			

* The information for this table was obtained by the rapid technique of Blankhart (personal communication, 1965).
[a] One child only.

The questionnaire should cover the number and timing of meals and the following aspects related to the usual limiting factor, protein intake, both from breast-milk and from other foods:

Breast-feeding: still carried on or not; complete or partial, i.e., night only.

Largely carbohydrate foods : types (e.g., part of adult foods, or specially prepared gruels or pastes); quantities; times.

Protein foods—animal milk : type (e.g., fresh or boiled liquid from cow, goat, etc., sour-milk products; tinned—powdered, condensed or evaporated); quantities (daily and monthly); cost; number, approximate timing and volume, dilution and other ingredients (e.g., sugar) in feeds; method of feeding (e.g., bottle, cup and spoon, indigenous feeding vessel, etc.).

Other animal proteins : types (e.g., eggs, fish, meat, etc.); quantity; frequency.

Vegetable protein foods : types (e.g., legumes,[1] green leafy vegetables); quantity; frequency; method of cooking.

Household studies of food consumption in early childhood have been performed only rarely; they are extremely difficult to carry out. Investigations by household visiting and direct observation of foods eaten by young children have been undertaken by Oomen & Malcolm (1958) in Papua, by Flores & Garcia (1960) in Central America, and by Blankhart (1965) in Indonesia.

More recently, Flores et al. (1964) carried out three-day family food-consumption studies in three Indian towns in Guatemala, at yearly intervals for four years. The pattern of food consumption was constant. Pre-school children received the general family diet, though with smaller amounts of protein.

Assessment of the quantity of breast-milk produced can be attempted in either of two ways, both of which require observation for several days.

First, test-feeding may be carried out, in which the child is weighed before and after a feed, although this shows only the amount of milk taken rather than the amount secreted. If the child is at home and if (as is usually the case) permissive breast-feeding is being practised, this presupposes a continuous surveillance in the house and, because of the often small quantities taken at irregular intervals, an extremely accurate weighing machine. If carried out with a set feeding schedule in hospital, there may be an inhibition of the let-down reflex.

Secondly, following the period of observation of food intake by the young child, a period can be allocated when the breast-milk can be expressed manually or mechanically by the investigator at 3-4 hour intervals,

---

[1] An assessment of the value of various legumes for infant feeding has to be based on a knowledge of protein content, cooking properties, digestibility and other factors (Aykroyd & Doughty, 1964).

measured and then fed to the child with a cup and spoon. It may be more convenient to do this is at a nearby health centre or hospital, in which case the mother may require compensating for her trouble. Again, a disturbance of the let-down reflex is likely.

A further problem with regard to the measurement of dietary intake in this age-group is that infant feeding is, or should be, a progressive, dynamic process, quite different from the relatively static and monotonous (though seasonally variable) diet of the average adult in the tropics. To achieve accurate results, longitudinal studies by direct observation would be required on a number of children.

Cultural Influences [1]

Knowledge of the local culture pattern is essential for the successful conduct of the field investigation, for an understanding of the local etiology of malnutrition, and for the ultimate implementation of any programme aimed at improving the situation. Ideally, such knowledge should include an understanding of the leadership structure, kinship systems, religion (including attitudes towards life, death and disease), and the cultural philosophy concerning life-goals and values. However, certain aspects of the culture pattern have a more direct bearing on the problem, and only these will be touched upon.

Cultural patterns

Food attitudes

Very seldom does man eat all the potentially edible materials available to him. More often his culture pattern, learned from his parents and associates by subconscious observation and by explicit instruction, classifies for him items as appropriate or inappropriate as food.

The food classifications employed, which usually have no relation to scientific divisions (e.g., protein, vitamins, etc.), are often extremely complex, but appear natural, normal and correct for the particular community. The more important and commonly found classifications of nutritional importance include the following:

(a) *Food and non-food*—those of the potentially edible local items that are viewed as food and those which are not eaten.

(b) *Age-group, or sex-linked, foods*—items regarded as suitable, or forbidden, for various age-groups or sexes, in particular for young children or women, and during pregnancy, the puerperium or lactation.

---

[1] Detailed consideration of cultural factors and nutrition has been given by Mead (1953), Burgess & Dean (1962), Jelliffe (1955b, 1957, 1962, 1964) and by Jelliffe & Bennett (1961, 1962a, 1962b).

(c) *Celebration foods*—items especially associated with culturally defined holidays or periods of rejoicing.

(d) *Disease-linked foods*—items deemed to produce illness in some circumstances (e.g., eggs and fish are believed to cause intestinal worms if given to young children in Malaya), or items to be avoided in certain diseases (e.g., the restriction on " hot " *(garam)* foods in illnesses of the same classification in India).[1]

(e) *Cultural " super-foods "*—often the main staple (e.g., rice in much of South-East Asia, and plantains for the Baganda of East Africa), having great historical, psychological and emotional significance to the particular community and tending to dominate the local dietary.

(f) *Modern prestige foods*—relatively newly introduced foods, most often in towns, which may have become symbols of prestige and modern living (imitation of socio-economic " superiors "; influence of advertising). They may include various forms of tinned milk, milk-carbohydrate powders, aerated bottled drinks, etc.

A consideration of food attitudes must also include methods of food preparation (e.g., cooking practices, types of pots, stove and fuel, domestic measures) and meal patterns, including times, usual dishes, family order of eating, special dishes for children, way of taking food, use of cutlery, chopsticks, fingers, etc.

Disease causation

Local concepts of the causation, cure and prevention of disease are extremely important. Illnesses, especially diarrhoea, are often treated by dietary changes, mainly of a restrictive nature, as well as with herbals and appropriate magical ritual.

The advanced, and therefore more obvious, syndromes of malnutrition are often recognized and classified by uneducated indigenous peoples. The terms used usually refer descriptively to some striking feature, or to the presumed causation—for example, the Luganda word *obwosi* (synonymous with kwashiorkor), which means " disease of the displaced child "—but show no connexion with the actual dietary etiology.

Child rearing

The general pattern followed in rearing young children must be known, especially with regard to the following:

(a) *Obstetrical*—prenatal maternal diet, immediate procedure with placenta (e.g., draining of blood).

(b) *Neonatal*—" pre-lacteal " feeds, laxatives, discarding of colostrum.

---

[1] Disease-linked food classifications are often related to local concepts of body physiology (Foster, 1952, 1966), as, for example, the ancient Indian view that health or ill-health are related to the balance in the body of three *dosha* (humours) (Jelliffe, 1957).

(*c*) *Breast-feeding*—when started, techniques of nipple preparation, indigenous tests of breast-milk, duration of complete and partial breast-feeding, local galactogogues, diet of the mother (normal, restricted, increased).

(*d*) *Animal milk*—type, quantity, dilution, additions, feeding method (e.g., cup and spoon, bottle, local feeding-vessel, etc.), milk preparations (e.g. yoghourt, cheese).

(*e*) *Feeding orphans and twins*—wet nurse, induced lactation, artificial feeding and method.

(*f*) *Supplementary foods*—age introduced, type, quantity, method of feeding (e.g., spoon, finger, tongue).

(*g*) *Other protein foods* (animal and vegetable)—age introduced, type, quantity, method of feeding.

(*h*) *Method of stopping breast-feeding* (weaning)—age, abrupt or gradual, sent away or not, child prepared or not, the use of deterrent substances on breast, " compensation " or not, apparent reasons for weaning.

(*i*) *Food preparations for children*—special foods and their preparation; if none, which part of adult dietary used, recipes, number of meals daily, methods of child feeding.

(*j*) *Person responsible for feeding*—mother, grandmother, older sibling, etc.

(*k*) *Attention to sex of child*—preferential treatment of male or female child.[1]

Food production

Important aspects of the local culture pattern will be concerned with food production and will include customs relating to methods of cultivation, animal husbandry and food storage.

Cross-cultural survey problems

While many problems may arise in both prevalence and long-term survey work as a result of cross-cultural misunderstandings, the following difficulties have been observed commonly in various parts of the world:

(*a*) *Local concept of modesty*, which often limits the extent of the clinical assessment by restricting the examination of women to female team members.

(*b*) *Specimen collection*, which may be misunderstood and resisted through fear that the blood or urine may be used for occult purposes, or that its loss may weaken the donors.

---

[1] In a Beirut hospital, McLaren, Ammoun & Houri (1964) reported twice as many female admissions with marasmus, although the general paediatric admission ratio was 1 girl : 2 boys.

(*c*) *Difficulties with names and numbers*, which arise when the culture forbids that one's own name or that of one's husband or child, or the number of children in the family, should be mentioned before strangers.

Collection of information

Background data. Library research into cultural factors is difficult because in most countries anthropological publications are not generally available to nutritionists, and are seldom directly concerned with aspects of the culture immediately relevant to nutrition.

Special survey data. Detailed information can be obtained only through prolonged and intensive investigations on the part of a trained cultural anthropologist. Such studies do not fall within the scope of a cross-sectional nutritional prevalence survey. Yet the results of intensive investigations " in depth " are of great value in the selection of the areas or population groups for a nutrition survey, and in the planning of programmes for the solution of the nutrition problems revealed.

Exceptionally, an anthropologist may already be working in the survey area, in which case collaboration is obviously indicated. Alternatively, if there are several culturally and ecologically similar groups in an area, it may be possible to select one in which an anthropologist is already at work. If so, the ideal time for collaboration between nutritionist and anthropologist is late in the second year or early in the third year of the latter's field study, by which time he will speak the vernacular fluently, be accepted by the community and be deeply versed in at least some aspects of its culture.

Furthermore, by that time, the social anthropologist may be expected to welcome the further insight into the community that can result from study by a group with different technical knowledge and skill.

It may often be found that while the anthropologist has been concentrating principally on a particular aspect of the local culture pattern, —for example, the clan system or kinship relations—he has also acquired a great deal of information useful to the nutrition worker, although he may not appreciate its public health significance. Conversely, the deeper subtleties of the causation of behaviour that so greatly influence nutrition may be obscure to the non-anthropologist until the fundamental concepts of a group's attitudes to all aspects of life have been explained and discussed.

General survey data. Generally, however, this type of collaboration with a trained anthropologist is not possible, and the nutrition team must be prepared to collect as much information as possible concerning the culture pattern in the course of the prevalence survey. This is obviously difficult to do in the short time usually available, and care should therefore be taken to avoid drawing anything but the most broad and tentative conclusions.

Nevertheless, guided by such background information as is available, and by knowledge of the ways of " parallel groups " with similar modes of life, the nutrition team can obtain some information on the local culture pattern at the survey site and in the course of rapid ecological visits.

It is particularly valuable to have a daily meeting of all staff after the survey has been completed for the day, when impressions of the local way of life can be pooled and possible clues to relevant features of the culture pattern discussed. For example, it may be noticed that certain types of charms or amulets are commonly worn, or that certain medicinal scar patterns are frequent in some age-groups, or that differences of costume or physical adornment exist in different age-groups. Such clues are always to be found and can be followed up subsequently by further directed observation, and by discreet and friendly indirect questioning at the survey site or in the homes.

Socio-Economic Factors

The socio-economic circumstances of a community are particularly difficult to assess quantitatively, because people are understandably reluctant to reveal their income and other wealth to strangers—often, indeed, fearing that these inquiries may lead to increased taxation. Also, the relevance of earning capacity to human nutrition is usually less obvious when the particular community's food supply is principally home-grown.

Socio-economic data of nutritional relevance

It is convenient to consider socio-economic data relating to nutrition in their separate aspects rather than in combination. The following is a list of items in each group:

Social data

(*a*) Population of community—number, age and sex distribution, geographical distribution.

(*b*) Family details—size, relationships, stability, intervals between children.

(*c*) Education—literacy of men and women of parent and grandparent age-groups, presence of books and newspapers, children attending school (type of school, classes, examinations passed).

(*d*) Housing—type, floor, roof, walls, lighting, ventilation, furniture, provision for sleeping, number of rooms, population per house, owned or rented.

(*e*) Kitchen—building, location, stove, fuel, type and condition of cooking utensils, rubbish disposal.

(*f*) Food storage—size, contents, pest-proofing.

(*g*) Water supply—source, distance from house, purity, approximate amount of water available per person.

(*h*) Latrine—type (if any) and condition (cleanliness, fly-proofing).

Economic data

(*a*) Occupation—primary (e.g., farmer), secondary (e.g., home industry, seasonal unemployment).

(*b*) Family income—wages, home industries, cash crops, non-cash income (e.g., foods grown), debts, intrafamilial distribution of goods or cash.

(*c*) Tangible wealth—land, number of livestock, boats, modern status symbols (e.g., sewing machine, bicycle, motor-scooter, radio).

(*d*) Budgeting—expenditure on food, clothes, rent, fuel, light, education, transport, domestic services, charitable contributions, recreation (including tobacco and alcohol).

(*e*) Prices of foods—shops and markets, seasonal variation (with special reference to protein foods suitable for young children).

Collection of Information

Background data. Figures for national *per capita* income, sometimes broken down on a regional basis, and legal minimum wages may be available in the appropriate government departments and should be ascertained.

Special survey data. For detailed information, careful, tactfully conducted surveys will have to be carried out by appropriate experts.

General survey data. Most often, approximate data have to be collected by observation at the survey site and in the course of the rapid ecological visits.

However, any attempt to assess socio-economic circumstances by tangible western yardsticks, such as clothes or type of house, may be difficult because in some cultures these are of less importance. Wealth and status may be measured by the number of cattle (whether healthy and productive or not), or by gold ornaments owned by women, which will certainly not be displayed for the investigator. The local " indicators " of wealth must be discovered, and—if easily identifiable by observation—carefully noted.

It is useful, while the survey is proceeding, to make notes on the clothes and ornaments worn, provided that it is also known whether, in the particular culture, the population would or would not tend to wear their best clothes for the occasion.

Items selected from the foregoing points can be looked for during the rapid ecological visits. In particular, the houses can be noted (e.g., bamboo or mudbrick construction, thatched or metal roof) as well as their furnishings and the type of household water supply, e.g., natural (pond or stream) or man-made (roof-drainage to barrel or tank, or bore-hole and pump). The type of transport available is also easily observed (buffalo cart, canoes or boats, bicycle, motor scooter, etc.), as well as other relatively expensive items, such as radios.

In the cultivation area, the amount of land available should, if possible, be observed. This may be complicated where a family has multiple small cultivated areas in various places, and where the land may or may not be suitable for the growing of particular crops. Approximate areas devoted to high-protein vegetable foods, particularly legumes and ground-nuts, can be noted, and also the extent and type of cash crops grown (the area under cultivation with cotton, coffee, tea or cocoa) or the number of coconut palms.

The number of stock and poultry also should be estimated, if possible, due account being taken of the local cultural significance of various animals that may be kept as symbols of wealth—for example, cattle for some African pastoralists—or as sources of food for the household (e.g., the buffalo for its milk in India), or as celebration food (e.g., pigs in the New Guinea Highlands), or as beasts of burden (e.g., the buffalo in Thailand), or as producers of saleable products (e.g., chickens and their eggs), or for a combination of these reasons.

Visits to markets and nearby shops may disclose another important socio-economic factor, namely, the cost of the major, nutritionally significant foods, particularly the animal and vegetable protein foods suitable for young children. These are best made unobtrusively by a junior team member, preferably one belonging to the local community, otherwise the prices quoted are likely to be higher than usual.

Family size and structure must also be ascertained: they constitute a basic factor in the interpretation of the socio-economic data referred to above. This may be very difficult to undertake in the course of a field survey. Many peoples are suspicious of family enumeration or regard it as inauspicious. Also, with large families, relationships may be complex and confusing to the foreigner because of a completely different system of nomenclature and classification of kinship relations. A further complicating factor may be the practice of " borrowing " children or sending them to stay with relatives.

Food Production

The assessment of food production in a country or region has ultimately to be considered in terms of the availability of the production to families. It is therefore dependent upon such factors as preservation, distribution, marketing and economics.

Data of nutritional relevance

All aspects of food production and supply are relevant to the assessment of the nutritional status of the community. Among the important aspects are the following:

(*a*) Family food supply: home produced, purchased, wild (collected, hunted, fished), obtained by barter; seasonal variation.

(*b*) Farming methods: hoe, plough, mechanized; bush clearing, rotation, double-cropping; irrigation; drainage; fertilization; insect and pest control; availability of modern extension services.

(*c*) Land: tenure, area per family, suitability (for different crops, pasture, infertile, etc.), actual utilization (especially staples, vegetable protein foods, cash crops); number of agricultural workers (family, labourers).

(*d*) Livestock and fishing: number of livestock (cattle, sheep, etc.), milk production (yield, milk not used), fishing facilities (freshwater, ponds, sea, methods, yields).

(*e*) Finance: capital available, facilities for credit, purchasing power, stabilization of prices, co-operatives, indebtedness.

(*f*) Distribution: communications (roads, transport); storage, preservation and processing (home, industrial); marketing (local, regional and world trade, prices and availability of foods).

Collection of information

Background data. In some countries, national food-production figures are available, usually from the Ministry of Agriculture. These data include information on imports and exports, and may need to be corrected for potential human food produced but not intended for human consumption (e.g., soya press cake used for cattle feed).

FAO has recommended techniques for the presentation of production figures in a standardized form. Though of value in indicating national production figures for certain types of food (especially animal and vegetable protein foods) and—if revised at intervals—in demonstrating production trends, these data have the disadvantage of being approximate: they usually make no distinction between the diverse geographical, ethnic, socio-economic and agricultural regions within a country, and give no indication of the distribution of food to vulnerable groups.

Specific survey data. As in the case of surveys, detailed information concerning the production of food and its availability to families calls for a lengthy and specialized investigation by agricultural nutritionists. Such an investigation is not normally possible in the course of most surveys. FAO has, however, been encouraging governments to participate in a world-wide agricultural census scheme, and more figures may become available for certain regions in the future.

A small-scale study of food production and other ecological factors may be practicable for a limited sample of homesteads, as shown by the surveys carried out by Collis, Dema & Omolulu (1962a, b) in Nigeria.

In this type of study, at least one investigator will have to spend several weeks in making a detailed investigation on a statistically selected sample of households. Where there is a considerable seasonal variation, as is usually the case, it will be necessary to repeat the investigation at appropriate times within the year.

General survey data. In the course of rapid ecological visits to cultivation sites and markets, some outline information can be obtained concerning food production and availability. The approximate areas under cultivation with different types of crop (especially vegetable protein-foods and cash crops), the number of livestock and methods of agriculture can be noted.

In the event that an agricultural nutritionist cannot be attached to the team, any details of local methods of food production, preservation and storage that cannot be understood should be noted, for discussion with experts after the team's return to base. Similarly, if any food plants, cultivated or wild, cannot be recognized by the team, the complete plant, i.e., leaves, fruit etc., should be brought back, together with a record of the indigenous name, for exact identification.

Health and Educational Services

Although not " ecological factors " related to the development of malnutrition, information can sometimes be usefully collected at the same time concerning existing health and educational services in the area, since programmes concerned with bettering the nutritional status of the community will often be in part related to the improvement of these services and in part channelled through them.

Hospitals and health centres

Full information should, if possible, be gathered on the following points:

General : number of hospitals and centres, distribution, number of beds (total, paediatric, maternity), record keeping

Admissions : number, age-groups, diagnoses, results of treatment (cured, improved, not improved, died, proportion of autopsies to deaths), mothers admitted with children, maternity admissions (rooming in), percentages of births to prenatal attendances

Out-patients : number, age-groups (including prenatal attendances and " young child clinics "), diagnoses

Follow-up system : home visiting

Staff : doctors, medical assistants, nurses, and assistant nurses, midwives, and assistant midwives, laboratory technicians, domestic staff

Buildings : wards, outpatients, laboratory, offices, kitchens, accommodation for relatives

Equipment : transport, drugs, food supplements (especially dried skimmed milk)

Training programmes : medical and paramedical personnel

Miscellaneous : methods of prevention and treatment of malnutrition (especially use of dried skimmed milk), use of nutrition rehabilitation units, immunization.

Educational facilities

The following data are useful:

Schoolchildren : number, type, distribution, percentage in school, nutrition education (formal curriculum, school meals, school gardens)

Young people : clubs (Young Farmers, Scouts, etc.)

Adults : literacy (percentage, sex distribution), parent-teacher associations, clubs, etc. (community development, voluntary organizations)

Mass media : radio, press, television.

Collection of information

Background data. These will be available, in varying degree of completeness, at the Ministries of Health and of Education and at the headquarters of other relevant agencies—for example, Community Development, Ministry of Information, and voluntary organizations.

General survey data. Concurrently with the gathering of information on conditioning infections from hospitals and health centres in the area, data concerning the medical and educational services should be assembled. This will be a full-time job occupying a senior team member for some days, either before or after the survey is carried out.

Conclusion

It is evident that any assessment of ecological factors in the course of a nutritional prevalence survey must vary greatly in complexity, depending upon the type and number of staff, the time available, and the purpose of the investigation. Obviously, as much information as possible is desirable to give a complete picture of the existing situation and of the scope for improvement. Nevertheless, rapid screening surveys using a limited number of clinical signs and, possibly, basic anthropometry can give useful preliminary information as to prevalence of malnutrition. The economical use of limited staff and opportunities enables data on causative ecological factors to be assembled, which will indicate any more-detailed studies, including special investigation of selected aspects of the ecological background, that may be necessary.

TABLE 16. GUIDE LIST OF FEATURES OFTEN IDENTIFIABLE DURING RAPID ECOLOGICAL VISITS

	Home
Family size :	number, relationships, ages, sex, interval between children
Occupations :	primary, secondary
Education :	adult literacy, presence of books and newspapers, children at school
House :	type and construction (roof, walls, floor), number of rooms
Economic :	furniture, clothes, radio, transport (bicycle, wagon, motor scooter, car)
Kitchen :	stove, fuel, cooking utensils, dishes in preparation
Feeding pattern :	meals seen, foods not used, breast-feeding, modern " prestige " foods
Food storage :	size, contents, pest-proofing
Water supply :	type, distance, purity
Latrine :	type, state
	Cultivation site
Land :	area, utilization with different crops (including cash crops)
Farming methods :	tilling procedure, irrigation
Livestock and fishing :	number of beasts and poultry, fish pond
	Markets and shops
Food and weaning equipment :	availability and prices of foods (especially protein foods for children), advertising, availability of bottles and nipples

In many surveys conducted in developing countries, the size and training of the team and the time available will both be limited. In such circumstances it may sometimes be possible for a sample of homesteads to be investigated in some detail (Collis, Dema & Omolulu, 1962a, b). If, as is often the case, even this is not feasible, information on major ecological factors can be gauged only roughly during the actual survey. Factors that can be noted in practice will obviously include only some of those in the lists given earlier in each section. Those chosen for observation on the particular prevalence survey will depend on various local circumstances and especially on their probable relevance to nutrition and their ease of identification in the course of rapid ecological visits (Table 16).

5 Nutrition Surveys

TYPES OF SURVEY

The nutritional status of a community can be assessed directly by two types of field investigation: longitudinal incidence studies, and cross-sectional prevalence studies (Gordon, 1963).

Longitudinal Incidence Studies

In the longitudinal incidence study, selected members or families in a community are kept under continuing systematic surveillance for a prolonged period " in the setting of prevalent social customs, economic vitality, nutrition and pathology " (McGregor, 1964).

Frequently these studies are undertaken on children, when environmental variables can be assessed, particularly the diet, infections, socio-economic circumstances and cultural practices, and their effect evaluated longitudinally in so far as growth, development and physical and mental health are concerned (Stewart & Acheson, 1964). They are, in fact, general health surveys, with particular emphasis on nutrition (Phadke & Panda, 1965).

This type of approach owes much to the initial work of Spence and his colleagues in Newcastle upon Tyne (Spence et al., 1954; Miller et al., 1960), and recently longitudinal studies have begun to be undertaken more frequently in developing tropical regions.[1]

The advantages of longitudinal incidence studies

Longitudinal investigations are usually carried on for at least one year and thus not only permit the true annual incidence of malnutrition and

---

[1] Longitudinal studies of child health have been carried out, or are under way, in many parts of the world, including the following places: *Eastern Mediterranean*—Beirut, Lebanon (J. Harfouche—personal communication, 1965); Jordan (Pharaon et al., 1965); *Asia*—rural Hyderabad, India (Jyothi et al., 1963; Swaminathan et al., 1964); *Africa*—Keneba village, Gambia (McGregor, Billewicz & Thomson, 1961); Sukuta village, Gambia (Marsden, 1964); Durban, South Africa (Kark & Steuart, 1962); Imesi village, Nigeria (Morley, 1963); Akufo village, Nigeria (Gilles, 1964); Lagos, Nigeria (N. Rea—personal communication, 1965); Ibadan, Nigeria (M. Janes—personal communication, 1965); *the Americas*—joint INCAP-ICNND Guatemala study (W. Unglaub—personal communication, 1965); Guatemala (W. Ascoli & N. S. Scrimshaw—personal communication, 1965); Mexico City (Ramos-Galvan, 1966); Cali, Colombia (C. Canosa—personal communication, 1965); Bogota, Colombia (R. Rueda-Williamson—personal communication, 1965); *West Indies*—rural Jamaica (Standard & Miall, 1965).

disease to be determined, but show the seasonal variations caused by the climate, the availability of food, community activities and other factors.

Most illnesses in early childhood are short-term episodes, and in longitudinal studies the incidence of such severe diseases as infantile beriberi and measles, or such minor conditions as impetigo, can be discovered and correlated both with one another and with other environmental circumstances. This contrasts with the short-term cross-sectional prevalence surveys, which miss most of the acute conditions and tend to overemphasize chronic diseases (Williams, 1964).

Another advantage is that the ages of children born during the study will be known with accuracy, together with the dates and causes of death. Growth can be compared with standards for age, and such vital statistics as the mortality rates and causes of death in infants, in the 1-4-year age-group, and in the perinatal period, can be assessed.

Above all, longitudinal studies permit of an understanding of the dynamic interplay of factors at work, and in particular enable an identification of locally important causes of malnutrition to be made (Williams, 1964).

Finally, the prestige attaching to the research aspect of this type of work may help to attract young doctors to work in rural districts, while the detailed knowledge gained of the particular area may ultimately lead to its use for the field training of medical and paramedical personnel, and, above all, help to plan long-term medical services adapted to local problems.

The disadvantages of longitudinal incidence studies

Long-term incidence studies are not easy to organize. They can be expensive, and are by their nature time-consuming. Also, by the time the results of a longitudinal study are completed and analysed, they may be out-of-date because the community itself may have changed.

Constant standards and methods of examination and interview have to be maintained over the whole period and not be altered with experience.

The ethical question of the degree of clinical responsibility to be assumed will have to be decided in advance, clearly defined and adhered to throughout. This will have to be judged according to the circumstances of the particular study. In some surveys, it may be justifiable to limit the therapy and advice given to the use of placebos and emergency medical care; in many others more than this will be necessary. Moreover, " any survey inevitably alters both the observer and the observed " (Williams, 1964).

Preparation of the population to be surveyed calls for careful thought and explanation, obviously much influenced by the type of clinical care to be offered to parents.

Many practical difficulties may arise—for example, the seasonal or other movement of people between the town and rural villages, or a high incidence of defaulters due to indifference or suspicion.

Lastly, suitably trained staff may be difficult to recruit, and still more to retain. A large measure of patience, dedication and team-spirit is needed on the part of the survey group—well exemplified in the Newcastle upon Tyne study (Spence et al., 1954).

Techniques

In the longitudinal surveys being undertaken in different parts of the world (p. 132), numerous variations in technique and procedure are applied; these are often dictated by local circumstances and the special aims of the particular study, which must be clearly defined at the outset. Nevertheless, certain general principles seem to be common to many such investigations.

Sampling. Statistical guidance will be required with sampling regarding the number to be covered, the frequency of examinations, the length of study and the selection of families. Allowance must be made for a probable decrease in the total during the observation period due to defaulting and to deaths.

In view of the present-day interest in the nutritional problems of early childhood, many longitudinal surveys aim at observing a selected group of full-term babies, born by normal delivery, through the first 2-5 years of life. If—as is rarely the case—the ages of children are known with precision, an alternative may be the surveillance of a group of infants and pre-school children (N. Rea—personal communication, 1965).

Selection of area. The area selected should be as typical of the particular ecological situation as can be judged on the available evidence. Frequently, a simultaneous survey may be made of contrasting socio-economic groups [1] (R. Rueda-Williamson—personal communication, 1965; N. Rea—personal communication, 1965) or ethnic communities (J. Harfouche—personal communication, 1965). In the INCAP-ICNND Guatemala long-term study, another major factor in area selection has been the varying levels of infant mortality rates (W. Unglaub—personal communication, 1965). In such cases also the advice of a statistician and an anthropologist should be sought.

Selection of places of examination. Usually three examination sites have to be planned: a regular clinic for the survey children, systematic home-visiting, and some form of emergency morbidity clinic service for the acutely ill.

Home visits are essential for the assessment of environmental and socio-economic circumstances, for the coaxing of defaulters and for the investigation of any deaths that may have occurred.

It is also important to arrange for transport, for those attending the regular clinic, for home-visiting staff and for emergency cases.

---

[1] If one of the contrasting groups consists of children of the local élite, it may be possible to use the results obtained as a basis for local standards for growth and development.

As pointed out by Kark & Steuart (1962), useful, though incomplete and biased, longitudinal information exists already in many parts of the world in the records of such health centres as have an adjacent defined area and sufficient staff to permit home-visiting. The disadvantage of this information is that it is necessarily influenced by the health centre's activities, and hence not typical of areas lacking similar facilities.

Selection and training of staff. A full-time staff is needed for continuous employment throughout the whole survey period, preferably headed by a doctor with paediatric and public-health experience.

An adequate preliminary period must be devoted to the selection and training of auxiliary staff and to pre-testing methods, in particular the techniques of interviewing and home-visiting, often culminating in a pilot study.

Type and frequency of investigations. Although the detailed arrangements vary, a longitudinal survey commencing at birth may often start with regular examinations held monthly for three months, and thereafter at three-monthly intervals. Care should be taken to ensure that children are seen within a defined number of days of their scheduled appointment —for example, three-monthly intervals: $\pm$ 7 days (C. Canosa—personal communication, 1965).

Data collected during longitudinal surveys

Longitudinal surveys of children often include the serial collection of some of the following data:

(*a*) *Anthropometric measurements*—weight, height (length), circumference of the head, chest and arms, skin-fold thickness

(*b*) *Clinical characteristics*—general, nutritional stigmata, physical development (milestones, sometimes radiological bone-age), psychological development

(*c*) *Biochemical data* [1]—haemoglobin, haematocrit, plasma proteins

(*d*) *Parasitological data*—results of examining stools for ova, etc., thick film for malaria

(*e*) *Tuberculin test results*

(*f*) *Health history*—type and duration of illnesses since last visit (e.g., diarrhoea, respiratory-tract infection), immunization

(*g*) *Dietary history*—types and approximate quantities of food given in previous period (often 24 hours).

Data on socio-economic circumstances of the family and cultural attitudes also have to be collected. Some may be obtained by questionnaire

---

[1] Biochemical tests are usually carried out at less frequent intervals than the clinical examination and anthropometry. Special local problems may suggest other biochemical tests as a matter of routine—the serum alkaline phosphatase if rickets is prevalent, or urinary thiamine if beriberi is common.

initially, but usually more-personal details will only be learnt later either by questioning when rapport has been established or by observation during home-visiting.

If practicable, a brief study of other family members should be undertaken, including the obstetrical history of the mother and a clinical and anthropometric examination of the parents and siblings.

Items of information collected in this type of survey require to be carefully pre-defined and graded numerically, so that they may lend themselves to analysis on punch cards. Precise criteria for the retrospective diagnosis of illness must be laid down—for example, diarrhoea may be defined as six or more loose watery stools in 24 hours. Likewise, the grading of socio-economic data must be defined—for example, various degrees of overcrowding, types of water supply, or social groups.

Subsampling techniques may be employed to obtain more-detailed information on a percentage of those being studied. It is particularly valuable if family food-consumption studies, made by actual measurement of foods cooked and eaten, can be carried out on a statistically selected subsample. Similarly, more-detailed biochemical tests, such as serum levels of vitamin A or the amino-acid imbalance test may be carried out on a subgroup.

Conclusion

More longitudinal health surveys are needed in representative rural and urban areas of the world, and the nutrition of the community must form a major aspect of all such studies.

Unfortunately, in many places such long-term incidence studies will not be feasible, principally because of cost and shortage of staff. In addition therefore to longitudinal studies in selected areas, the assessment of the nutritional status of the community will often have to be evaluated by short-term cross-sectional prevalence studies.

Cross-Sectional Prevalence Studies

These studies can be single examinations of populations undertaken in a specified short interval, usually of a few days or weeks, when they are known as point prevalence surveys, or they can be repeated on the same groups at prescribed intervals, when they are termed periodic prevalence surveys.

The advantages and disadvantages of cross-sectional prevalence studies

Short-term prevalence surveys offer the obvious advantages of being relatively inexpensive, requiring few staff and taking little time to carry out.

The limitations and disadvantages of these surveys are again clear. They are brief in duration, and, unless supplemented by information from health services, reflect conditions during only one season of one year.

They are short episodes and thus afford extremely limited opportunities for gaining a real insight into the way people live and the causes of their nutritional problems.

They provide accurate figures only for relatively chronic conditions, such as fluorosis or protein-calorie malnutrition; they are misleading with regard to important acute conditions of short duration, such as infantile beriberi.

Lastly, it is a frequent and at times valid complaint that surveys can easily become sterile academic exercises that fail to better the conditions in the community. Plainly, surveys are not carried out solely to satisfy scientific curiosity, but to define problems and suggest logical means of improving the situation.

Accordingly, point prevalence surveys are not the complete answer for the nutritional assessment of the community. Their results must be carefully weighed against the evidence from other sources, particularly local health statistics and against information derived from long-term incidence studies, if these become available.

Alternatively, an attempt may be made to cover possible seasonal differences in nutrition and to obtain a rough estimate of probable disease incidence by carrying out periodic cross-sectional prevalence surveys at selected periods of the year representative of the annual climatic and agricultural cycle (Collis, Dema & Lesi, 1962; Collis, Dema & Omolulu, 1962a, b; Pharaon et al., 1965).

Types of prevalence survey

Nutrition prevalence surveys can vary greatly in complexity, scope and purpose. The term may cover a wide range of activities, from small, unelaborate teams with limited objectives, relying mainly on rapid screening by clinical assessment, to large multi-disciplinary groups, including doctors, non-medical nutritionists, biochemists and dietitians, disposing of ample funds and extensive laboratory facilities and working in an area for longer periods.

Surveys of all the different types can yield valuable information. The most appropriate type for a given situation depends on the aim of the survey and the local resources in skilled staff, money and time.

In addition to obtaining information on the nutritional condition of the community, surveys can have other useful by-products. They provide valuable opportunities for the testing of new or modified methods suitable for field conditions. They can be most helpful in the teaching of professional and non-professional personnel, concerning survey techniques, and in fostering an appreciation of the ecology of malnutrition in rural areas. Moreover, they may involve the people of the community themselves, especially those assisting in the planning and carrying out of the survey, and prompt them to study practical ways of improving their own nutrition.

Special groups

Prevalence surveys can be carried out on certain special groups within a community, including schoolchildren, personnel in the armed forces, prisoners, and other groups subject to some form of discipline and, by that token, more easily accessible and organized for nutritional survey work. These are, however, selected samples with particular problems and with nutritional advantages and disadvantages. The results obtained refer solely to the group examined and are not necessarily typical of the community at large.

Organization of prevalence surveys

Careful, detailed consideration must always be given to the planning of the particular survey in question, and, while each will be unique in purpose and scope, the principles involved can often be usefully considered in the following stages: planning (preliminary planning, field reconnaissance, technical planning, team training), field work, analysis, interpretation, and action.

PLANNING

Preliminary Planning

Purpose of the survey

Basic to the planning of a survey is a clear definition of its purpose. The decision will be influenced by various factors, including available background data, and the potential scope of the survey team. This, in turn, will determine whether the survey should be general or specific, whether it should consist mainly of simple clinical signs, used as a preliminary screening, or should include more elaborate biochemical investigations on a research basis.

Consideration of the purpose of the study may also suggest the geographical area and population groups to be included, and possibly the desirability of restricting the investigation to a particular age-group or sex.

It is often not sufficiently appreciated that time devoted to careful planning represents a saving of time and the avoidance of confusion and failure in the field.

Preliminary plan of action

At an early stage, a written preliminary plan of action must be drawn up. Of necessity this will be a tentative outline based on available information and background data.

Field Reconnaissance

Approach to local people

The success of a community survey depends largely on the thoroughness of the planning, which will be guided by available information concerning the local environment and culture patterns and by statistical considerations.

Usually, several months have to be given over to communication with various categories of officials and people in the area. These will normally include government departments and officials and local community leaders who may be traditional, political or religious, or all of these.

At an opportune moment, a senior member of the survey team must make a preliminary visit or field reconnaissance to the area in order to meet the local public health workers, community leaders and administrators, to assess the situation with regard to accommodation and transport, and to make a preliminary inquiry into the pattern of malnutrition, food habits and general mode of life.

Careful prolonged explanations in simple, non-technical language, and a full discussion concerning the purpose of the survey and the methods envisaged are essential. It cannot be stressed too much that these are the people who must be convinced, since they will, in most cases, be primarily involved in telling the community of the team's visit and intentions, and in attempting to ensure co-operation and attendance. Without local understanding, success in a community nutrition survey is unlikely.

It is vitally necessary to provide a stimulus whereby to ensure the attendance of the population. To this end, an undertaking to treat any sickness found is helpful. A knowledge of possible local reactions to the techniques and methods to be employed is important—for example, the willingness of women to undergo clinical examination, or anxiety that samples of blood, faeces or urine may be misused for occult purposes. Frank discussions with local leaders may help to clarify ideas and suggest ways of obviating cross-cultural misunderstandings.

Apart from explaining the purpose of the survey, and so allaying fears and misconceptions, preliminary discussions and correspondence will lead to the arrangement of a survey time-table. At this point practical problems, such as the selection of the most useful collecting points, seasonal travel difficulties and social problems resulting from periods of widespread community activity (related to agriculture, religion or ritual) should be borne in mind.

Involvement of local health workers

It is particularly important that local health workers should be associated as team members in every activity, from the planning stage to the actual field work. Clearly, they cannot remain mere bewildered spectators, since it will probably fall to them to try to implement any action suggested.

Practicability of preliminary plan

Information and advice obtained during field reconnaissance also permit of an assessment of the extent to which the theoretical preliminary plan of action is suited to the conditions in the area.

Technical Planning

Once the purpose of the survey and its extent and depth have been decided, technical planning can be undertaken. This will probably be based on the preliminary plan of action, influenced by observation during the field reconnaissance and by the advice given by local leaders.

Technical planning may be considered under four headings: selection of methods, statistical guidance, selection of equipment, and training of personnel.

Selection of methods

As noted earlier, three main categories of methods of assessment are available for use in a community nutrition survey: direct assessment of human groups; indirect assessment of human groups; and assessment of ecological factors.

Direct assessment of human groups

Reference has already been made to the four methods of assessing the nutritional status of groups of individual human beings in a community directly: clinical signs; anthropometric measurements; biochemical tests; and biophysical methods. Usually, a combination of these methods will be favoured.

The range of practicable clinical signs, anthropometric measurements and biochemical tests is listed elsewhere. In all surveys, the selection of tests and methods to be used depends upon various factors, in particular the age-groups to be covered and the nutritional public health problems likely to be encountered. For example, tests for serum-alkaline-phosphatase levels would not normally be included in a nutritional survey of young children in a tropical community, in a sunny rural area, where rickets was known to be a rare clinical problem.

Surveys almost always include examination for clinical signs. In general surveys, the signs to be looked for should include a selection of the stigmata listed earlier. For research purposes, less certain or newly recognized signs may also have a place, in an attempt to assess their significance. In rapid screening surveys, covering large numbers and often employing junior staff, only certain selected signs are noted, on the assumption that, if necessary, suggestive findings may be followed up with more-detailed investigations in affected areas.

The clinical signs looked for will also have to be adjusted to suit a particular age-group. Thus, a survey of young children, among whom protein-calorie malnutrition is the main problem, would not be concerned with testing the ankle jerks.

Finally a rapid survey may, though rarely, be undertaken without clinical signs being included. For example, haemoglobin estimations may be carried out to screen for iron deficiency, or the urinary thiamine for deficiency of this nutrient.

Basic anthropometric measurements will usually be carried out and may consist, for all age-groups, of weight, height (or length), triceps skin-fold and arm circumference. When young children are being studied, the circumference of the head and chest should also be measured.

It is difficult to generalize concerning the range of biochemical tests to be applied, as these will depend on the purpose of the survey, the age and sex of the group under investigation, and, above all, the available laboratory facilities. In most surveys, where tests are employed, they are normally limited to a sample of those attending, as they are often expensive, time-consuming and difficult to perform, collect and interpret. Often the selected tests are related to possible deficiencies suggested by a general knowledge of the local diet and disease pattern, or, by analogy, to findings from some other ecologically similar area. A haemoglobin estimation should always be included, both as a screening test for iron deficiency and other types of nutritional anaemia and because of its relationship to malaria and hookworm infection—both important conditioning diseases.

As described elsewhere, biophysical tests usually play little part in nutrition surveys but may be required for certain specific investigations, such as the dark-adaptation test for avitaminosis A, or radiological examination of the wrists for rickets.

In practice the individual assessment of groups in most nutrition prevalence surveys is based on the use of clinical signs, associated with basic (or more extensive) anthropometric measurements and selected, locally appropriate and practicable biochemical tests (always including a haemoglobin estimation) usually carried out on a sample of the population that has been examined clinically.

Indirect assessment of human groups

In addition to the health statistics obtained from background data, it should be possible to collect further information during the survey period from local medical service records, from data on birth and death registration, and by means of a questionnaire concerning the mortality and morbidity rates of different age-groups relating to malnutrition and nutritionally relevant infections.

Assessment of ecological factors

Apart from evaluating the nutritional status of the community by clinical, anthropometric, biochemical and other means, nutrition surveys must also attempt to collect as many data as possible concerning the epidemiology of the malnutrition found. Information concerning ecological factors—conditioning infections, food consumption, cultural influences, socio-economic factors and food production—may be drawn from background data and special surveys (e.g., family food-consumption studies), or by means of observation and questionnaire at the survey site, together with rapid ecological visits to homes, cultivation sites, etc.

Statistical guidance [1]

Statistical guidance is of importance at every phase of survey work, but especially at the planning stage and in relation to sampling, design of survey forms, and evaluation of results.

Sampling

If statistically sound sampling procedures based on probability are not followed, the significance of survey results will at best be uncertain, and possibly biased and incorrect. By contrast, with correct sampling, investigations can provide accurate information on an examination of only a portion of the population, with a consequent saving of time, money and staff and with less disruption of the local community (Woolsey et al., 1954).

However, sampling problems are far from simple and usually require the specialized skill of the statistician. Some understanding by the nutritionist of statistical principles is valuable in order to bridge the gap between the two technical fields of knowledge.

It is neither possible nor necessary to examine all members of the population; the basis of sampling is to select a random sample of sufficient size to give accurate, unbiased and representative results for the community as a whole (Witts, 1964).

Sampling will be based on checked local census figures (if available), or other community lists, preferably those including population numbers, age-groups and household distribution, and on a knowledge of variable factors, such as those related to the yearly meteorological and agricultural cycle, to migrations of population, etc.

Random sampling may be achieved by two main selection methods (Reh, 1962)—systematic procedures, which are based on the selection of house numbers from the census at specified numerical intervals, and unrestricted procedures, in which the sample is chosen by lottery or from standard printed tables of random numbers.

The size of the sample for each individual survey is determined by the size of the population-group, the probable prevalence of the characteristic sign or syndrome to be measured, and the degree of precision required in the results. Attention must also be given to the practical, non-statistical errors (e.g., inter-observer, experimental, etc.) inherent in the measurement.

In practice, in the selection of the sample size, a balance will have to be struck between statistical requirements and local field realities, such as difficulties of travel in certain terrain or the absence of a local census. Also,

---

[1] Further detailed consideration is given by Reh (1962), Swaroop (1966) and Schaefer (1961).

provision should, if possible, be planned for any adjustments necessitated by unforeseen changes in the field.

The combination of methods and approaches usually adopted in nutrition surveys will call for different sample sizes and, possibly, different sampling techniques, using the multiphase method. For the more general measurements, such as clinical assessment, weight and height, a large sample may be manageable, while for the more complicated biochemical determinations and time-consuming food-consumption studies, a smaller sample will have to suffice. Statistical advice will also be required concerning the number of rapid ecological visits to be made in the course of the survey.

The ICNND survey procedure is based on the practical application of subsampling. All persons attending are given an " abbreviated clinical examination ". A sample of them are given a " detailed clinical examination " and selected biochemical tests. Finally, a smaller proportion undergo special biochemical investigations (Wilson et al., 1964).

If biochemical tests are carried out on a random subsample and on subjects selected because they show marked clinical signs, the two groups must be clearly differentiated (Sinclair, 1964).

Unfortunately, in some circumstances, expert guidance from a statistician may not be available on the spot. At times advice may be sought by correspondence; otherwise, every effort should be made to ensure that representative areas are included, if the region under study is not homogeneous. Variations in age structure, ethnic groups, geography, agriculture, food patterns, economic level, religion, occupations, levels of modern education, health facilities and known disease patterns must be taken into consideration.

Survey forms

Forms employed must be easily identifiable—for example, through the use of coloured paper or card. They must show the items to be filled in clearly and unambiguously.

Two main types of composite survey form are in widespread use in varying sizes and degrees of complexity: the single sheet and the punch-edge card.

All newly designed forms need an accompanying guide sheet listing exactly what is wanted under each heading, with definitions. They should be tried out on a small scale before use in an actual survey.

(*a*) *Single sheet*. This can be of paper or cardboard, and examples are shown in Figs. 46 and 47. They are not presented as ideal patterns, nor do the signs and other data listed necessarily coincide with suggestions made in the present monograph. They are, however, forms that have been found useful in practice.

(*b*) *Punch-edge cards*. These are cardboard rectangles of various sizes, with space in the centre for recording data in the field, and with holes punched round the edge (Fig. 48). Two widely used brands are the McBee

**FIG. 46. ABBREVIATED SURVEY SHEET USED AT NSAMBYA, KAMPALA
(ALSO LISTING OTHER NON-NUTRITIONAL DISABILITIES)**

NSAMBYA URBAN CHILD HEALTH SURVEY

NO: **52**   NAME: **HERINA ADHIAMBO**   SEX: **F**

ADDRESS: **Plot 72**   BIRTHDAY: **18/7/63**   AGE: **16** mo.

CLINICAL

Nutrition   + dyschromotrichia / + sparse hair / — oedema / — moon face / — other (state)

Remediable complaints   chronic otitis media / + conjunctivitis / spleen / — other (state)

Congenital or other abnormalities   — club foot / — harelip / — polio / — other (state)

Skin disease   sepsis / + scabies / — tinea / — burn scars / — molluscum

Medicinal   + vaccination scar / — charms / — incisions / + other (state)

ANTHROPOMETRY

Wt.	**9·37** kg.	Wt/age	**+80** % level
Length	**74·1** cm.	Wt/ht	**+90** % level
Head Circ.	**46·0** cm.	Wt/hd	**+90** % level
Chest Circ.	**48·0** cm.	Chest/head ratio:	(over one)/under one
Arm Circ.	**14·0** cm.	Arm circ.	**+80** % level
Skin fold	**9·1** mm.	Skin fold	**+90** % level

LABORATORY

Hb.   **9·5** gm %

Stool   negative / + Ascaris / — Hookworm / — Giardia / — E.histolytica /
     — Strongyloides / other (state)

Thick B.F.   negative / + MT / — QT

FIG. 47. DETAILED CHILD HEALTH AND NUTRITION SURVEY FORM USED BY ICNND

(a) Front of card

Pediatric Card for Children Ages 0-4 years.   READ INSTRUCTIONS BEFORE USING.

DATE	NAME		☐ Boy ☐ Girl	AGE ___yrs___mo	CARD NO.

LOCATION	AREA OF ORIGIN		☐ Rural ☐ Urban	☐ Other siblings examined	☐ Informant not mother

LENGTH	in / cm	STD	%	WEIGHT	lb / kg	STD	%	1	2	3	4	5	6

MOTHER AGE yrs / U M R	If now pregnant mos	Number of PAST PREGNANCIES___ ___liveborn ___stillborn ___abortions / MULTIPLE BIRTHS	Of the liveborn: ___now living ___now dead	Of those dying: ___died at < 1 yr ___died at 1-4 yr ___died at 5+ yrs	Mother's age at: term. 1st preg. yrs / term. last preg. yrs

THIS CHILD:	Age U R M	Birth order	Premature? YES NO	Walked ___mos	DIARRHEA ☐ Current ☐ Recent ☐ Recurrent	RESPIRATORY ☐ Current ☐ Recent ☐ Recurrent	☐ Pica_____ ☐ Parasites_____ ☐ Malaria_____ ☐ Other_____

GENERAL IMPRESSIONS
- ☐ Apathy
- ☐ Pallor
- ☐ Irritability

HAIR
- ☐ Dry staring
- ☐ Dyspigmentation
- ☐ Thin
- ☐ Easily pluckable

EYES
- ☐ Conjunctival dryness
- ☐ Conjunctivitis
- ☐ Bitot's spots
- ☐ Xerophthalmia
- _____

LIPS
- ☐ Angular lesions
- ☐ Cheilosis

GUMS
- ☐ Swollen red papillae (diffuse)
- ☐ Bleeding

TONGUE
- ☐ Filiform papillary atrophy
  - ☐ Mild ☐ Mod. ☐ Severe
- ☐ Glossitis

GLANDS
- ☐ Thyroid enlarged (visible)

SKIN, GENERALLY
- ☐ Inelastic
- ☐ Petechiae
- ☐ Dermatitis, with desquamation or crazy pavement type
- ☐ _____

ABDOMEN
- ☐ Hepatomegaly
- ☐ Splenomegaly
- ☐ Pot-belly

LOWER EXTREMITIES
- ☐ Bilateral edema
- ☐ Calf tenderness

SKELETAL
- ☐ Cranial bossing ☐ Frontal ☐ Parietal
- ☐ Craniotabes
- ☐ Costochondrial beading
- ☐ Enlarged joints
- ☐ Bone tenderness
- ☐ Muscle wasting
- ☐ _____
- ☐ _____

OTHER
- ☐ 1._____
- ☐ 2._____

CLINICAL IMPRESSION
- ☐ Marasmus
- ☐ Pre-kwashiorkor
- ☐ Kwashiorkor

REMARKS:

PHOTOGRAPH #_____of

G   F   P

EXAMINER'S INITIALS_____

☐ URINE sample #_____   ☐ BLOOD sample #_____   ☐ FECES sample #_____

URINE DATA
Urine volume_____ml, during_____hours
Creatinine_____mg/ml or_____mg/ hrs

Thiamine - - - - - - - - _____ ___
Riboflavin - - - - - - - _____ ___
N'methylnicotinamide - - _____ ___

Other,#1_____ - - _____ ___
Other,#2_____ - - _____ ___
Other,#3_____ - - _____ ___

PARASITOLOGIC FINDINGS
1___,2___,3___,4___,5___,6___,7___

BLOOD DATA
Total plasma protein - - - - - _____ ___
Albumin - - - - - - - - - - - - _____ ___

Hemoglobin - - - - - - - - - - _____ ___
Hematocrit (PCV) - - - - - - _____ ___
M.C.H.C. = 100 Hgb/PCV - - - - _____ ___

Serum Vitamin C (mg/100 ml) - - _____ ___
Serum Vitamin A (mcg/100 ml) - _____ ___
Serum Carotene (mcg/100 ml) - _____ ___
Alkaline phosphatase - - - - - _____ ___
Other,#1_____ - - _____ ___
Other,#2_____ - - _____ ___

FIG. 47. DETAILED CHILD HEALTH AND NUTRITION SURVEY FORM USED BY ICNND (*continued*)

(*b*) Reverse of card

DIETARY   Information obtained by:

CHILD – – BREAST FEEDING	CHILD NOW FED: (one or more) ☐ Breast milk ☐ Other milk ☐ Other foods	IF CHILD NOW NURSES: ___feedings/day ☐ Self-demand OR ☐ Schedule ___hrs	IF NURSING TERMINATED: ☐ Abruptly at___months ☐ Gradually___to___mos ☐ NEVER breast fed	FACTORS IN TIME OF WEANING: Maternal / Infant ☐ Illness ☐ Illness ☐ Work ☐ ___ ☐ Pregnancy ☐ ___

CHILD – – INITIAL NON-MILK FOODS	1 2 3 4 5 6

CHILD – – PHARMACEUTICAL SUPPLEMENTS	☐ Iron from ___months to ___months or ☐ PRESENT ☐ Regularly ☐ Occasionally ☐ Vit A & D from ___months to ___months or ☐ PRESENT ☐ Regularly ☐ Occasionally ☐ Vitamin C from ___months to ___months or ☐ PRESENT ☐ Regularly ☐ Occasionally ☐ ___ from ___months to ___months or ☐ PRESENT ☐ Regularly ☐ Occasionally

CHILD – – MILK FEEDING (not breast)	Fresh milk: ☐ Cow ☐ Water buffalo ☐ Goat ☐ ___ ☐ Sheep ☐ Camel	Processed milk: ☐ Dry skim ☐ Dry whole ☐ Evaporated ☐ ___	PRESENT intake: ___(vol)/day ___(wt.)/day ___(times)/day	Is formula water boiled? YES NO Is drinking water boiled? YES NO

CHILD'S PRESENT DIET

Do you give this child any special foods or juices other than the family diet?   YES   NO

If YES, what kinds? _____

Usual present diet:

Food type	Food	Quantity/Day	Times/day OR times/wk	Age this food first started
MILK				
GRUELS,CEREALS				
VEGETABLES				
FRUITS				
MEAT,FISH,FOWL				
EGGS				
OTHER				

MOTHER'S DIET during LATEST PREGNANCY			MOTHER'S DIET during LATEST LACTATION		
Foods avoided Why?	Special foods Why?	Supple- ments Why?	Foods avoided Why?	Special foods Why?	Supple- ments Why?
1 Salt ___	1 Milk ___	1 Iron ___	1 Salt ___	1 Milk ___	1 Iron ___
2 ___	2 ___	2 Calcium ___	2 ___	2 ___	2 Calcium ___
3 ___	3 ___	3 Vitamins ___	3 ___	3 ___	3 Vitamins ___
4 ___	4 ___	4 ___	4 ___	4 ___	4 ___
5 ___	5 ___	5 ___	5 ___	5 ___	5 ___
6 ___	6 ___	6 ___	6 ___	6 ___	6 ___

At what age do your children begin to drink...   Coffee?___yrs   Wine?___yrs   Soft drinks?___yrs (kind_____)   Tea?___yrs   Beer?___yrs   Other?___yrs (kind_____)

Cards, employed by ICNND, and the Cope-Chat Cards. They offer the advantage that positive findings can subsequently be marked by slotting the appropriately numbered edge-holes, and the cards may then be needle-sorted by hand.

In both types of form, if it is proposed to transfer the information to punch cards, such as those of IBM or ICT, for mechanical sorting and analysis, it is necessary for each item to have a code-number. This can be done with a list of items and their corresponding punch-card code numbers, or, alternatively, by means of an entry against the appropriate item on the sheet or card (Fig. 48); the transfer of information is thereby facilitated.

Design of survey forms

The designing of the most useful forms for a particular survey (including the size and material) is a complicated task and will be influenced by personal preference and by the purpose of the investigation. The guidance of a statistician is helpful in order to ensure that the relevant data are recorded in a form that can be easily analysed, preferably by transfer to punch cards.

Common types of form. Large numbers of different types of form have been employed in nutrition surveys all over the world, and the locally most suitable system will have to be developed for each survey. Basically the following types of information have to be recorded: data on individuals (identification, clinical assessment, anthropometry, laboratory tests); dietary information; findings of rapid ecological visits; and, if possible, food-consumption data.

Composite survey forms. These are commonly used, and each lists some or all of the data for the survey, and sometimes dietary information as well. A form is issued to each individual being examined, to be kept by him until the field assessment is completed, when it is collected. Personal data concerning identification, clinical assessment, anthropometry and recent diet are filled in as the person moves from " station " to " station ", while laboratory results are added later. Forms for children must show the state of dental eruption, recorded by the standard visual coding (see Fig. 32).

Identification data will consist of at least the date, location, survey day, number, name, age, and sex, and also such other details as may be necessary in the particular community (e.g., " son of ", or home village). It may be useful to have spaces for both stated and verified ages (or birth-dates).

Whatever the form used, it is important that *both* positives *and* negatives should be marked appropriately ($+$ or $-$); otherwise, uncertainty will exist later as to whether a clinical sign has been looked for or not. As noted earlier, the classification of physical signs into degrees of positivity (i.e., $+$, $++$, $+++$) is not usually recommended (except for the degree of thyroid enlargement), because grading of this kind is difficult to define objectively.

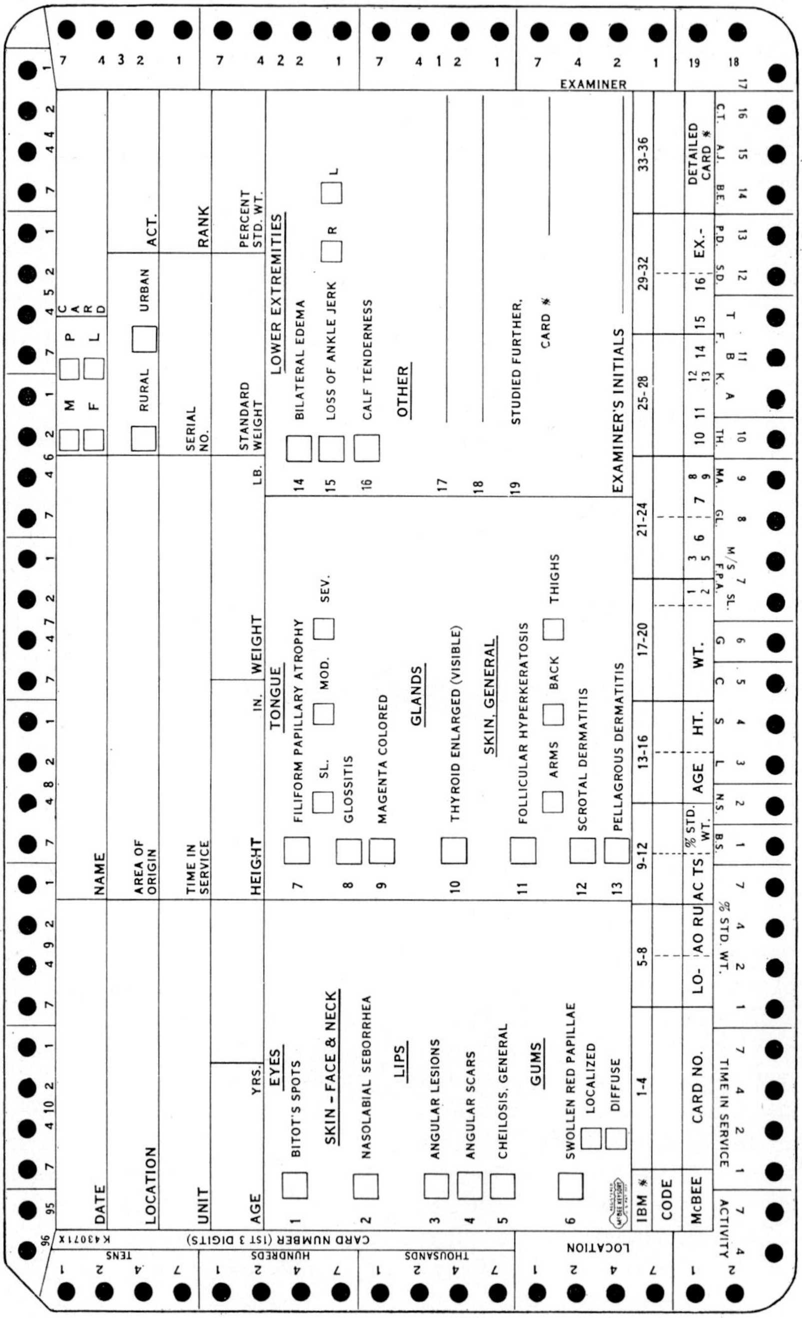

FIG. 48. ABBREVIATED PUNCH-EDGED SURVEY CARD USED BY ICNND (McBEE CARD)

The recording of past histories is not usually advisable in prevalence surveys in developing countries (e.g., " recent attacks of diarrhoea ") as the resulting information is not sufficiently reliable to justify the time and effort involved.

Forms for rapid screening surveys. In addition to detailed clinical assessment schedules, abbreviated simplified forms will be required for rapid screening surveys.

Dietary questionnaire forms. These may be used at the survey site or in the home. The inquiries should be condensed, precise, in logical order and should try to avoid leading questions. They should be concerned with only a short preceding period—often of no more than 24 hours. A system of ticks or check marks should be used for the answers, and space should be allowed for comments. The detailed construction of the questionnaire will obviously depend on local dietary habits and food resources and will be based on background data and information obtained during field reconnaissance. Approximate quantitative information may be obtained if local measures of content and utensils, such as bottles and spoons, and even cooked servings, of dishes are available to the questioner.

The dietary questionnaire may be a separate form or may be included as part of the composite form.

Rapid ecological visit forms. These will be used by the small mobile group visiting homes, cultivation sites and markets. Suggested data that may be included are given in Table 16.

Food-consumption forms. These have been fully discussed by Reh (1962) and will not be considered here.

Expression and evaluation of results

Statistical assistance is needed for the evaluation of results, and in particular for testing the significance of various findings.

Selection of equipment

The type of equipment will vary widely, depending not only on the scope and purpose of the survey, but on the terrain in which it is being carried out. Maintenance in the field must not be overlooked.

Transport and accommodation

The more remote the community the more comprehensive and carefully planned the details of transport and accommodation will have to be. Road conditions as well as financial considerations will determine whether standard cars, or four-wheel-drive utility vehicles (e.g., Land-Rover, Jeep), or even a mobile field laboratory, housed in a lorry with an electrical generator for refrigeration, etc., and with a gas supply for Bunsen burners, should be used.

In less developed parts of the world, questions of fuel and water for vehicles, which may have to be carried by the team itself, call for special attention. A strong trailer, sufficiently sturdy to be towed by a utility vehicle over rough roads, may prove a very useful and economical way of transporting water and heavy equipment.

In some areas, part of the journey may have to be made on foot, or by bicycle, dog sled, boat, or canoe, in which case some form of water-proofing of equipment must be provided. Also, in remote roadless areas, porterage of equipment may be necessary. Advance arrangements may have to be made for porters, money in a convenient form and the packaging of equipment in bundles suited to the local method of carrying.

Accommodation and food for the team have to be planned. During the field reconnaissance, a senior team member will have gauged the situation. The type of accommodation, and hence the degree of organization and planning, necessary in connexion with sleeping, washing, toilet and cooking arrangements will vary according to whether an hotel, a rest-house or tents are to be used. The amount and type of food, drink and cooking utensils to be taken or bought locally must also be planned ahead. Easily carried packaged meals and bottled soft aerated drinks are often the most convenient for lunch, which will usually be eaten in the field. Some extra food should always be carried, because local volunteer assistants and helpers may have to be included.

Team members will be wise to adopt a perhaps unduly cautious attitude to food and drink while carrying out the field part of a survey. Apart from serious illness, bouts of " traveller's diarrhoea " may disrupt the team's efforts, and are in any event difficult to deal with in the often closely scrutinized circumstances in some rural village areas. All food should be freshly cooked, if possible, and always thoroughly cooked. Drinking-water should be boiled, while milkless tea or coffee, or bottled carbonated soft drinks may be used instead of dubious " boiled " water.

Anthropometric equipment

The types of scales and equipment for measuring weight and height or length will have to be decided. If both young children and adults are to be included, two types of each apparatus will probably be needed. Other items, such as tape measures and skin-fold calipers will also be required.

All this equipment must be carefully packed to minimize damage incurred on a jolting journey over bad roads. Items may also be needed for the setting up of the equipment (e.g., a table as a level surface for a length-board), together with weights for testing the scales through the full weight-range envisaged.

Laboratory equipment

This will depend on the range and number of biochemical and other tests envisaged. The amount carried should exceed the estimated need by 20%.

The collecting apparatus for blood samples will consist of cutting needles or commercially pre-sterilized paper-wrapped lancets for capillary blood, as well as sterile syringes or vacuum tubes for venous samples. The more expensive disposable blood lancets and dry disposable syringes are most useful, and should be chosen if funds permit.

The quantities of other items needed for taking blood samples must be calculated, including material for cleaning the skin (e.g., gauze swabs, spirit or merthiolate), tourniquets, etc.

For the collection of urine, routine screw-capped glass, or preferably plastic, bottles can be used.

Containers for blood samples may be capillary tubes; if so, material for sealing the ends must be available, either a flame (from a Bunsen burner with gas from a portable cylinder), or clay or plasticine brought for the purpose. For larger samples, screw-capped flat-bottomed bottles—if necessary containing an appropriate preservative—will be required. If various samples are taken for different purposes, the requisite number of each type of container must be estimated.

Haematology. For haematological purposes, blood may be taken directly with a pipette into Drabkin's solution in flat-bottomed, screw-capped bottles, a haemoglobin examination being carried out with an electric photometer at the end of the survey.

Thick blood films for malaria are made on a glass slide; with care and practice, up to five films can be made on each slide, which is pre-labelled and divided into sections by transverse lines drawn with a grease pencil. These will require to be stained in the field with Giemsa (or other) stain. Thin blood films, for subsequent examination for red-cell morphology, can be made one per glass slide, fixed by immersing in methyl alcohol, and stained on return to base.

For these haematological tests, sufficient lancets, bottles with Drabkin's solution, labelled glass slides and staining equipment (including Giemsa or other stain, staining racks for the thick films, and wide-mouthed vessels for spirit for fixing thin films) are required.

Stools. For stool samples from adults and older children, screw-cap glass containers can be used with a small quantity of stool preservative. For young children, the small stool sample can best be obtained through the use of an anal tube. Equipment needed will consist of sufficient small 2-ml screw-capped containers containing 1 ml of 10% formol-saline, open-ended glass anal tubes (0.5 cm × 7.5 cm) and wooden applicators, for poking out the core of the stool obtained by inserting the tube into the rectum.

Packing. Containers must be as unbreakable as possible and flat-bottomed, so that they can be packed upright into boxes ensuring the minimum of rattling. If possible, specially designed boxes, trays or shelves of the correct size should be constructed from the cheapest local materials.

Glass slides are dried after fixing or staining in the field and made into convenient-sized packets of about 50, wrapped in labelled white paper.

Refrigeration. Biochemical specimens requiring refrigeration pose special problems depending upon the degree of cooling required and the local facilities. Large, ice-containing thermos flasks may be adequate, with ice brought each day from a near-by hotel, rest-house or local hospital, and the specimens may be kept thereafter in these flasks. More rarely, dry ice may be available and necessary. An electric refrigerator can be fitted into a four-wheel-drive utility vehicle or mobile laboratory.

Special care may have to be taken with particular specimens in order to avoid exposure to sunlight or excessive shaking.

Apparatus may be required for centrifugation. This may be carried out using a low-r.p.m. hand machine or a fast electric centrifuge, which can be operated off a car battery, depending on the particular specimens.

Labelling. This is of paramount importance, and much confusion and waste of effort will be avoided if strict attention is paid to this aspect of the survey. The numbering system must be clear and understood by every member of the team. A simple alphabetical list of days (A, B, etc.) and the consecutive numbering of those attending are often advisable. Specimen containers can then be pre-labelled with the appropriate letter and number (e.g., C1, C2, etc.) if specimens are being taken from all those attending, or with blank labels if random sampling is to be used. The labels used should be waterproof and should not smudge or smear.

Whenever possible, specimens should be taken that can be preserved or refrigerated in the field, and brought back to base at the end of the survey. In some circumstances, however, a field laboratory may be set up at the survey site or in a near-by building or town. Problems of transport between the survey site and the laboratory will, in that case, have to be worked out in regard to vehicles, drivers, time, fuel, etc., if the specimens taken have to be examined before the survey team returns to headquarters.

Drugs and inducements

The treatment of illness found in the course of a survey, or its appropriate referral, is often a major incentive to attend, and especially for mothers to bring children. Sometimes it may be felt necessary to issue a minor " medicine ", such as a few tablets of inexpensive ferrous sulphate, to the mothers of all the children. In addition, cheap, effective, easily administered drugs must be carried in quantities roughly estimated beforehand for the treatment of those actually found to be sick.

Drug lists will vary from region to region. The following is a simple and economical basic list of drugs routinely used in community child-health surveys in East Africa (Jelliffe & Jelliffe, 1963):

Eye infections :	small tubes of sulphacetamide (10%) and tetracycline (1%) eye ointments.
Skin disease :	gentian violet (1%) aqueous solution, sulphur ointment, benzoic acid ointment.
Ear infections :	boric and spirit ear drops.
Sepsis and miscellaneous infections :	disposable syringes of benethamine (long-acting) penicillin (1.2 mega units) for intramuscular injection, sulphathiazole tablets, small quantity of chloramphenicol capsules.
Malaria :	chloroquine tablets.
Intestinal helminths :	piperazine tablets, bephenium packets.
Miscellaneous :	iron tablets, dried skim milk, dressings, bandages, etc.

In addition, paper is needed to wrap up the tablets, and squares of newspaper can be prepared beforehand, or small, inexpensive envelopes purchased. A packet of wooden tongue depressors should be available for dispensing ointment, together with a limited supply of small bottles and boxes.

Other inducements may be advisable, especially for children. Thus, the issue of a cheap sweet or lump of sugar to children after the laboratory specimens have been taken is well worth while. In less sophisticated communities, e.g., the Karamojong pastoralists of Uganda, more " classical " gifts of tobacco, matches and ornaments for parents and elders were found to be helpful (Jelliffe et al., 1964).

General equipment

In a mobile survey, it may be necessary to take chairs and tables: lightweight, folding aluminium chairs and collapsible wooden tables of various sizes are preferable.

Shelter from the rain and sun may be required. Sometimes sticks and string are useful as a fence around each " station " to create an orderly line of flow.

Clothes should be practical, cool, easily washable and culturally acceptable to the local community and, where necessary, should include raincoats and umbrellas.

Training of personnel

Some weeks before the survey begins, the complete team must meet on several occasions. The purpose of the survey should be outlined and available background data discussed, preferably with a senior team member who has already made a field reconnaissance and can report on accommodation, transport problems and recent news from persons on the spot with whom the team will be co-operating.

The planned " lines of flow " to be followed on the survey should be discussed in detail—move by move—with the person responsible for each particular aspect. A complete set of equipment should be available, including anthropometric apparatus and all types of record forms, which can be displayed in appropriate numbered " stations " as they will be used on the survey. As procedures are described, the actual materials should be employed for purposes of demonstration. The techniques and forms to be employed by the group engaged in rapid ecological visits to homes, cultivation sites and markets should also be demonstrated and discussed.

A lengthy discussion is desirable, and an adaptation of forms, equipment or procedure to the circumstances of the particular survey may result.

To ensure a standardization of techniques of measurement and clinical signs, the team should study descriptions and illustrations, such as those given in the present volume. At a subsequent meeting, the clinical signs should be presented one by one, if possible with accompanying colour slides, followed by a full exchange of views and a practical demonstration of the anthropometric measurements to be employed. It is also necessary to demonstrate the correct method of recording results on appropriate forms, and to afford an opportunity for practice.

At a further meeting, a " mock survey " may be organized, with children attending and with the " stations " set up as they will be in the field. It is important that the entire team, including senior members, should understand the complete operation and be capable of carrying out all the component tests and examinations. At this stage the composition of the groups to work at each station can be decided upon and their duties clearly defined.

The importance of ensuring an orderly flow of subjects and of labelling needs to be stressed, for an apparently minor error in the course of a survey day may upset the clinical and laboratory results and nullify the day's work.

In a new area or with newly recruited staff, it may be necessary to carry out a preliminary pilot project.

Types of staff. The types of staff required will vary with the survey methods to be employed. In the field, specially trained staff will be needed to cover the following activities: assessment of clinical signs, anthropometry, taking samples for laboratory tests, completing questionnaires on diet and during rapid ecological visits, as well as for the various techniques required for household food-consumption studies.

A variety of persons, including doctors, non-medical nutritionists, public health nurses and medical students, can be trained to do any of these tasks. The active participation of members of the local public health services in the survey teams is strongly recommended.

In all cases, there must be a clear definition of the duties and functions of the team members. It is useful if the members are trained to be interchangeable, to allow for absence due to illness or accident, and because a variation of duties prevents staleness.

Laboratory technicians, supervised by a biochemist, will be needed at local or base laboratories, if biochemical tests are taken.

While carrying out the actual field work, local untrained volunteers will be required. In most cases they can be engaged for a small remuneration, and are invaluable for interpreting, directing and keeping the line of flow intact and moving steadily.

FIELD WORK

Household surveys

Ideally, prevalence surveys should be carried out by means of house visiting, which offers the advantage of seeing the family together in their domestic setting, of not missing sick individuals, such as children with kwashiorkor, who may be kept at home, and of causing the least disruption of normal life and behaviour.

In general, surveys by systematic home visiting are usually not practicable owing to the difficulty of transporting equipment and the time taken to see a limited number of persons. However, if time permits and few laboratory specimens are to be taken, and also, if the people live in villages or in large family units, household nutrition surveys can contribute greatly to an understanding of the domestic background of malnutrition, as shown by the studies of Oomen & Malcolm (1958) in New Guinea. Moreover, a survey by house visiting may be necessary where it is not culturally permissible for the population, particularly for women, to attend a public meeting-place.

In some parts of the world, no villages exist, and people live instead in scattered homesteads with adjacent cultivation areas. In such circumstances, the population to be surveyed has to be assembled on a selected day at a suitable point, which should be so situated as to enable everyone, including mothers with children in their arms, to attend with a minimum of inconvenience. Clearly, this cannot be arranged without the full co-operation of the local authorities.

Great difficulty in this respect arises with nomadic or pastoralist peoples, and still more with hunter-food gatherer groups, such as the Hadza of northern Tanzania (Jelliffe et al., 1962b).

Surveys at collecting points

In a community nutrition prevalence survey, as distinct from a study of " ready-made " groups such as schoolchildren and armed forces, the major problem often is how to collect the entire population of the particular age-range under investigation from the circumscribed geographical or administrative unit that has been selected statistically.

If villages or similar population groups exist—as on small islands—there may be little difficulty, provided that the community leaders understand and support the project. Suitable assembly points may be arranged at the health centre, the chief's compound, the community hall or other socially familiar focal point, such as the village square.

However, in countries where there is a shortage of doctors, the prior announcement of the survey team's arrival may mean that sick persons, including those suffering from malnutrition, will be brought into the villages from the surrounding countryside, thus giving a false impression of the health situation. In such a circumstance, the village mayor, headman or other official who can recognize, and exclude from the main survey, persons from outside the area can help greatly. He may have a census list of the population or, at least, know whether all of his people have attended or not.

Frequent movements of village populations, such as those occurring during market days in Haiti (Jelliffe & Jelliffe, 1960), also create problems. In every case all persons who may be absent, whether visiting relations or working in industry or agriculture at distant points, must be taken into consideration. It should also be borne in mind, in the assessment of malnutrition and disease prevalence, that sick persons may have been admitted to local hospitals or hidden at home; they must be sought for and included in order that the findings in the community may be complete.

Poorer areas in cities are often difficult to survey, unless low-cost housing estates exist and are treated as population units.

Slum areas are of increasing relevance in the urbanizing tropics, but present peculiar difficulties. Understandably, the inhabitants are often uncooperative or, at best, indifferent. Furthermore, because of the sprawling, overcrowded nature of slum districts it is not easy to concentrate on a limited, circumscribed area, and it may therefore be necessary to carry out the survey, at least in part, by means of home visiting—an unduly lengthy method yielding a slender return for the time spent. The collection of laboratory specimens is particularly difficult.

Essentially, the problem is to collect the entire population of the selected age-groups in the given area, to exclude persons from other areas, and to ensure that the examination is not limited either to the relatively healthy or to the very sick.

In every case, surveys carried out at collecting points must be complemented by visits to homes, kitchens, cultivation sites, shops, etc.—i.e., rapid ecological visits.

Stations and line of flow

It is indispensable, though difficult when dealing with rural people, to organize a smooth, continuous line of flow. Without this, the team's field work will become progressively more confused as the day advances—to the point where the results may have to be abandoned.

To help in the preliminary organization and to supervise its continuation throughout the day, the co-operation of a schoolteacher, the chief, the village mayor or analogous official, accompanied by his assistants, is essential.

Before the day of the survey, the local authorities must know how many stations will be required, where they should be situated, and what each should comprise.

The stations may be set up in rooms in a single building or adjacent buildings, or in the open, in the shade of a tree. The site chosen will depend on local circumstances, including the probable degree of wind, rain or sunshine. If shade is available, some stations, including those for the clinical examination and anthropometric measurements of children, may best be located out of doors. They will be cooler and have better light than a dark crowded room. If necessary, the open-air stations can be surrounded by a rough " fence " of string and sticks brought by the team for the purpose. It is usually better to set up the laboratory station, where blood samples are taken, in an enclosed room so as not to frighten children waiting their turn.

Problems of modesty arise in connexion with the clinical examination and anthropometric measurement of adults or older children. As already noted, weighing is best carried out with subjects lightly clothed or nude, but since this is not usually possible, adults may have to be weighed in their clothes, subject to an appropriate adjustment.

Clinical examinations of entire populations can be carried out either by setting up one station for men and older boys and another separate one for girls, women and their young children, or by making a combined visit to a family group. In either case, examinations will have to be carried out in rooms or, in some parts of the world, in *ad hoc* screened-off areas of thatch or palm-leaf. Of these two methods, the visit to the family group is often preferable, as the family composition can be observed and only one station is required, making for greater simplicity in the line of flow. Whichever is chosen, undressing rooms or screened-off areas are required. In the family-group examination, two to three rooms are needed in order to ensure a continuous flow.

Even where privacy has been arranged, the examination of the genitals for scrotal or vulval dermatosis may be resisted. A further problem will arise if urine samples are collected. Either separate urine-passing rooms or screened-off areas will be needed for each sex; collection may be attempted at the time the clinical examination is made.

The requisite number of stations and the line of flow will have been determined in the planning phase. The degree of simplicity of each station will depend upon its function and on the facilities available, and improvisation will clearly be called for. A certain amount of basic furniture will be necessary, such as four chairs (two for the team, one for the person to be examined, and one for the local assistant/interpreter) and one or more tables (e.g., a small table for the clinical examination and one or two large tables for laboratory specimens).

Stations should be so placed that they are in the actual line of flow. They should not be near enough to one another to cause possible confusion and noise, or too far apart to give rise to difficulties in directing people. Thirty metres normally represents a reasonable distance. It will probably be found advantageous to place the station at which most time has to be spent close to the start of the line of flow.

Example of lines of flow: community child health surveys in East Africa

As an example, the line of flow normally applied in the community child health surveys in East Africa will be described. These surveys are carried out on young children, so that questions of modesty do not enter into the clinical examinations, which can, if necessary, be undertaken in the open air.

Five stations are ordinarily employed, in the following sequence: (i) identification; (ii) anthropometry; (iii) clinical assessment; (iv) laboratory specimens; (v) dietary inquiry.

(i) *Identification station*

At the first station, a survey form is issued to each person on which is listed the survey date and number, the person's name (and, if this is not culturally specific, other data, such as " child of "), sex, age, group or tribe, religion, if relevant, and village, town or area.

This form has to be kept by the individual, or the child's mother, until the last station has been reached; it is then collected. It is most important to ensure that the data obtained at each station are consistent—i.e., that they refer to the same subjects. At each station the form must be checked before examination, in order to obviate any confusion with the numbering, which can occur very easily and, once it has developed, prove difficult or even impossible to sort out in a crowded rural survey.

The station can be manned by one team member, assisted by one or two clerks who have been shown the routine but who will need to be supervised closely if errors in numbering are to be prevented. A local policeman or other responsible person can sometimes be persuaded to control the flow of persons so that they present themselves one at a time. A local schoolboy or other volunteer can carefully direct the person to the next station after the form has been completed.

If it has proved difficult to make an accurate age-assessment, this may be attempted by means of an " events calendar " (Table 3, p. 60) at the first station, in which case an additional team member familiar with the local language will be required. Alternatively, the assessment may be made later

—on a sample of the persons seen—either at a separate station, or in conjunction with the dietary inquiry station.

If some of the team members do not speak the local language, those who do should be deployed where they will be most needed (e.g., age-assessment and dietary inquiry). In addition, where language problems exist, as many as possible of the local volunteer assistants should be bilingual.

(ii) *Anthropometry station*

At the second station, anthropometric measurements are carried out. Again, two local volunteers will be required, the one to direct the line of persons waiting, and the other to guide people to the next station.

Weighing machines and length-measuring apparatus should be set up on flat surfaces. A length-board for young children may be placed on a large table.

For the measurement of adults, two persons are needed: a team member to do the measuring and a trained clerk or assistant to record it. For young children, two more volunteer assistants are needed, to hold the child while the measurements, etc. are being taken. The results should be announced clearly, occasional checks being made to ensure that they have been correctly recorded. They are recorded in the appropriate spaces on the survey form.

In addition to anthropometric instruments, two tables (one small for the recorder, one large for the length-board) will be required, with 3 or 4 chairs.

(iii) *Clinical assessment station*

Again, two local volunteers are used, for controlling the queue and directing people to the next station.

Clinical assessment is carried out by one of the team physicians, who has at hand a list of the signs to be looked for. These will have been typed, in the order in which they are to be sought, on a piece of paper affixed to a sheet of cardboard and covered with cellophane. The examiner can then check through the list (e.g., oedema—negative; Bitot's spots—positive, etc.). Each sign and its result are read aloud by the physician and marked appropriately as positive or negative on the clinical assessment sheet (see Fig. 46) by a trained clerk or assistant, whose work must be continuously scrutinized.

The person being examined should be in a good light and wearing as few clothes as possible. In the case of adults and school-age children, this will usually consist of shorts or drawers; young children should be examined naked. An approximately head-to-toe sequence of inspection is best followed, with palpation (e.g., liver, spleen, muscle wasting, pre-tibial oedema, etc.) done after this. Auscultation is not usually needed, and, in any case, it is difficult to hear sounds such as cardiac murmurs in the noise attending most surveys. However, the physician should wear a stethoscope in case it is needed for a particular sick person who may be discovered—for example, a child with respiratory tract infection, and also as a token that the team is a genuine medical one, with a doctor present to examine and treat the sick.

Whilst most signs should be reported as " positive " or " negative ", and the recording of grades of positivity is not recommended, certain signs may sometimes be given some qualitative definition. For example, in the East African child health surveys the shade of dyspigmentation of the hair is stated, e.g., RB = red brown.

In addition, unexpected findings may be briefly noted in the space reserved for this purpose. The clinical assessor should also carry a small notebook for the recording of his observations.

In the case of young children, the state of eruption of the teeth should be recorded according to correct dental convention (Fig. 32), as this may help in confirming the estimated age.

A minimum of equipment is needed. Apart from a stethoscope, only the check list of signs, pencils, one small table and three or four chairs are usually required. A pocket torch and a box of wooden tongue depressors should be at hand for the examination of the mouths of recalcitrant young children. It is useful to have a reference book, such as the present volume, available at the station, with descriptions and illustrations of clinical signs. It may also be helpful to have a chart of local hair colours at hand.

(iv) *Laboratory station*

At the fourth station, samples are taken for subsequent biochemical or other tests. It is at this station that cross-cultural clashes are most likely, as the taking of a " piece " of the body, especially blood, may be considered, in some rural groups, to be intended for an occult purpose, particularly if blood is taken by a woman wearing lipstick. However, misunderstanding may sometimes help, as in Haiti, where finger-prick blood collection for thick-film examination for malarial parasites was equated with a popular and highly successful penicillin anti-yaws campaign that had been carried out in preceding years (Jelliffe & Jelliffe, 1961).

It will be found expedient in the first place to examine, and take samples from, the local dignitaries—in Africa, the chief's family—and educated people, such as the schoolteacher, both as a matter of courtesy (especially as they will usually be helping the survey team) and as an example. Should any of the procedures prove unacceptable, especially the collection of blood samples, they may have to be deleted and the programme modified. The taking of venous samples from young children cannot be recommended, for the insertion of a needle into the jugular vein in the neck or the femoral vein in the groin, though safe, routine procedure in hospital practice, is understandably alarming to rural mothers.

The taking of samples for laboratory tests should, wherever possible, be carried out in the privacy of a room, partly to allay the fear of waiting children and parents. A sweet or a lump of sugar should be given to each child at the end; otherwise the fear experienced is likely to be communicated to other children waiting in line and to intensify their anxiety and resistance.

Flies, which can rapidly ingest a blood sample from a slide may complicate the taking of specimens, as can wind-blown dust. Appropriate measures must be taken.

Whatever the number and type of samples taken, the collecting apparatus —needle or syringe and correct containers—must be at hand in the proper place on the table used in the field as a laboratory bench. Similarly, equipment for sealing or closing tubes or containers, items for labelling (e.g., grease-proof pencil, ball-point pen), and boxes or thermos flasks for specimens must be available in selected places.

The detailed routine for taking specimens cannot be discussed here. In fact, it is necessary for those carrying out the sampling to devise a routine based on time-and-motion studies carried out before leaving for the field. Minor differences in practical technique can mean an increase in efficiency, as judged by the fatigue of those engaged in collecting the samples and by the numbers that can be dealt with in a given period.

Each member of the laboratory group must know his detailed function and how to carry it out speedily, with economy of movements and a minimum of interference with his co-workers.

Ideally, two laboratory workers are needed, one to take the sample and the other to have the container ready and seal it, to label it and place it in the appropriate box or thermos flask, and to record the tests taken from the person, both on the survey sheet and in a record-book.

As noted earlier, blood samples from adults and older children are collected from venous blood with a Vacutainer (vacuum tube) with a disposable needle attached to a plastic tube or with a syringe, or from capillary blood by finger-prick. The latter technique is the only one for young children in field circumstances. A heel-prick is found to be more suitable by some workers.

Stool samples may be brought in by families in containers that have been distributed at least the day before. With illiterate groups there is the difficulty that the containers cannot be labelled in advance by the survey team or by educated local volunteer assistants, nor can they be labelled by the subjects themselves. There may thus be confusion in identifying the samples.

There may also be a lack of co-operation, so that few stool samples are brought in. This may be due to misapprehension, suspicion of witchcraft, distaste for the task, or a cultural prohibition on contact with excreta. On receipt, the stool samples must be correctly labelled, and without delay—in any event on the same day—stool preservative (10% formol saline, MIF, etc.) can be added, if only a small specimen has been brought. If too large a sample has been submitted, a small portion will have to be transferred to another container and preservative added. Plainly, it is better merely to add preservative to the initial sample. For this, a small specimen of stool the size of a pea or other locally known object of similar size should be requested in clear terms.

For young children, a stool sample is best obtained by means of the anal-tube technique. This is not advisable in the case of infants, especially in the first six months of life, as the stool is too liquid or semi-solid. In pre-school-age children, a practised operator can obtain samples from about 75% of the children. The disadvantage of the method is that the sample is very small. After removal of the tube from the anus, the core of stool is poked out of the tube with a wooden applicator into a small flat-bottomed screw-capped vial, containing 1 ml of 10% formol saline.

Urine sampling is always difficult. As noted earlier, random samples may be collected from adults in the privacy of the clinical assessment. special rooms may be set aside, or an available latrine used for the purpose, For young children, special collection techniques may be employed, particularly for males, but they are very difficult to apply at a crowded survey site; alternatively, mothers may be asked to " catch " a specimen in a plastic jar supplied to them at the survey site. Fasting samples of urine are usually impossible to guarantee with any certainty.

The laboratory samples taken from each subject can be checked on the survey form by means of ticks at the side of the appropriate space. The laboratory results can be filled in later when they are available.

Apart from the two laboratory workers and the two local volunteers for directing and controlling the flow, a further local assistant, preferably bilingual, will often be required for explaining, reassuring and, in the case of frightened young children, assisting the mother to restrain the struggles of her child.

One or two large tables will be required, together with a minimum of four chairs. A plastic basin, soap, towels and, if necessary, a light plastic jerry-can of water should be brought by the team to the station.

(v) *Dietary inquiry station*

In the East African child health surveys, the last station deals with the questioning of mothers about the diets of their young children. This has to be done by a relatively senior team member, fluent in the local language and preferably belonging to the same community.

As the task calls for unhurried care, not all the mothers can be questioned, and some system of statistical sampling has to be adopted. A suitable form for this rapid dietary inquiry will be required, and will have to be based on some background knowledge of local foods and cooking practices. It is useful to have a range of local measures and utensils at hand—spoons, cups, bottles and gourds—to help the mothers to reply accurately.

Mothers should be asked solely about their children's present diet, without reference to the dietary progress in the past. Direct questions should be avoided. Replies are likely to be approximate and inaccurate, and the item that can be verified by observation at the survey site, at least in some traditional societies, is whether the child is still breast-fed or not.

In addition, at this station drugs are issued according to the written instructions of the physician at the clinical assessment station. The survey form is collected from each person and placed in a large envelope.

The staff for this station will consist of one team member and a junior medically-trained assistant to dispense drugs and give other treatment. Both will have to speak the local language. One local volunteer assistant will be required to direct the flow. Apart from dietary inquiry forms and medicines, one or two small tables will be required and three chairs.

Rapid ecological visits

Concurrently with the prevalence survey, rapid ecological visits will be carried out, and information obtained from local hospitals and health centres, and from collection points for vital statistics.

General remarks

It is evident that the stations and line of flow will vary in detail from one survey to another. In planning the line of flow, it should be borne in mind that the activities at certain stations (e.g., collection of laboratory samples; dietary inquiry) take much longer than at others (e.g., clinical assessment). The time required at each station should be tested in advance of the survey. A selective system may have to be introduced, whereby only a proportion (e.g., 20%) of those attending go to the stations at which the examinations, etc. are protracted.

The question of operator fatigue is of importance. Where practicable, team members should have rest periods or, if qualified to do so, move from one station to another.

Public relations

Adequate preliminary explanations to the local authorities and leaders, the provision of medicine for the sick, a sympathetic and friendly approach, and—not least—the unusual " circus " appeal of the team's visit to rural areas are normally sufficient to ensure attendance.

Nevertheless, cross-cultural problems may arise, as, for example, among the San Blas Indians of Panama who consider disease to be due to " soul abduction ", with the result that a survey based on modern concepts was neither easily acceptable nor relevant (Jelliffe et al., 1961b).

Regard must, of course, be had to local conventions and customs in the matter of social salutations and greetings, behaviour during home visits, and the choice of clothing. The families of local leaders and dignitaries should be the first to be examined, both as a matter of courtesy and as a means of inducing wavering members of the community to follow their example. Luncheon should be arranged for some of the local volunteer assistants, and possibly for the local leader also, at which the organization of the survey could be discussed, and queries about local customs raised in a discreet and friendly manner.

Finally, on completion of a survey, an abridged report drafted in general terms should be sent to the local authorities (subject to the concurrence of the central authority concerned). The customary letters of thanks will, of course, go to all who have assisted.

Daily programme

The day's programme obviously should start as early as possible. The hour chosen will depend upon the distance of the collecting point from the team's quarters and the time needed for the population to travel, often on foot, to the survey site. The local leaders should be consulted.

In the evening, the laboratory workers must ensure that samples are packed or, if necessary, stored in a refrigerator, as well as attend to other work that has to be done in the field, such as staining thick blood films with Giemsa and checking the next day's supplies.

Finally, the whole team should meet to exchange impressions, discuss problems and decide upon any necessary changes in procedure. A member of the team should be detailed to make the day's entry in a survey log book or field diary: this should list the place visited, the number seen by age-group and by examination (e.g., clinical, laboratory tests), the names of the principal persons met, the number of houses visited by the rapid ecological visit group, general impressions and organizational problems. Cultural practices observed may also be discussed and a précis included in the field diary.

ANALYSIS, INTERPRETATION AND ACTION

The purpose of this phase of survey work is to determine, through analysis of the data obtained, whether or not the nutritional status of the community is satisfactory. The analysis of the facts gathered is followed by their collective interpretation in relation to the local ecology.

Forms of malnutrition of local importance as public health problems can then be defined, together with the probable causative factors. Finally, plans for remedial action must be suggested. The data and the conclusions drawn therefrom must be presented logically and clearly to ensure the understanding, co-operation and support of the administration.

The present section deals with broad principles. The problem of expressing results for certain special groups (e.g., young children) will be considered.

Analysis

Analysis of the data will be easier if the forms have been prepared with the assistance of a statistician.

Some results can be worked out by hand, in particular the simpler data such as the percentage of a population with a given physical sign. This is, however, time-consuming, even with the aid of logarithm tables, slide-rule or calculating machine. There is also the risk of mathematical error.

If punch-edge cards of the Cope-Chat or McBee type are used, findings will be recorded in the field in the centre of the card. Later, positive findings can be marked on the same card by slotting the suitably numbered edge-holes, and then sorted by hand with a special knitting-needle.

Where practicable, data may be transferred from the survey forms to punch-cards of the IBM, ICT or similar type. The task is greatly facilitated if the survey forms bear the punch-card code numbers, against each item recorded, when the punching operation can be carried out with no intermediate step. Sorting and analysis can then be done by an electrical counter-sorter.

If a very detailed analysis is required, including, for example, multiple correlations, data on IBM or ICT cards can be used for analysis by a digital computer. While the actual analysis of data is extremely fast, highly specialized programming is required before it can be carried out. This is likely to be time-consuming, especially as many computers have only one programmer dealing with a flow of projects of many types.

If mechanical sorting, with either an electric counter-sorter or an electronic computer, is the process chosen, the programme must be planned in advance with the machine operators.

Grouping of results. The data may be analysed for the whole population, if desired; they should, however, be grouped in various ways according to the local circumstances. Results may be analysed by age-group, sex, socio-economic standing, ethnic group, religion or other classification.

Age considerations

There are four principal problems with regard to age in the analysis of survey data:

(*a*) *Age estimation.* The difficulties with regard to estimating age, especially of children in developing countries, have been discussed on page 58.

(*b*) *Age standards.* The need for anthropometric standards appropriate to the stage of life is self-evident. What is less appreciated is that different biochemical and haematological standards are also needed. In some cases, these are not available : adult standards may have to be used tentatively. As some of the standards given cover age intervals that are longer than those required in practice, interpolation will be necessary for the intermediate age-levels—for example, an assessment of the significance of the triceps skin-fold of a 5-month infant will be based on interpolation between the standards for a 3-month infant and those for a 6-month infant (Annex 1, Table (5)).

(c) *Age abbreviation.* If ages are grouped broadly, the question of method of " age abbreviation " has to be considered. It is suggested that this should be to the nearest unit, e.g., 12 years and 5 months should be recorded as 12 years, and 4 years and 9 months as 5 years. Ages at the half-way point should be recorded to the next higher unit (e.g., 7 years and 6 months should be recorded as 8 years).

(d) *Age-groups.* Certain well-recognized, broad age-groups can be used: infants (birth to 11 months); pre-school-age children (1-4 years; 12-59 months); school-age children (5-15 years); young adults, 16-35 years; adults, 36-55 years, old adults over 55 years. The term " young children " is used in the present work as a convenient, if approximate, term to include both infants and pre-school-age children.

Results in children are often given—depending upon the investigation— in 3-month age-groups for the first year of life, in six-month or yearly groups for children of 1-5 years, and in yearly groups for school-children.

Within these groups, the degree of differentiation by smaller age intervals depends on the type of examination, the standards available for comparison and the need to pin-point the age-incidence of a given type of malnutrition. For example, for the identification of infantile beriberi as a public health problem, mortality in the first year of life, if recorded with sufficient accuracy, may be broken down into monthly intervals in order to assess the number of deaths occurring in the characteristic 2-5 month period. Similarly, it is most valuable to consider the first years of life year by year, and to view the second year of life (12-23 months) in isolation with regard to clinical signs and anthropometric measurements in protein-calorie malnutrition, as this is usually the main danger period for this condition.

Expression of results

Data from nutritional surveys are largely concerned with the prevalence of certain clinical signs, or with the results of biochemical tests or anthropometric measurements, both of which are expressed as figures. Special attention is given later to the problem of the presentation of data for protein-calorie malnutrition (page 198).

Clinical signs

The positive clinical signs found should be reported initially as " percentage of positives " for each sign in the total population examined, and in each broad age-group, e.g., infants, pre-school-age children, school-age children and adults. A further break-down of results into smaller age-groups and by sex will often be required, especially for adults, because the cumulative strain of continuous reproduction often results in severe malnutrition in women.

As noted earlier, no diagnostic conclusion can usually be drawn from the high prevalence of a single sign. However, in order to assist interpretation, positive signs may be considered together in two ways. First, the positive signs present should be listed together in accordance with the grouping of signs suggestive of various deficiencies (see page 43). Secondly, the percentages of the total population, or of specific age-groups, which show combinations of three or more suggestive signs listed in the different groups should be calculated. Thus, the pre-school-age segment of a population surveyed might be found to have 23% positive with a combination of three or more signs regarded as suggestive of protein-calorie malnutrition of early childhood (see page 43).

Nutritional anthropometry

Results from nutritional anthropometrical measurements should be reported in two ways: (*a*) mathematically; and (*b*) in relation to standards of reference.

(*a*) *Mathematical reporting.* Measurements in figures should always be given for each relevant age-group and sex as the mean plus or minus twice the standard deviation ($\pm$ 2 S.D.).[1] These mathematical figures are required in order to ensure an understanding of the results by other workers, and, if need be, to permit further interpretation (including construction of percentile levels), and analysis or comparison of the findings to be made in the future.

The reporting of results in relation to percentiles of the standards is not recommended because this mathematically correct procedure is not easily understood by junior health personnel or administrators, while in less-well-fed communities a high proportion will fall without differentiation into the " below 3rd percentile " level.

(*b*) *Reporting in relation to standards of reference.* Anthropometric measurements must also be expressed in terms of standards of reference. As noted earlier, it is recommended that each measurement be compared with two standards—a general standard of reference and a local standard of reference.

If no local standards are available, comparison can be made only with the general standard. The advantages and problems of using this somewhat

---

[1] Falkner (1962a) gives an excellent simplified account of mathematical considerations of anthropometry.

arbitrary yardstick are discussed on page 56. Sometimes a regional standard—from a near-by country with a population of similar genetic composition—may be available in place of a strictly local standard.

With the exception of the problem of obesity in more privileged parts of the world, the anthropometric assessment of malnutrition in the community is concerned exclusively with enumerating those who fall in varying degrees below the standard measurements.

The method of expressing the degree of inadequacy has to be easily understandable to junior staff and simple to calculate. It must also permit of easy comparability between one group and another, while, at the same time, precluding the drawing of unduly broad conclusions.

For these reasons, it is suggested that anthropometric measurements in community prevalence surveys should be reported in relation to 10% categories below the standard. Suggested general standards of reference[1] in metric measurements are set out in the 19 tables in Annex 1.

By the use of the appropriate table, the percentage below standard can be read off, and results for a community expressed as percentages in the suggested 10% categories.

For example, in a community survey the weight for age of pre-school-age children might be found to be distributed as follows:

over 90% standard 30%
90-81% standard 35%
80-71% standard 20%
70-61% standard 10%
60% standard and below 5%

This type of classification has one obvious disadvantage. It does not record the normal range of distribution of anthropometric measurements, and will therefore include some non-malnourished but genetically small persons in the lesser degrees below the standard. Nevertheless, it is simple, practical and easily understood, and it is recommended that the anthropometric results of field surveys of communities should be expressed both mathematically and in this manner, in relation to the general standards of reference given and to the local standards of references, where such exist.

Biochemical tests

The results of biochemical tests should be presented for the total population investigated, if appropriate, and also broken down into the main age-groups and for both sexes, especially for adults.

---

[1] The general standards of reference have been derived from the following sources:
   Young children : Harvard Standards (Stuart & Stevenson, 1959), except for triceps skin-fold (Hammond, 1955a), arm circumference (N. Wolanski—personal communication, 1964), and weight-for-height figures (Stuart & Stevenson, 1959);
   School-age children : Baldwin-Wood Standards (Baldwin & Wood, 1923), except for triceps fat (Hammond, 1955b) and arm circumference (O'Brien, Girshik & Hunt, 1941);
   Adults : Actuaries Standards (Society of Actuaries, 1959), except for triceps fat (Brozek, 1956) and arm circumference (Hertzberg et al., 1963; O'Brien & Shelton, 1941).

The results should be expressed mathematically as the mean plus or minus twice the standard deviation. In addition, they should be presented as percentages falling into different ranges of values. These may be given tentative labels (e.g., " low ", " deficient "). However, with the exception of a low haemoglobin, the labels given must be interpreted with extreme care in view of the inadequate state of knowledge concerning possible variability in different ecological circumstances, especially in relation to prolonged adaptation to dietary patterns. Suggested guides to the interpretation of biochemical and haematological findings are given elsewhere.

Dietary assessment

Where detailed food-consumption studies have been carried out, Reh (1962) recommends that the results should be given as the difference for the group between observed consumption and the suggested allowances for all nutrients, expressed as percentages. She advises against the labelling of groups as " undernourished " or " malnourished " in respect of one or more nutrients on the basis of food-consumption studies alone.

If outline information has been obtained by means of a questionnaire and observation during rapid ecological visits, the results can be expressed as percentages of persons or families stating that they eat certain foods. In young children, analysis can often be made in three-month groups for the first year (e.g., birth to 3 months; 4 to 6 months, etc.), and in six-monthly periods thereafter. In all cases, it must be stressed that this information is at best only qualitative, giving an extremely approximate outline of the general dietary pattern.

Other ecological data

Similarly, other information concerning the ecological background, including conditioning infections, cultural influences, socio-economic factors and food production, gathered by means of observation and questionnaire, can be expressed as percentages of families or people in different age-groups having certain characteristics. Again, the superficial and approximate nature of findings obtained in this way must be stressed.

Results with regard to malaria (e.g., parasite and spleen indices) permit the degree of endemicity to be expressed.

Interpretation

Nutritional surveys—both prevalence and incidence studies—are epidemiological investigations into the nutritional status of a population by various direct and indirect methods, together with an evaluation of the determinant ecological factors in the environment.

They are attempts to make a community diagnosis, and, as with the diagnosis of illness in an individual, information obtained by several

12

methods is usually required. Thus, while in clinical medicine a diagnosis may very occasionally be made on the basis of one pathognomonic sign, such as the rash in herpes zoster, more usually information obtained by several means is required, including the history, clinical examination, radiology, biochemical and haematological tests.

Similarly, the diagnosis of certain limited types of malnutrition in the community can occasionally be strongly suggested on the basis of one clinical sign only, as with iodine deficiency and goitre, or of one test as with a low haemoglobin and iron deficiency. Yet, even with these examples the possibility of factors other than nutritional deficiency, including goitrogenic substances in the diet and malaria (respectively), has to be considered. Moreover, at times, advanced syndromes of a particular deficiency may be readily identifiable, such as kwashiorkor and nutritional parasmus, but give no idea of the prevalence of more common, less advanced forms of protein-calorie malnutrition of early childhood.

All the methods that can be used for the assessment of the nutritional status of a community are individually imperfect, inaccurate and subject to their own technical errors. It is therefore particularly important to avoid drawing sweeping conclusions based on limited evidence. The literature is full of examples of the unwarranted use of survey results.

The assessment of the nutritional status of a community must, then, be based on a thoughtful consideration of all available findings and information (Table 17).

Although valuable information can certainly be obtained with less than the complete range of methods, which usually cannot be applied on many small-scale prevalence surveys, the probability of obtaining a valid picture of the nutritional condition of the community in its widest sense increases if various approaches can be employed in conjunction. The different methods are aimed at assessing quite diverse aspects of human nutrition, ranging from food production to cellular metabolism. Not only do they permit of a wider understanding of the causes and effects of malnutrition in the area, but the results obtained by the different methods can be used collectively to confirm or diminish the probability of a particular deficiency's being present in the community (Krehl & Hodges, 1965).

The evaluation of the combined information gathered from the various methods of assessment should be aimed at delineating, as thoroughly as the complexity of the survey warrants, the following:

(a) the principal deficiency diseases in the community in different age-groups, and their priority;

(b) the probable causative factors.

In the more usual short-term cross-sectional surveys with which this monograph is principally concerned, prevalence figures will be obtained, together with approximate incidence data at hospitals and health centres,

TABLE 17. INFORMATION USEFUL FOR ASSESSMENT OF NUTRITIONAL STATUS *

Sources of information	Nature of information obtained	Nutritional implications
(1) Agricultural data Food balance sheets	Gross estimates of agricultural production Agricultural methods Soil fertility Predominance of cash crops Overproduction of staples Food imports and exports	Approximate availability of food supplies to a population
(2) Socio-economic data Information on marketing, distribution and storage	Purchasing power Distribution and storage of foodstuffs	Unequal distribution of available foods between the socio-economic groups in the community and within the family
(3) Food consumption patterns Cultural-anthropological data	Lack of knowledge, erroneous beliefs and prejudices, indifference	
(4) Dietary surveys	Food consumption Distribution within the family	Low, excessive or unbalanced nutrient intake
(5) Special studies on foods	Biological value of diets Presence of interfering factors (e.g., goitrogens) Effects of food processing	Special problems related to nutrient utilization
(6) Vital and health statistics	Morbidity and mortality data	Extent of risk to community Identification of high-risk groups
(7) Anthropometric studies	Physical development	Effect of nutrition on physical development
(8) Clinical nutritional surveys	Physical signs	Deviation from health due to malnutrition
(9) Biochemical studies	Levels of nutrients, metabolites and other components of body tissues and fluids	Nutrient supplies in the body Impairment of biochemical function
(10) Additional medical information	Prevalent disease patterns, including infections and infestations	Interrelationships of state of nutrition and disease

* Adapted from WHO Expert Committee on Medical Assessment of Nutritional Status (1963).

while long-term studies will reveal the incidence in the community itself.

Statistical guidance will be needed for the assessment of the findings. At the same time, it is salutary to note the comment of Gordon (1963): " Modern methods of machine tabulation, computer analysis and statistical manipulation have obvious value in dealing with long-term projects with many data, but the interpretation of results remains rooted in the value judgements of workers in the field."

Presentation

The presentation of data may often be organized at two levels. First, in order to speed up any action that may be considered necessary, a short, lucid typewritten synopsis of the main findings should be sent as soon as possible to the appropriate authorities in the country. The analysis of data always takes time, and, if a preliminary report is not presented, further extensive delays will occur before the final draft, with tables, graphs, etc., is ready, and one or two years may pass before the report is finally published and reprints made available.

Secondly, a fuller and more detailed report of the survey is needed, whether published or not. This main report should be clear and logically developed, with figures for the most part kept out of the text and incorporated in tables, graphs or histograms. It should be as detailed as possible, although editorial policy usually insists on limiting the text to the essentials.

Obviously, the method of presentation will vary with the purpose and scope of the survey, with the object and range of the report, and with individual preference regarding style and emphasis.

In general, however, the report should contain the sections described in the following paragraphs.

Background data

These will comprise a brief account of the area, often illustrated with a map, containing information about the particular community, including its culture pattern and ethnic groups, the geography and climate, including communications, the social development, including level of education, schools, information on economic status, food production, including processing and storage, health facilities and demographic data, including the population and its age and geographical distribution, and morbidity and mortality statistics.

Purpose of survey

A general definition of the purpose of the survey is required, perhaps with an explanation of the reasons for carrying out the particular study in the area.

Methods employed

This section will contain a description of sampling procedures, practical methods used in field work, including pilot projects, and the details of the techniques employed in the clinical assessment, including definitions of signs looked for and control of observer error, in the biochemical estimations (with references to the published accounts of the techniques), in the anthropometric measurements, including the instruments used, in the dietary investigations, including food-composition tables used, in the assessment of ecological factors, and in the gathering of information concerning local health statistics. Copies of questionnaires used should be attached.

Results

These are usually best presented in tabular form under the heading of the particular method of assessment (clinical, biochemical, etc.) broken down by broad age-groups and by sex, where necessary.

The tables showing the results of the clinical examination should show the numbers examined and the percentages positive with different signs. These can be more meaningfully presented in the "groupings of signs" suggestive of various deficiencies given earlier. If necessary, a separate table may be required for a presentation of three or more suggestive signs in combination.

Both biochemical and anthropometric results are shown in figures (e.g., units, grams, centimetres). These can be presented in a table giving the numbers examined and the mean (average) result plus or minus twice the standard deviation ($\pm$ 2 S.D.) for each group.

The biochemical findings should also be given as percentages falling within certain specified levels. Thus, with haemoglobin findings in pregnant women, where the standard is 10 g/100 ml, levels should be given as: 10 g to 8 g, 17%; 8 g to 6 g, 21%; etc., or if space permits, presented as a histogram. Sometimes it may be feasible to show biochemical findings that fall below the standard of reference in tentatively labelled groups, e.g., "low", "deficient". The uncertainty regarding the universal correctness of these labels is emphasized by the inverted commas.

Anthropometric measurements should also be expressed in a simple, understandable way by means of percentages of the population examined that fall in various 10% levels below the standard of reference, e.g., 90%–81%; 80%–71%; 70%–61%; 60% and below. As suggested earlier, presentation should, if possible, be given in relation to two yardsticks—the general standards of reference and the local standards of reference. To emphasize the differences between the results obtained and the standards, graphic presentation, though not essential, may be helpful.

Data on ecological factors may be presented in tables. Much of the information is, however, semi-qualitative and can be given descriptively.

Photographic illustrations in the report may be of value in describing various ecological circumstances, showing examples of the types of malnutrition, and illustrating techniques and methods. Their reproduction is, however, costly, and they take up considerable space. Perhaps the main value of a limited number of photographs is in supplementing the descriptive account of the local people and their way of life, and ensuring that the reader receives a clear impression of the subjects and the site of the survey.

Discussion

(*a*) *Correlation of evidence.* Essentially, this will be concerned with a consideration of the positive findings and the collective evidence they provide of the presence of different types of malnutrition in the several age-groups in the community. At times it may prove impossible to attempt anything beyond a forecast requiring fuller investigation—for example, therapeutic trials or additional biochemical tests.

(*b*) *Ecological diagnosis.* The deductions must be correlated with the ecological factors that appear to be etiologically relevant in the particular region. From the analysis of all the data available, suggestions can be made for future action.

(*c*) *Recommendations for future action.* The aim of public-health investigations is to improve the health of the public. They should not become mere academic exercises undertaken in a spirit of scientific curiosity. Responsible officials and administrators should therefore be associated with the investigations at an early stage, and a summary of findings, interpretations and suggestions should be sent to them without delay.

Action

Follow-up surveys may be necessary to note the development of certain nutritional trends (e.g., in infant feeding or in an apparent increasing incidence of some form of malnutrition) or to assess the effects of recommended preventive measures.

Apart from follow-up surveys, further investigation may occasionally be desirable in order to clarify some of the results obtained. Therapeutic trials or more detailed and specific biochemical tests on selected groups may be indicated. The etiological factors may have to be identified with greater precision, or the value of the preventive measures investigated scientifically.

Specific recommendations for action must be realistic in terms of needs, cultural, social and economic considerations, existing and potential resources and health and educational services. They should be clearly set forth in strict order of priority. Thus, the prevention of doubtful subclinical deficiencies should not receive undue emphasis if severe forms of malnutrition with a high incidence and mortality are common in some age-groups; it is obviously incorrect to give prominence to a recommendation for an expensive and difficult campaign to iodize salt in a rural tropical community where goitre is moderately prevalent as a largely cosmetic clinical entity, when a high percentage of pre-school-age children in the same region are dying of kwashiorkor.

Obviously, the range of recommendations may vary widely. They should be aimed at the most important potentially preventable etiological factors responsible for the particular forms of malnutrition. Detailed study of possible recommendations is beyond the scope of the present monograph, but the following are likely to merit consideration: improvement of health services, especially for mothers and children; agricultural improvements, including increased production of protein foods, storage, processing, distribution and marketing; health education (MCH services, schools, etc.); legislation, including fortification of foods, rationing and minimum wage-levels; supplementary food programmes for young children, pregnant and lactating mothers, and schoolchildren; and the prevention of infective diseases, through immunization, improved water-supply, anti-malaria measures, etc.

6 Special Problems in Different Groups

YOUNG CHILDREN

In developing regions of the world malnutrition makes its principal impact on young children. These children are at a stage of life when growth is rapid, nutrient requirements are high, and the diets likely to be given are inadequate, because of poverty, lack of suitable foods, parental ignorance or fallacies in the form of food prejudices and restrictive taboos. It is also a period of continuous stress from bacterial, viral and parasitic infections.

Malnutrition in Early Childhood

Although there is no precise dividing-point, it is helpful to consider the types of malnutrition seen in young children in developing countries in the two usual age-groups—infants and pre-school-age children (1-4 years).

Infants

The nutritional status of children in the first year of life depends on the local methods of infant feeding and, through the foetal stores, on the maternal diet in pregnancy and on the mother's own nutritional status. However, the principal practical determinant is often whether the baby is breast-fed, as is traditional, or whether, as is increasingly the case in urban areas, attempts are made to feed it artificially.

Breast-fed infants

While it is difficult to generalize, the nutritional status of the breast-fed baby is usually excellent in the first 5-6 months. Growth is well sustained as sufficient protein, calories and vitamins are supplied by breast-milk. The only common exception to this is infantile beriberi, which usually occurs in exclusively breast-fed babies of mothers in areas of Asia where diets are largely composed of thiamine-deficient polished rice, the peak incidence being at 2-5 months of age (Aykroyd & Krishnan, 1941). It is essentially maternal malnutrition " transmitted " to the suckling by the mother's thiamine-deficient breast-milk. The condition is difficult to diagnose before the full clinical picture has developed, since the mother may appear healthy and the infant well-nourished, as judged by weight and development of muscle and subcutaneous fat. Neither incidence nor prevalence of the condition can be ascertained by survey methods. It can be gauged approximately by the age-specific 2-5 month mortality rate (if such can be obtained), or by hospital data concerning acute cases of infantile beriberi responding dramatically to parenteral thiamine.

Generally, in traditional rural circumstances in developing tropical regions, infants in the second half of the first year of life will continue to be breast-fed, usually with inadequate supplements of largely carbohydrate gruels or pastes. Severe malnutrition is usually not seen at this stage, although avitaminosis A (as with keratomalacia in Indonesia), or early rickets (as in Ethiopia) may occur, where for dietary and social reasons these forms of malnutrition are prevalent.

More commonly, the second semester of infancy is characterized only by an inadequate weight gain, as shown by a somewhat flattened growth curve, and sometimes by a degree of iron-deficiency anaemia.

Artificially fed infants

At the present time, there is a world-wide trend towards urbanization, partly planned, but largely haphazard. Among these new townspeople, there is an increasing decline in breast-feeding, partly because mothers have to seek employment in jobs where breast-feeding is no longer culturally acceptable, and, to an increasing extent, because of the unfortunate influence of advertised infant foods and the example of socio-economic " superiors ".

For the majority of families in tropical regions, artificial bottle-feeding is not practical—economically, educationally or hygienically.

Specially imported animal milks and processed products designed for babies are too expensive for parents to be able to buy in sufficient amounts, so that token, homeopathic doses are normally used. Mothers ordinarily have not had sufficient education to follow the necessary routine of preparation, dilution and protection from contamination. Lastly, conditions in the home with regard to supplies of water and fuel, kitchen facilities, and the means for storage protected from insects and dust make the preparation of uncontaminated feeds an impossibility.

In these circumstances, the majority of non-breast-fed infants reared artificially on the bottle receive very dilute, highly infective feeds, resulting in most cases in protein-calorie malnutrit on, sometimes associated with infective diarrhoea, and often leading to death.

The type of resulting malnutrition depends on the artificial feeds the child has received. Usually, this will be over-diluted milk, supplying wholly inadequate protein and calories. Infective diarrhoea occurs frequently, and ultimately nutritional marasmus develops.

If the baby is fed on liquid, largely carbohydrate preparations, instead of diluted animal milk, and avoids severe diarrhoea, infantile kwashiorkor is likely. This situation has already developed in Trinidad, where poorer, less educated mothers may use a gruel of arrowroot starch as the sole food, so that the peak incidence of kwashiorkor is found to be at 5 to 7 months of age (Jelliffe, Symonds & Jelliffe, 1960). A lowering of the age-incidence of kwashiorkor is also found, though in lesser degree, in many areas of developing countries in the process of urbanization.

Furthermore, because of the increasing use of prepared animal-milk products, certain vitamin deficiencies may be expected to occur more frequently. A rise in the incidence of infantile scurvy is likely, whereas, at present, this condition is rare among breast-fed, traditionally reared infants, who receive adequate ascorbic acid through breast-milk.

If, as is probable, cheaper milk preparations will often be used, including skim-milk in powdered or condensed form, severe avitaminosis A, including keratomalacia, will occur more frequently and become a nutritional public-health problem of increasing importance.

Pre-school children (1-4 years)

This period of childhood, especially the second year of life, is notoriously fraught with risk. The young child is " transitional " as regards diet, immunity to infections and psychological dependence. This is a period of rapid growth with high nutrient needs, particularly of protein for swiftly increasing muscle tissue. It is a time when several meals a day are required and when foods should be easily masticable and digestible.

It is at this time also that the non-immune child comes in contact with a succession, or more often an accumulation, of bacterial, viral and parasitic infections. Lastly, it is often the occasion for the psychological trauma that occurs as a result of the sudden separation from the mother—after a prolonged period of continuous intimate contact and permissive breast-feeding—frequently caused by a further pregnancy.

Certain vitamin- and mineral-deficiency diseases occur with varying frequency in pre-school-age children in different parts of the world, including, for example, avitaminosis A, rickets and iron-deficiency anaemia. The incidence varies greatly from place to place, depending upon the local dietary and social factors. Thus, rickets in sunnier parts of the world may be related to lack of exposure to available ultraviolet light due to overcrowding in urban dwellings, as in old-style walled cities or in slums, or to a deliberate sheltering of young children from the sun for various cultural reasons, e.g., to prevent their acquiring a darker complexion or to escape the " evil eye ".

However, the principal forms of malnutrition seen during this transitional period are those now termed " protein-calorie malnutrition of early childhood ", including kwashiorkor. In one form or another, these are common in most developing countries, and represent the principal nutritional public-health problem in the world. Thus, in Haiti in 1960, it was found that 7 000 per 100 000 of the pre-school-age population in the country as a whole were suffering from kwashiorkor (Jelliffe & Jelliffe, 1960), while in Kampala, Uganda, 10% of admissions to the children's wards at Mulago Hospital demonstrated this advanced syndrome (Musoke, 1961), and more than 50% of those attending local child-welfare clinics showed clinical and anthropometric evidence suggestive of mild to moderate malnutrition of this type (Welbourn, 1954).

Owing to the important and wide prevalence of this type of malnutrition, the present section deals mainly with current views on nomenclature, etiology, clinical features and appropriate survey methods.

Protein-Calorie Malnutrition of Early Childhood

The nutritional status of young children as regards protein and calories may be viewed as an uninterrupted downward gradient running from " normal ", through mild and moderate degrees of malnutrition, to severe syndromes, including kwashiorkor and nutritional marasmus (Jelliffe, 1959).

Suggested terminology

The label " protein-calorie malnutrition of early childhood " (PCM) has been suggested as a generic term to cover the whole range of mild to severe, classifiable and unclassifiable manifestations, including the two main severe clinical syndromes of kwashiorkor and nutritional marasmus.

The reasons advanced in favour of this term are:

(*a*) It emphasizes that kwashiorkor is *not* the only clinical end-result associated with protein-shortage in young children. In fact, lesser manifestations of protein-calorie malnutrition are at all times far more frequent, while in some countries nutritional marasmus is the most common severe form (Graham & Morales, 1963; McLaren, Ammoun & Houri, 1964; Mönckeburg, 1966).

(*b*) It stresses the need for consideration of calorie intake as well as protein, not only in infant-feeding in tropical regions, but in the treatment of all syndromes, including kwashiorkor (Dean & Skinner, 1957).

(*c*) All the syndromes can be related to a diet low in protein, but with different levels of intake of calories in the form of largely carbohydrate foods.

(*d*) The term " early childhood " is appropriate, as the various syndromes may occur commonly from the early months of life up to late pre-school age.

The two major, severe syndromes of protein-calorie malnutrition of early childhood are kwashiorkor and nutritional marasmus, and any

FIG. 49. KWASHIORKOR, SHOWING OEDEMA, MISERY, WASTED MUSCLES WITH PRESENCE OF SUBCUTANEOUS FAT, FLAKY-PAINT RASH AND HAIR CHANGES

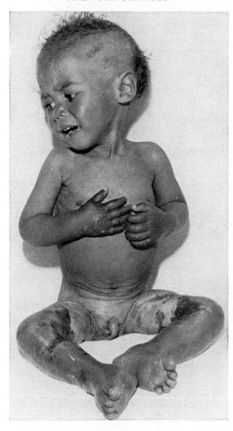

attempt to assess the signs found in less severely affected children will be based on a clear definition of the clinical picture in these advanced cases.

Kwashiorkor (Fig. 49)

Nomenclature

Williams (1933) introduced the socially descriptive West African word "kwashiorkor"[1] to scientific medical literature, but a variety of other terms have been used for this dramatic, severe malnutrition syndrome.

Some of these terms are listed below:

(*a*) Clinically descriptive: enfants rouges, culebrilla,[2] bouffissure d'Annam, syndrome dépigmentation oedème

(*b*) Pathologically descriptive: fatty liver disease

(*c*) Suggested nutritional etiology: dystrofia pluricarencial, syndrome pluricarencial (multiple-deficiency disease); mehlnährschaden (flour malnutrition), nutritional oedema syndrome, malignant malnutrition

(*d*) Vernacular name: *obwosi*[3] (in Luganda).

Terms previously used are listed in various publications (Trowell, Davis & Dean, 1954; Waterlow & Scrimshaw, 1957; De Silva, 1964), but today these are largely of historical interest, since, by unofficial international agreement, the term kwashiorkor is currently used almost universally for this particular extreme form of protein-calorie malnutrition of early childhood, even though there is disagreement about minimum diagnostic criteria.

---

[1] Meaning a disease occurring in a young child displaced from his mother by a subsequent pregnancy.

[2] "Snakeskin", referring to the flaky-paint rash sometimes found.

[3] As with many vernacular names for the condition in African languages, *obwosi* has the same meaning as kwashiorkor.

Etiology

Kwashiorkor can occur in infancy or in later childhood, and even, though rarely, in adult life. However, in classical circumstances, it has its main incidence in the second year of life. Thus, of 1141 cases analysed by Trowell, Davis & Dean (1954), 45% were between 1 and 2 years of age, and 69% between 1 and 3 years of age.

Kwashiorkor is never exclusively dietary in etiology. Infective, psychological, cultural and other conditioning factors, either singly or in combination, are also operative. Nevertheless, the principal cause is always a nutritional imbalance in early childhood, that is, a diet that is low in protein, but that contains carbohydrate calories. A similar syndrome can be produced experimentally by feeding a low-protein, mainly carbohydrate diet to piglets (Platt, 1958).

Descriptions of the clinical features of kwashiorkor have been much confused by workers in one country or region arbitrarily assuming that the clinical picture with which they are familiar is necessarily identical in detail in other parts of the world. Kwashiorkor is a variable syndrome with certain constant features. Details of the clinical picture will vary with the following factors:

(*a*) the degree of deficiency and the ratio of carbohydrate calories to protein intake;

(*b*) the velocity of onset;

(*c*) the age at which the patient is affected; [1]

(*d*) the duration;

(*e*) conditioning factors—e.g., infections, psychological trauma; and

(*f*) genetic characteristics—e.g., skin colour, type of hair.

Thus, the infantile kwashiorkor of Trinidad, with its peak incidence between 5 and 7 months of age, almost never shows hair changes and consistently has an enlarged liver (Jelliffe, Symonds & Jelliffe, 1960). This contrasts markedly with the usual classical textbook tropical African case (Trowell, Davis & Dean, 1954).

In addition, Gopalan (1961) has shown that in two parts of India the clinical picture of kwashiorkor varies. In Hyderabad, affected children are much lighter in weight than those observed in Coonoor, because of a lower-calorie staple food and because of a later introduction of semi-solids. Similarly, obese variants of kwashiorkor are well recognized in Jamaica, where they are known as " sugar-babies " (Waterlow, 1948; Jelliffe, Bras & Stuart, 1954).

---

[1] The importance of the age at which malnutrition occurs has been emphasized in experimental malnutrition by Widdowson & McCance (1963), who have shown that different species have their own vulnerable periods in so far as the potential for subsequent recovery is concerned.

Despite these variations of detail in different parts of the world, it seems justifiable to divide the clinical features of kwashiorkor into three categories: constant, usual, and occasional (Jelliffe & Dean, 1959).

Constant signs of kwashiorkor

There are four constant features in kwashiorkor, which, though normally accompanied by other signs, can be regarded as diagnostic if found in early childhood in regions where the diet in infancy is predominantly carbohydrate. These are oedema, growth failure, muscle wasting with retention of some subcutaneous fat, and psychomotor change.

(a) *Oedema.* This is the cardinal sign of kwashiorkor and the syndrome should not be diagnosed in its absence. It can be detected initially in the pretibial region by the production of a definite pit as a result of moderate pressure for three seconds with a finger or thumb over the lower end of the tibia.

In tropical circumstances, the oedema occurring in hookworm disease, which is associated with severe anaemia, or in beriberi, or in the nephrotic syndrome, when it is accompanied by a heavy albuminuria, may require differentiation. Particular difficulty may be encountered with hookworm disease, as it can itself be a conditioning factor in the development of kwashiorkor.

(b) *Growth retardation.* The growth retardation of kwashiorkor has been demonstrated in an analysis of certain anthropometric measurements of a large group of affected children admitted to the Infant Malnutrition Research Unit (IMRU), Kampala (Table 18). A low body weight (68% of the standard) and a low mid-arm circumference (77%) are the main abnormal features, with body length (91%) much less affected. The fact that weight is proportionally much more affected than length has also been shown by Sénécal & Aubry (1958), McFie & Welbourn (1962), and Moncada (1963).

The interpretation of weight in untreated kwashiorkor is complicated by the presence of oedema fluid and, especially in the so-called " sugar baby " variants in some parts of the world, by a relatively thick layer of subcutaneous fat. Also, as Dean (1960) has shown, in Kampala, the severity of kwashiorkor, as measured by the clinical picture or by the mortality rate, is not always proportional to the degree of weight loss, even if the weight is taken after oedema has subsided.

(c) *Muscle wasting with retention of some subcutaneous fat.* Muscle wasting is a constant feature of kwashiorkor, both clinically and at autopsy, and a reduction in the circumference of the upper arm is usually particularly evident. It is much less obscured by oedema than the forearm or leg, although minimal oedema may occasionally be detectable, especially over the dependent triceps. However, even when none can be found, there is a further decrease in arm circumference when body oedema subsides, indicating the constant presence of subclinical oedema and an increased water content of muscle and skin (Frenk et al., 1957). Nevertheless the mid-arm circumference has the advantage of being both simply measured and roughly circular.

This reduction in arm circumference has been confirmed as one of the main features of the syndrome by anthropometric measurements on a large series of children with kwashiorkor (Table 18). Clinical palpation suggests

TABLE 18. CERTAIN ANTHROPOMETRIC MEASUREMENTS IN CHILDREN WITH KWASHIORKOR, EXPRESSED AS PERCENTAGES OF LOCAL STANDARDS *

Measurement	Proportion of locally accepted standard value (%)
Weight	68
Arm circumference	77
Calf circumference	78
Length	91
Sitting height	92

* Data supplied by the Infant Malnutrition Research Unit, Kampala.

that it is principally due to muscle wasting, and this can be demonstrated both at autopsy and during life by surface measurements and radiology (Jelliffe & Jelliffe, 1960; McFie & Welbourn, 1962).

Muscle wasting can also be demonstrated functionally by testing the infant's ability to hold up his head when gently pulled from a lying to a sitting position (Smythe, 1958).

The relatively thick layer of subcutaneous fat can also be observed on both the body and the limbs. It can be palpated during clinical examination, and confirmed by using skin-fold calipers. Its presence in part reflects the child's calorie intake in the form of largely carbohydrate foods.

(d) Psychomotor change. The child with kwashiorkor is apathetic, miserable, inert, withdrawn and anorexic. His motor development is retarded and has usually regressed in recent weeks.

The causation of this psychomotor change is complex. In some cultures the psychological trauma due to the maternal withdrawal associated with " weaning " from the breast, sometimes including actual geographical separation from the mother, often plays a part. The possibility of bio-chemical change affecting the brain is suggested by changes in the electro-encephalogram (Nelson & Dean, 1959), while physical components include a lowered basal metabolic rate, and the weakness and hypotonicity due to severe muscle wasting.

Usual signs of kwashiorkor

Certain signs, though not necessary for diagnosis, are common and are usually present either singly or in any combination:

(*a*) *Hair changes.* Although varying greatly from one part of the world to another, some degree of hair abnormality is usually found, although kwashiorkor can occur with wholly normal hair. The hair changes may comprise lightening in colour (dyspigmentation), straightness (if the normal hair is curly, as in African children), silkiness, and loosely attached roots, as shown by sparseness and " easy pluckability ".

Of the hair changes, dyspigmentation, if present, can be the most striking. It appears to occur most readily in African children. It is absent in cases of acute onset and, conversely, most marked in chronic syndromes of gradual evolution, such as with some of the " sugar baby " cases in Jamaica.

Dyspigmentation of the hair can occur from non-nutritional environ-mental and genetic causes. In some regions it is not uncommonly found in children without kwashiorkor.

However, if genetic and environmental causes can be excluded, the correlation of dyspigmentation of the hair in pre-school children with a community diet, for this group, of largely carbohydrate, low-protein foods is suggested by (*a*) its absence in African children who are not protein-deficient (as among the Hadza hunters of Tanganyika) (Jelliffe et al., 1962b), as compared with the very high incidence among the children of the Baganda, whose diet is based on steamed plantain (Welbourn, 1954); (*b*) its maximal occurrence at age 1-3 years, when, in most tropical regions, the child's diet is low in protein and high in carbohydrate calories (Jelliffe, 1955a); and (*c*) the fact that African children in the Congo with dyspigmentation of the hair have been shown to have a lower weight curve, especially in the second year of life, than children with normal black hair (André & Hole-mans, 1955).

However, this subject calls for further investigation; its complexity is indicated by the range of abnormal hair colours that can be found in kwa-shiorkor—light brown, reddish-brown, blonde, etc.

(*b*) *Diffuse depigmentation of the skin.* Probably with the same patho-genesis as dyspigmented hair, and usually paralleling it, light-coloured skin is a common feature of kwashiorkor, although with the genetic range of coloration found in any population, it may be difficult to gauge with cer-tainty. It is most easily seen in darker pigmented groups, especially children of African descent, and, in the same way as dyspigmented hair, it is often most pronounced in chronic cases of gradual onset.

(c) *Moon-face.* The full, well-rounded, somewhat pendulous and blubbery cheeks, known as moon-face, are often present in kwashiorkor. The pathogenesis of moon-face is uncertain. It occurs particularly in obese variants of kwashiorkor, and is presumably the result of increased fat, with possibly some degree of oedema. However, in addition to its probable relationship to the intake of carbohydrate calories, the effect of endocrine dysfunction also merits consideration, as the appearance can be similar to the Cushingoid face of pathological or steroid-induced hyperadrenalism.

(d) *Anaemia.* Again, this varies in commonness, and even more in precise etiology from country to country; thus in Jordan, some cases are vitamin-E responsive (Majaj et al., 1963). It is usually not severe unless other causes, such as a heavy hookworm infection, malaria or kala-azar, are also present.

Occasional signs of kwashiorkor

The various signs that are occasionally present include the following:

(a) *Flaky-paint rash.* This well-known lesion has been described elsewhere (Trowell, Davis & Dean, 1954; Jelliffe, 1955b) as occurring in advanced cases. It varies in commonness in different parts of the world. If present, it is virtually pathognomonic.

(b) *Hepatomegaly.* Although extreme fatty infiltration is a constant pathological finding, a considerably enlarged liver, sometimes extending down to the level of the umbilicus, is a feature of the kwashiorkor syndrome in only certain parts of the world, especially in the infantile cases of the West Indies (Waterlow, 1948; Jelliffe, Bras & Stuart, 1954), and in parts of Indonesia (Oomen, 1957b; Blankhart, 1958). From a world standpoint, hepatomegaly should be viewed as an occasional manifestation, and in some tropical communities the large livers found in late infancy and in the preschool age-group are often associated with splenomegaly and are principally the result of malaria (Walters & McGregor, 1960).

(c) *Other skin lesions.* Children with kwashiorkor may sometimes show indolent sores, fissures (as behind the ears), and a " moist groin rash " (Trowell, Davis & Dean, 1954).

(e) *Associated vitamin deficiency.* A variety of signs possibly due to associated vitamin deficiency may be found, including keratomalacia and angular stomatitis. Their commonness varies from one part of the world to another.

(f) *Associated conditioning infections.* These may include chest signs of tuberculosis, severe anaemia in hookworm infection, and dehydration, even when peripheral oedema is present, from diarrhoea.

Nutritional marasmus (inanition) (Fig. 50, 51 and 52)

Nomenclature

The term at present used for this second severe syndrome of protein-calorie malnutrition is imprecise, but clinically descriptive, referring to a person, usually a young child, showing severe wasting, principally due to a grossly inadequate diet. Older terms include athrepsia, cachexia, decomposition, infantile atrophy, denutrition, and inanition.

Etiology

Nutritional marasmus is principally due to severe under-nutrition, that is, a diet very low in both protein and calories—so-called " balanced starvation ". While it can occur at all ages, including adulthood, it is seen most commonly in the first year of life—in contrast to kwashiorkor, which occurs mainly in the age-group 1-3 years—frequently as a result of attempted artificial feeding with very dilute milk, and also often associated with infective diarrhoea and sometimes with tuberculosis. A late form of childhood nutritional marasmus can occur in the pre-school period as a result of prolonged breast-feeding not supplemented with other foods, so-called " breast starvation ".

Once again a clinical picture similar to nutritional marasmus can be produced in piglets by feeding them a diet low in both protein and carbohydrate calories (Platt, 1958).

The clinical signs of nutritional marasmus can be divided into two groups: constant and occasional.

Constant signs of nutritional marasmus

The two constant features of nutritional marasmus are growth retardation and wasting of muscle and of subcutaneous fat.

(*a*) *Growth retardation.* This is extreme. Weight retardation is much more marked than that of length: the child is usually below 60% of the standard weight.

(*b*) *Wasting of muscle and of subcutaneous fat.* This can be detected by clinical inspection and by palpation. The arm feels thin and the skin is loose (Gongora & McFie, 1959), and measurements of the circumference and the skin-folds of the upper arm, and subsequent calculation of muscle circumference are all very low. It is also clinically apparent in the wizened " little old man " or " monkey " face.

Occasional signs of nutritional marasmus

(*a*) *Hair changes.* Minor abnormalities of the hair may be seen occasionally. These are never marked, although light-brown, somewhat sparse hair may be found. The conspicuously dyspigmented hair occurring in many children with kwashiorkor never occurs.

FIG. 50. NUTRITIONAL MARASMUS, SHOWING EXTREME WASTING OF MUSCLE AND FAT

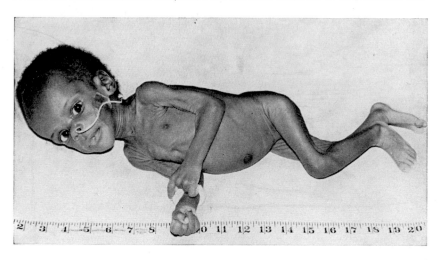

FIG. 51. NUTRITIONAL MARASMUS AND RECOVERY

(a) Nutritional marasmus, showing extreme wasting of muscle and fat, large-seeming head and small chest

(b) Same child after nutritional recovery. Note change in body proportions

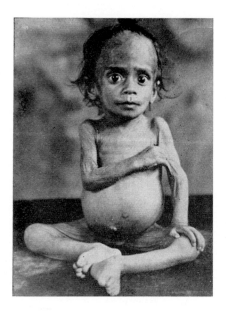
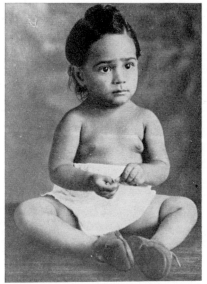

FIG. 52. NUTRITIONAL MARASMUS IN YOUNG SCHOOL-AGE CHILD, SHOWING SEVERE WASTING OF MUSCLE AND FAT

The condition is more common in infants but can occur in older children and adults

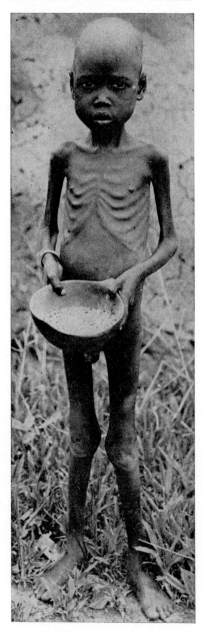

(b) *Associated vitamin deficiency.* In particular, angular stomatitis and keratomalacia may be present.

(c) *Associated conditioning diseases.* These may include the dehydration resulting from infective diarrhoea, oral moniliasis (thrush), and chest signs due to tuberculosis. In contrast to kwashiorkor, oedema is absent and the child seldom exhibits psychomotor change, such as apathy or anorexia.

Intermediate severe syndromes

The term " protein-calorie malnutrition of early childhood " has been introduced in an attempt to attach a tentative etiologically helpful label to the group as a whole. Yet even with advanced forms there will be frequent cases which are intermediate between the two clinical " mountain-peaks " of kwashiorkor and of nutritional marasmus, and which cannot be defined in precise terms.

In addition, the interrelationships between the two major syndromes are such that changing circumstances may result in a transition from one clinical picture to another. A child with early kwashiorkor can be forced into nutritional marasmus by severe infective diarrhoea and ill-advised, prolonged " therapeutic " starvation, or an infant with nutritional marasmus due to inadequate breast-feeding may fall ill with kwashiorkor during the second year of life when carbohydrate foods are given.

Mild-moderate protein-calorie malnutrition

Lesser degrees of protein-calorie malnutrition of early childhood,

FIG. 53. LINES OF DEVELOPMENT IN PROTEIN-CALORIE MALNUTRITION
OF EARLY CHILDHOOD

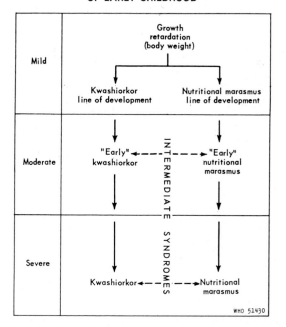

The diagram is a schematic attempt to correlate the development of mild, moderate and severe protein-calorie malnutrition in the two main lines of development—i.e., leading to kwashiorkor and to nutritional marasmus as well as to indeterminate, atypical, intermediate syndromes. The dotted lines stress the potential convertibility from one line of development to the other (Jelliffe & Welbourn, 1963).

sometimes termed " latent ", " hidden " or " marginal ", are far more common than the advanced syndromes, and in order to assess the full extent of the problem, these mild-moderate forms must also be enumerated in a nutritional assessment of the community (Jelliffe, 1963).

The problem is complicated by the variability of the clinical picture, by difficulties in regard to the objective definition of some of the signs, such as psychomotor change, and by the fact that a continuous gradient exists between the obvious severe case and the well-nourished, healthy child (Fig. 53 and 54 (a), (b), (c)).

As judged by the records of children attending clinics who subsequently develop kwashiorkor, and by the common flattening of weight curves in the second year of life in regions where kwashiorkor is widespread, the first clinical indication of protein-calorie malnutrition appears to be growth failure, attested in particular by a low body weight or an inadequate weight gain.

In general terms, the clinical picture of mild-moderate protein-calorie malnutrition (Fig. 54 (b), (c)), is of an underweight disproportionate child, with a long-seeming body, thin limbs, a head that appears too large (Dean,

FIG. 54. DEGREES OF PROTEIN-CALO-
RIE DEFICIENCY IN EARLY CHILDHOOD
(a) Normal healthy well-fed child

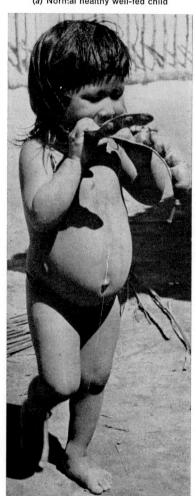

1960; Hassan, 1960; Moncada, 1963), and feet that seem unduly elongated (Thomson, 1960).[1] The buttocks are flattened and the scapulae appear " winged ". The chest is small, especially in contrast with the abdomen, which is often somewhat distended because of thin abdominal muscles, a bulky, fermentable, largely carbohydrate diet, sometimes associated with heavy burdens of roundworms and enlargement of the liver and spleen, often on a malarial basis.

Other signs in the grouping suggestive of protein-calorie malnutrition will be present in varying combinations, depending, among other things, on whether the child is in the kwashiorkor or marasmus " line of development " (Fig. 53).

In the kwashiorkor " line of development ", hair changes, including dyspigmentation, straightness, sparseness and easy pluckability, moon-face, psychomotor change and other signs in the suggestive grouping will be found in different combinations, together with a clinically obvious layer of subcutaneous fat. These cases—when marked— have been termed: " prekwashiorkor ", " early kwashiorkor ", " subclinical kwashiorkor ", or " latent kwashiorkor ".

By contrast, in the marasmus " line of development ", the principal clinical signs will be low weight and diminished subcutaneous fat and muscle, sometimes with minor hair changes.

As with severe syndromes, children with less advanced protein-calorie malnutrition may fall intermediately between these two " lines of development ".

---

[1] Historically, the characteristically lesser effect of malnutrition on skeletal growth has been recognized for many years, resulting in " the body being elongated and the head large " (Jackson, 1925). Similar results are also found in piglets experimentally subjected to severe undernourishment, which develop heads that are too large, legs that are too long and bodies that are too small (McCance, 1964).

FIG. 54. DEGREES OF PROTEIN-CALORIE DEFICIENCY IN EARLY CHILDHOOD *(continued)*

(*b*) Mild protein-calorie malnutrition. The child on the left is 18 months old and weighs the same as the 6-month-old baby on the right

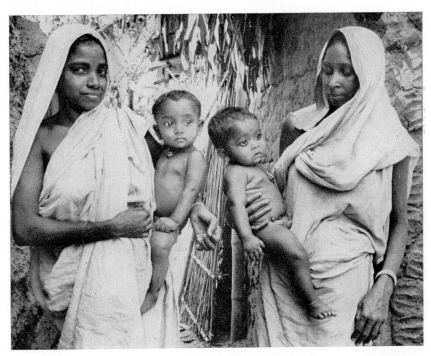

From the anthropometric point of view, mild to moderate cases show abnormal measurements that might be expected from findings in the advanced syndromes of kwashiorkor and nutritional marasmus and are suggested by the clinical picture described above (Fig. 54 (*b*), (*c*)).

The principal anthropometric abnormality is a low weight for age, approximately paralleling the severity of the malnutrition. Despite early interference with bone metabolism (Jones & Dean, 1956), there is much less interference with linear growth, as indicated by measurement of body length (Dean, 1964), unless mild-to-moderate protein-calorie malnutrition is prolonged, when stunting, or " nutritional dwarfing " can result, with children both undersized as well as underweight.

The head circumference, though affected, is much less so than the weight, especially if malnutrition occurs in the second year of life. This is because 50% of extra-uterine skull growth occurs in the first year of life. The apparent largeness of the head is due to the contrast between a relatively normal-sized skull with the thin limbs, the wasted face—in children in the marasmus " line of development ", and especially with the small chest,

FIG. 54. DEGREES
OF PROTEIN-CALORIE DEFICIENCY
IN EARLY CHILDHOOD (continued)

(c) Moderate protein-calorie
malnutrition in a pre-school-age child,
showing body disproportion
(large-seeming head, small chest,
thin limbs, long-seeming body and feet)

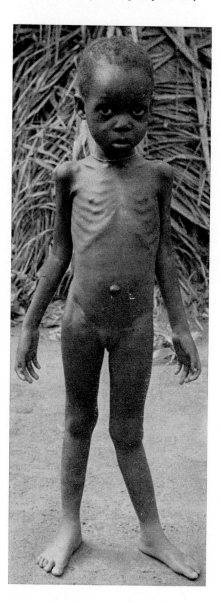

which is due in large part to wasted or poorly developed pectoral muscles, a finding which can be confirmed by a below-standard chest circumference.

Muscle wasting is clinically evident and can be calculated approximately from the measurement of arm circumference and of the triceps skin-fold. Recent field studies also suggest that the simply measured arm circumference *alone* parallels the underlying muscle wasting in the great majority of young children with all degrees of protein-calorie malnutrition (Robinow & Jelliffe—in preparation).

Attempts to classify the severity or degree of protein-calorie malnutrition have been made, on the basis of combined assessment of certain signs and measurements. Examples are the Oomen Malnutrition Index (Oomen, 1955; Trimmer, 1965) and the PCM Score (Jelliffe & Welbourn, 1963). The value of these classifications requires further investigation.

Nutritional dwarfing

In as yet ill-defined dietary circumstances, protein-calorie malnutrition—probably when mild-moderate and prolonged—results in nutritional dwarfing—that is, in children who are " considerably underweight and undersized, while at the same time appearing to have relatively normal body proportions " (Jelliffe, 1959). As Downs (1964) remarks, children with nutritional dwarfing are light in weight, short in stature, with relatively normal body proportions and subcutaneous fat appropriate to their weight; they are likely to be taken for healthy younger children.

This condition has received inadequate attention, but appears to be not uncommon in Peru (Graham, 1966) and in Arab refugee children in the Lebanon (Puyet, Downs & Budeir, 1963; Downs, 1964).

One important reason for knowing whether nutritional dwarfing is common or not lies in the lesser usefulness of weight-for-length measurements in community assessment, if this is the case.

Assessment in the community

An assessment of the prevalence of protein-calorie malnutrition of early childhood may form part of an over-all nutrition survey of a community. However, in view of its importance as a public health problem and the lack of factual knowledge,[1] it is suggested that specific surveys of this vulnerable age-group will often be indicated, both in rural and in urban areas, despite the recognized difficulties of collecting young children for examination.

Assessment will be directed at children from birth to 4 years (i.e., 59 months), using all available methods locally practicable. The data obtained from all sources are complementary and help to describe the situation from a different aspect.

All results should be reported for the entire young-child group (0-59 months). They should also be broken down into figures: (*a*) for infants (0-11 months); (*b*) for the pre-school-age group (12-59 months); and (*c*) for each year.

Direct assessment of prevalence in the community

Clinical signs

Signs in the grouping " suggestive " of protein-calorie malnutrition (see page 43) will be recorded, and the proportion presenting each individual sign calculated for each age-group. However, as noted earlier, they are difficult to define objectively and are variable in occurrence, so that their usefulness is limited, especially in some communities (Standard, Lovell & Garrow, 1966).

Percentages of children showing a combination of three or more signs in the " suggestive " grouping will be more helpful. Likewise the percentage in the different age-groups suffering from the two major syndromes— kwashiorkor and nutritional marasmus—should be analysed.

---

[1] Relatively few community surveys for protein-calorie malnutrition of early childhood have been carried out: New Guinea (Oomen & Malcolm, 1958); South India (Rao et al., 1959); Haiti (Jelliffe & Jelliffe, 1960, 1961); Trinidad (Jelliffe, Symonds & Jelliffe, 1960); the San Blas Indians (Jelliffe et al., 1961b); Ethiopia (Woodruff & Hoerman, 1960); Malaya (Dean, 1961); Java (Oomen, Prawirowinoto & Latuasan, 1954; Bailey, 1962); Nigeria (Collis, Dema & Omololu, 1962b); and in the East African community child health surveys: among the Bachiga (Jelliffe et al., 1961a); the Lugbara (Jelliffe et al., 1962a); the Hadza (Jelliffe et al., 1962b); the Acholi (Jelliffe et al., 1963); the Karamojong (Jelliffe et al., 1964).

Nutritional anthropometry

Basic measurements will consist of weight, length, triceps skin-fold, and the circumferences of the head, chest and mid-upper arm. The results should be reported in two ways: (a) mathematically, showing the mean (average) values and two standard deviations; and (b) compared with both the local standards, if available, and the general standards of reference. They can then be expressed as percentages of children in the four 10% levels below the standard—that is, 90-81%; 80-71%; 70-61%; 60% and below.

Single weight measurements

(a) *Weight for age.* For children seen only once in a field survey, the prevalence of malnutrition in the community has to be estimated from a single examination.

The significance of children with weight below the standard is complicated by the fact that this group will also include some who were born underweight, such as premature babies and twins, as well as some genetically in a low weight percentile. Moreover, it is not possible, on the basis of a single examination, to separate children recovering from infections or malnutrition from those who are deteriorating and in critical need of treatment.

The weights of actual clinical cases of kwashiorkor seen will be masked by oedema, and these children should be excluded from the weight classification.

However, these shortcomings are mitigated if single weight measurements are made on large numbers of children in a survey as part of the assessment of the approximate nutritional profile of a community.

If ages are known with certainty, the number of children in different degrees of " below-standard weight " for age are calculated.

Various methods have been suggested or used to express these findings. The Gomez system termed young children between 90% and 75% of the standard as first-degree malnutrition, between 75% and 61% as second-degree, and 60% and below as third-degree (Gomez et al., 1955). This classification has been used quite widely, especially in South America, and has proved extremely useful. However, the selection of levels below standard was based largely on clinical hospital experience in Mexico City.

Ford (1964) has suggested that 66% of the standard weight should be regarded as the " malnutrition line " but this has the disadvantage of including only obvious advanced cases.

Continental European schools of paediatrics have long used the general terms " dystrophia " or " dysthrepsia " for protein-calorie malnutrition of early childhood, and have, in fact, based the diagnosis of *degrees* of involvement on the percentage of standard weight—e.g., hypothrepsia 1, 90%-80%; hypothrepsia 2, 80%-60%, and athrepsia, below 60%.

The system here suggested, whereby weights are expressed in relation to the four 10% levels below standard, is thought to be more useful in that it does not draw diagnostic conclusions that may not be warranted in every case, and because it avoids labels that may be used in different ways by different authorities.

Should descriptive labels be needed for public health purposes, the following are suggested: 1st level underweight, 90%-81%; 2nd level underweight, 80%-71%; 3rd level underweight, 70%-61%; 4th level underweight, 60% and below.

(b) *Weight for length or for head circumference.* While age assessment must be attempted by all practicable means, an accurate estimate is often not possible. In such cases, as has been suggested, the weight may be expressed in relation to two measurements that are usually much less affected by malnutrition at that age—length and head circumference.[1]

As with other measurements, the weight-for-length and weight-for-head circumference should be expressed in percentages in the four 10% levels below the local and general standards of reference.

Such findings are plainly approximations, as both length and head circumference are, in fact, affected to some degree (Stoch & Smythe, 1963). They will probably be of most use in severe, relatively acute protein-calorie malnutrition, often seen in the second year of life, and less so in more chronically affected children in the later pre-school age when stunted height is also likely to be found.

Serial weight measurements

Where a more prolonged observation is feasible, failure to gain " significant " weight over an adequate period of observation may be an important indicator of protein-calorie malnutrition, although other factors must also be taken into account.

This method is only possible in special circumstances—for example in child health clinics or in longitudinal studies. It has the great advantage of not calling for accurate age assessment; but the measurements must be taken with care since the increments are small and the possibility of error greatly increased.

Because rates of growth vary, different periods of observation are needed for different age-groups (Table 19).[2]

If reliable records or graphic growth charts are available in child welfare clinics, it is suggested that the percentages in the various age-groups with different levels of " insufficient weight gain " should be recorded.

---

[1] In a survey of African pre-school children in Busoga, Uganda, whose ages were known, it was found that the weight for age correlated very strongly with the weight for length and with the weight for head circumference (Robinow & Jelliffe—in preparation).

[2] Marsden (1964) has introduced the more rigorous concept of " faltering ", which he defines as failure to gain ½ lb (226 g) over a period of three months during infancy.

TABLE 19. WEIGHT GAIN DURING THE FIRST TWO YEARS OF LIFE

Age (months)	Approximate average monthly weight gain	Minimum length of observation (months)	Weight gain that would be regarded as insufficient
0-6	1½ lb (679 g)	1	¾ lb (340 g) per month
7-12	1 lb (453 g)	2	1 lb (453 g) per 2 months
12-24	½ lb (226 g)	4	1lb (453 g) per 4 months

Single length measurements

Although, as noted earlier, linear growth is usually much less affected than weight, it is desirable, if practicable, to compare length for age with standards.

This is particularly important in order to detect whether " nutritional dwarfing " is common in a community—in which event, weight-for-length measurements will not be so helpful, as both weight and length are reduced proportionately.

Muscle depletion

This may be calculated from measurements of the upper-arm circumference and of the triceps skin-fold. Results can be expressed in relation to the four 10% levels below the standard.

In a field study of young African children in Busoga, Uganda, the arm circumference correlated very strongly with the calculated muscle circumference, as well as with weight for age (Robinow & Jelliffe—in preparation). It has also been found useful in field studies in rural Greece (X. G. Kondakis —personal communication, 1966), in Haiti (I. Beghin, W. Fougère & K. W. King—personal communication, 1966), and in Ankole, Uganda (R. Cook—personal communication, 1966).

As a simple approximation, therefore, the actual arm circumference can be used as a general anthropometric index of protein-calorie malnutrition and should also be expressed in relation to four 10% levels below the standard.

If precise age assessment is not possible, a further useful approximation, for both boys and girls, is that between 1 and 2 years of age the mid-upper arm circumference [1] is about 16 cm and the triceps skin-fold about 10 mm.

Chest/head circumference ratio

In well-nourished children, the circumference of the chest becomes larger than that of the head after the first six months of life. In protein-

---

[1] 100% 16 cm; 90% 14.4 cm; 80% 12.8 cm; 70% 11.2 cm; 60% 9.6 cm.

calorie malnutrition, the chest does not develop well, probably mainly because of wasting or poor growth of the pectoral muscles, and the head measurement is the larger of the two circumferences. The result is that the chest/head ratio is less than one (Hassan, 1960; Moncada, 1963; Dean, 1965). This simple test is of value for children between 6 months and 5 years of age, and does not need a tape measure; a piece of string will serve. It is suggested that the percentage of children in the different age-groups who have a chest/head ratio of below one should be calculated and reported.

Biochemical tests

Serum-albumin levels warrant reinvestigation in the field, in correlation with anthropometric measurements and clinical assessment, although the majority opinion at the moment is that they are not of value in identifying mild-to-moderate cases.

Tests of the urine may be carried out to measure creatinine excreted in a timed period as an index of muscle mass, or urea excreted, expressed per gram of creatinine, as a measure of protein intake. They are, however, inadequately evaluated as practical field methods. " Standards " are uncertain, and there arise the usual difficulties of urine collection from young children under field conditions.

The amino-acid imbalance test (Whitehead & Dean, 1964) holds out great promise, since it requires only a small amount of blood obtained by finger-prick, and the results are independent of age. It does, however, require the facilities of a well-organized central laboratory. Likewise, the hydroxy-proline excretion test, carried out on a random sample of urine, may prove of value in survey work (Whitehead, 1965).

The buccal-mucosa test of Squires (1965) appears to be simple to carry out, but needs further evaluation in the field.

Indirect assessment of prevalence in the community

Age-specific mortality rates

As noted earlier, age-specific mortality rates for 1-4 years of age, and in many regions for 1-2 years of age, should be sought. They can be expressed in various ways, but most simply as percentages of total mortality. They should always be interpreted in relation to the local setting. However, in many developing regions, such information will not be available or will be so inaccurate as to be meaningless.

Cause-of-death records

The specific death rates from malnutrition in ages 1-4 years should be collected, provided that sufficiently accurate local records exist, which is not usually the case.

Health-service statistics

Statistics concerning the major syndromes—kwashiorkor and nutritional marasmus—seen in out-patients and admitted to adjacent hospitals and health centres in the preceding year should be assembled, as well as the reported incidence of potential conditioning infections, including whooping cough, tuberculosis, measles, infective diarrhoea, intestinal helminths and malaria.

Assessment of ecological factors

Data relevant to the local epidemiology of protein-calorie malnutrition to be collected on the survey include the following:

(*a*) feeding practices with regard to young children, by detailed food consumption or rapid questionnaire;

(*b*) cultural influences;

(*c*) socio-economic factors;

(*d*) local food production and availability;

(*e*) incidence of conditioning infections, including the incidence of malaria and intestinal helminths as shown by laboratory tests, and of tuberculous infection, as indicated by the tuberculin test; and

(*f*) medical and educational services.

Priorities

While information has to be sought from as many useful sources as possible, relatively simple, practical surveys can be carried out, with limited personnel, on the basis of clinical assessment, anthropometry, available statistics from local health services and a largely qualitative investigation of causative ecological factors.

The apparent value of various methods of field assessment of protein-calorie malnutrition is given in Table 20, together with their probable feasibility in relation to the collection of samples or statistics, to laboratory services available and to age-estimation.

Methods for use in " direct assessment " in field prevalence surveys are given in Table 21 (where ages known) and Table 22 (where ages unknown).

Presentation

Although this topic is discussed in general terms elsewhere, further comments are pertinent at this point on the presentation of data likely to be collected in rapid prevalence surveys of young children (0-5 years).

Clinical assessment

A composite table will be required showing (*a*) single clinical signs (in the suggestive grouping); (*b*) combinations of three or more signs; and

TABLE 20. PROBABLE VALUE AND FEASIBILITY OF SUGGESTED INDICATORS
FOR THE COMMUNITY ASSESSMENT OF PROTEIN-CALORIE MALNUTRITION
IN YOUNG CHILDREN *

Indicators	Value of indicators			Feasibility of obtaining accurate data in developing countries	
	High	Medium	Low	Easy	Difficult
1. Specific mortality rate from malnutrition	*				*
2. Infant mortality rate			*		*
3. Mortality rate in children 1-4 years		*			*
4. Percentage of deaths of children below 5 years of age in relation to total mortality			*	*	*
5. Wills-Waterlow index (p. 100)		*			*
6. Specific mortality rate from diarrhoea and some infectious diseases (measles)			*		*
7. Prevalence of protein-calorie deficiencies					
(a) Clinical signs (grouped)				*	
(b) Weight for age	*				*
(c) Weight for length				*	
(d) Weight for head circumference		*		*	
(e) Arm circumference	*			*	
(f) Chest/head circumference ratio		*		*	
(g) Serum albumin		*		*	
(h) Urinary urea, expressed per gram of creatinine		*			*
(i) Amino-acid imbalance test	*				*
(j) Hydroxyproline excretion test	*				*

* Adapted by permission from Bengoa (personal communication, 1965).

(c) the major syndromes of kwashiorkor and nutritional marasmus (Table 23).

Nutritional anthropometry

Results should be presented showing percentages in different age-groups in four levels below standard: 90%-81%; 80%-71%; 70%-61%; and 60% and below.

The most important of these will be the weight for age (Table 24) (excluding kwashiorkor cases), but other anthropometric measurements, especially the arm circumference (Table 25), should be reported in the same tabular form, if ages are known in sufficient detail.

TABLE 21. TENTATIVE METHODS OF DIRECT ASSESSMENT OF PROTEIN-CALORIE MALNUTRITION OF EARLY CHILDHOOD AS A COMMUNITY PROBLEM (WHERE AGES ARE KNOWN)

Method of assessment	Remarks
Clinical signs	" Suggestive " group for protein-calorie malnutrition (single signs, combination of three or more signs)
	Major syndromes (kwashiorkor, nutritional marasmus)
Anthropometry:	
Weight for age	Using percentage of accepted standard [a] (e.g., 90 %-81 %, 80 %-71 %, 70 %-61 %, 60 % and below)
Height for age	Using percentage of accepted standard [a]
Mid-arm-muscle circumference for age	Using percentage of accepted standard [a] (calculated from mid-arm circumference and triceps skin-fold)
Mid-arm circumference for age	Using percentage of accepted standard [a]
Chest/head circumference ratio	One or above in well-nourished child over a year old
Biochemical:	
Amino-acid imbalance test	
Hydroxyproline excretion test	
Cytological:	
Buccal mucosa smear	

[a] Comparison should be made with both the general standards of reference and the local standards, if available.

TABLE 22. METHODS OF DIRECT ASSESSMENT OF PROTEIN-CALORIE MALNUTRITION OF EARLY CHILDHOOD AS A COMMUNITY PROBLEM (WHERE AGES ARE UNKNOWN)

Method of assessment	Remarks
Clinical signs	" Suggestive " group for protein-calorie malnutrition (single signs; combination of three or more signs)
	Major syndromes (kwashiorkor, nutritional marasmus)
Anthropometry:	
Weight for length [a]	Using percentage of accepted standard [b]
Weight for head circumference [a]	Using percentage of accepted standard [b]
Mid-arm circumference [a]	Using percentage of 16 cm (for 1-2-year-old children)
Chest/head circumference ratio	One or above in well-nourished child over a year old
Biochemical:	
Amino-acid imbalance test	
Hydroxyproline excretion test	
Cytological:	
Buccal mucosa smear	

[a] Probably most valuable at age 1-2 years.

[b] Comparison should be made with both the general standards of reference and the local standards, if available.

TABLE 23. METHOD OF REPORTING RESULTS OF CLINICAL ASSESSMENT
IN PREVALENCE SURVEY FOR PROTEIN-CALORIE MALNUTRITION
OF EARLY CHILDHOOD, SHOWING PERCENTAGES IN DIFFERENT AGE-GROUPS
WITH (a) SINGLE CLINICAL SIGNS, (b) COMBINATIONS OF THREE OR MORE SIGNS,
AND (c) MAJOR SYNDROMES

Age (months)	Number examined	Oedema	Dyspigmented hair	Easily pluckable hair	Thin, sparse hair	Straight hair	Muscle wasting	Depigmented skin	Psychomotor change	Moon-face	Hepatomegaly	Flaky-paint dermatosis	Combination of three or more signs	Severe syndromes	
														Kwashiorkor	Nutritional marasmus
0-3															
4-6															
7-11															
Total 0-11															
12-23															
24-35															
36-47															
48-59															
Total 12-59															
Total 0-59															

WHO 51481

If ages are not known, appropriate data (Table 22) can be reported in similar tables using broad groupings of " infants " and " pre-school children ", instead of small precise age-groups. These will particularly include clinical signs (single signs, combinations of three or more, major syndromes), weight for length, and arm circumference.

Statistics from local health services

Recorded attendances at hospitals and health centres are reported in the manner shown in Table 26. Again, if ages are not known with precision, the percentage attendances with both kwashiorkor and nutritional marasmus can be given for 0-11 months (or for " infants "), 12-59 months (or for " pre-school children "), and for 0-4 years (0-59 months) (or for " young children ").

Key findings in prevalence surveys

While detailed investigations of all possible sources are necessary and should be tabulated and documented, it is suggested that the simplest " key

14

TABLE 24. METHOD OF REPORTING RESULTS OF WEIGHTS FOR AGE
IN PREVALENCE SURVEYS FOR PROTEIN-CALORIE MALNUTRITION
OF EARLY CHILDHOOD, SHOWING PERCENTAGES IN FOUR LEVELS
UNDERWEIGHT FOR AGE

Age (months)	Number examined	Levels underweight for age[a]			
		Percentage in 1st level (90%-81% standard)	Percentage in 2nd level (80%-71% standard)	Percentage in 3rd level (70%-61% standard)	Percentage in 4th level (60% standard & below)
0-3					
4-6					
7-11					
Total 0-11					
12-23					
24-35					
36-47					
48-59					
Total 12-59					
Total 0-59					

WHO 51482

[a] Oedematous children with kwashiorkor should be excluded from this classification.

findings " gathered in rapid surveys for protein-calorie malnutrition of early childhood are those permitting of a rough assessment of the percentages in the community of (a) mild-moderate cases and (b) severe cases.

According to present evidence, the most useful practical definition of these two groups is as follows:

(a) *mild-moderate PCM :* total of 1st, 2nd and 3rd levels underweight for age (i.e., between 90% and 61% of standard weight);

(b) *severe PCM :* total of cases of kwashiorkor and 4th level underweight for age (which will include nutritional marasmus).

These can be tabulated according to age-group (Table 27), and in a more condensed, simplified form—with data reported for the groups 0-1 year, 1-4 years, and 0-4 years—may be regarded as the most fundamental community data for purposes of public health comparison, in the same way that the splenic index is used by the malariologist.

TABLE 25. METHOD OF REPORTING RESULTS OF ARM-CIRCUMFERENCE MEASUREMENTS FOR AGE IN PREVALENCE SURVEYS FOR PROTEIN-CALORIE MALNUTRITION IN EARLY CHILDHOOD, SHOWING PERCENTAGES IN FOUR LEVELS UNDER STANDARD FOR AGE

Age (months)	Number examined	Levels below standard arm circumference for age			
		Percentage in 1st level (90% - 81% standard)	Percentage in 2nd level (80% - 71% standard)	Percentage in 3rd level (70% - 61% standard)	Percentage in 4th level (60% standard & below)
0-3					
4-6					
7-11					
Total 0-11					
12-23					
24-35					
36-47					
48-59					
Total 12-59					
Total 0-59					

WHO 51482

TABLE 26. METHOD OF REPORTING TWO MAIN SYNDROMES OF PROTEIN-CALORIE MALNUTRITION IN YOUNG CHILDREN ATTENDING HOSPITAL OR HEALTH CENTRE

Age (months)	Number attending	Severe syndromes	
		Kwashiorkor	Nutritional marasmus
0-3			
4-6			
7-11			
Total 0-11			
12-23			
24-35			
36-47			
48-59			
Total 12-59			
Total 0-59			

WHO 51483

TABLE 27. METHOD OF REPORTING PERCENTAGES POSITIVE WITH
(a) MILD-MODERATE AND (b) SEVERE PROTEIN-CALORIE MALNUTRITION
OF EARLY CHILDHOOD FROM DATA COLLECTED ON A PREVALENCE SURVEY

Age (months)	Number examined	Mild - moderate [a] protein - calorie malnutrition (%)	Severe [b] protein - calorie malnutrition (%)
0 - 3			
4 - 6			
7 - 11			
Total 0 - 11			
12 - 23			
24 - 35			
36 - 47			
48 - 59			
Total 12 - 59			
Total 0 - 59			

WHO 51484

[a] Total of children in 1st, 2nd and 3rd levels underweight for age.
[b] Total of children with clinical kwashiorkor and children in 4th level underweight for age.

By these means, it will be possible to compare the prevalence of protein-calorie malnutrition in early childhood in communities in two regions or countries, as in the following example:

	0-1 year		1-4 years		0-4 years	
	Severe	Mild-moderate	Severe	Mild-moderate	Severe	Mild-moderate
Country A	1%	8%	3%	40%	2%	32%
Country B	0%	5%	1%	7%	0.5%	4%

Where the ages in only 50% or less of the children surveyed can be obtained, a similar classification can be used with weight-for-length in lieu of weight-for-age measurements, despite the greater difficulties in interpreting results (pages 193-195):

(a) *mild-moderate PCM :* total of 1st, 2nd and 3rd levels underweight for length;

(b) *severe PCM :* total of cases of kwashiorkor and 4th level underweight for length.

Avitaminosis A

Severe manifestations of vitamin-A deficiency are widespread in young children in some parts of the world, including Indonesia (Oomen, 1957b), while in other regions eye damage and blindness from avitaminosis A are public health problems at present unrecognized (McLaren, 1963; Oomen, McLaren & Escapini, 1964).

Etiology

The most dangerous manifestation, keratomalacia, principally affects young pre-school children, and is often associated with moderate or severe protein-calorie malnutrition. It is a disease of poverty and ignorance, with a diet economically and culturally restricted to exclude sources of vitamin A (e.g., milk, fish) and sources of carotene (e.g., green vegetables, papaya). In some communities, it may be precipitated by too early a cessation of breast-feeding (McLaren, 1956), and in urban areas, even among young infants, by artificial feeding with vitamin-deficient dried skimmed milk, in powdered or condensed form.

Poor storage may play a part, particularly in twins or premature infants, while infections—e.g., diarrhoeal disease and measles—act at times as the final conditioning factor (Oomen, McLaren & Escapini, 1964; McLaren, Oomen & Escapini, 1966).

Assessment in the community

Direct assessment. This may be gauged by the prevalence of clinical signs in the " suggestive " grouping, by low levels of serum vitamin A (after correction for low plasma proteins), and by dietary survey.

In addition, the presence of typically damaged eyes in older children and adults, showing phthisis bulbi, leucoma or staphyloma, may provide retrospective evidence of severe avitaminosis A in early childhood (Oomen, McLaren & Escapini, 1964; McLaren, Oomen & Escapini, 1966).

Indirect assessment. Hospital figures, both in the children's and ophthalmic wards, may furnish useful statistics concerning admissions with keratomalacia. However, these may represent an underestimate, because many classically trained paediatricians and ophthalmologists have not had much experience in diagnosing the ocular manifestations of vitamin-A deficiency.

Keratomalacia is so frequently a disease of the toddler that " weanling blindness " is an age-specific epidemiological phenomenon. Local records of age-incidence of blindness, if available, may disclose suggestive data (McLaren, Oomen & Escapini, 1966).

Ecological assessment. Cultural evidence suggesting that avitaminosis A is common may be indicated by vernacular names for various eye signs. Thus, in Indonesian, Bitot's spots are known as *sisikan* (" scaly like a fish "), and night blindness is termed *mata ajam* (" chicken's eyes "), referring to the inability of chickens to see well at night (Oomen, McLaren & Escapini, 1964).

Infantile Beriberi

Infantile beriberi is unquestionably a public health problem in parts of South-East Asia, where the diet consists mainly of polished rice. It is the only common form of malnutrition occurring in young breast-fed infants that is attributable to maternal dietary inadequacy, the mother's thiamine-deficient diet being matched by a low thiamine level in her milk.

Assessment in the community

Direct assessment. This is not possible in the course of a prevalence survey because the illness is usually an acute one—rapidly fatal if not treated with thiamine—or with rather non-specific features in the less frequent chronic cases. It is in connexion with this type of acute condition that long-term incidence surveys are particularly revealing.

Examination of pregnant women for " suggestive " clinical signs and for urinary thiamine levels will enable areas where infantile beriberi is a high risk to be defined, as may the estimation of thiamine in breast milk (Simpson & Chow, 1956).

Indirect assessment. If available, the age-specific mortality from 2 to 5 months will be helpful, as will statistics based on hospital admissions of typically affected infants responding dramatically to parenteral thiamine.

Ecological assessment. Knowledge of the local pattern of the feeding of infants and mothers will be suggestive.

Rickets

Rickets is common in some tropical and subtropical countries, where young children are given no vitamin D, either as food or as supplement, and where they are not exposed to sunlight because of crowded urban conditions or are purposely kept indoors for various cultural reasons—for example, to keep the skin fair or to avoid the " evil eye ".

Assessment in the community

Direct assessment. In view of the lack of specificity of many of the signs found in rickets (Winter, 1954), direct assessment is best based principally on the prevalence in young children of at least three of the " suggestive " groups of signs, preferably supported by high serum-alkaline-phosphatase levels and by radiological examination of the wrists in samples of those examined clinically.

Indirect assessment. Statistics of out-patient attendances and admissions of children with rickets may be useful, although the criteria used for diagnosis should be scrutinized.

Ecological assessment. Dietary patterns and cultural practices excluding children and women from irradiation with the ultraviolet light of sunshine may be relevant to the etiology of rickets in some areas.

Iron Deficiency

Anaemia is extremely common in young children in many developing countries. It is often due to a number of concurrent factors, including nutritional deficiencies (Wadsworth, 1959), bacterial and parasitic infections and genetic abnormalities, especially sickle-cell anaemia in children of African ancestry.

Iron needs are high in early childhood because of the rapid increases in the total number of red blood cells and in muscle mass which occur with normal development. Iron deficiency results when these needs are not met, as a result of dietary inadequacy (e.g., human and cow's milk; iron-poor staples) and iron loss (e.g., infection with hookworm or bilharziasis), often associated with suboptimal liver stores (e.g., twins, prematures, babies of iron-deficient mothers), and possibly with malabsorption.

Assessment in the community

Direct assessment. Haemoglobin estimations are the most useful screening test. Low levels must be investigated by (*a*) tests for iron-deficiency anaemia, e.g., thin blood films for cell morphology, microhaematocrit readings of packed cell volume; and (*b*) tests for common associated causes of anaemia, e.g., stools for hookworm ova and occult blood, thick blood film for malarial parasites, test for sickling in African children. Standards for the results of these investigations have already been indicated. Special research techniques for more-detailed haematological surveys may be required (Annex 2).

Indirect assessment. The number of children with iron-deficiency anaemia in the hospitals of the area must be investigated. Findings may be difficult to evaluate, as anaemia in young children in tropical regions is often due to multiple causes at a given time, and the necessary haematological laboratory facilities to ensure correct etiological diagnoses are not normally available.

Ecological assessment. Dietary studies are, of course, relevant, but they should also take account of the availability and absorption of iron present in the diet and also of iron ingested with food from the water supply, from the soil—as with laterite dust—and from ferrous cooking pots.

SCHOOLCHILDREN

Children of school age (usually 5-15 years) in developing regions do not normally show significant serious illness, still less mortality, from malnutrition. They have passed through the dangerous years of early childhood. They are growing more slowly, and are able to compete for, and digest, the full range of the adult diet. In rural areas, they may be able to supplement their diets with wild fruits, berries, insects and small animals. Ordinarily, they will have achieved a substantial immunity against at least some of the prevalent infections and parasites, particularly malaria.

On the other hand, schoolchildren in tropical regions are often undernourished, with positive clinical signs and subnormal anthropometric measurements, such as a low weight for height and thin subcutaneous fat, but without sufficient symptoms to warrant attendance at hospital or health centre. This is particularly likely to happen when children walk long distances to school with little, if any, breakfast, when no school meal is provided, and when assistance with heavy manual household chores, such as chopping wood or herding domestic animals, is expected of them when they return home in the evening.

Thus, while school-age children should be included in the total population sample examined in the course of a cross-sectional nutrition survey, it may be useful to carry out a survey of schoolchildren as such, since the planning of a school health service, in particular a school meals programme adapted to the local problems—nutritional, financial and practical—may thereby be expedited.

A survey of schoolchildren offers the advantage that the subjects are easily accessible, often in buildings equipped with tables and chairs that can readily be adapted to survey purposes. They can also be followed longitudinally, with the object of assessing growth. In fact, in the school health services, serial measurements of weight and height should be included in the pupil's health record. If such measurements are already available and are reliable, their analysis may yield valuable data.

The disadvantages of this type of survey are that it is directed at an age-group not markedly vulnerable nutritionally, and which may not even be representative of the school-age population as such. Often only a limited proportion of children will be attending school, with the remainder taking part in more traditional activities in the village, with somewhat different nutritional consequences.

Results must be assessed in relation to possible seasonal food variations and to the nutritional consequences of school holidays.

Nutritional assessment of schoolchildren

Methods of direct assessment are similar to those described by earlier workers (Patwardhan, 1961). However, certain features call for special attention.

Clinical assessment. While varying in different parts of the world, the following signs are likely to occur in this age-group and must be looked for carefully: Bitot's spots, conjunctival xerosis, anaemia, parotid enlargement, angular cheilosis, fluorosis, caries, goitre, tropical ulcers, hepatomegaly and splenomegaly.

Nutritional anthropometry. That the physique of schoolchildren is related to nutrition is suggested, for example, by the improvement in the heights and weights of well-to-do Indian children in South Africa as compared with those of the same genetic stock in India (Abramson, 1959). Likewise, Bakwin & McLaughlin (1964) have shown that the weights and heights of " privileged " American schoolchildren in 1936 are today matched by the measurements of children in the lower socio-economic groups.

Basic measurements recommended for schoolchildren are weight, height, triceps skin-fold and arm circumference.

Results are expressed separately for each sex and for age to the nearest year. In accordance with ICNND practice, results should be compared with Baldwin-Wood weight-for-height-for-age tables. Space does not permit of the inclusion in the tables of percentage levels under the standard for each of these, and results must be calculated for each individual as a percentage of the standard, so that results may ultimately be entered in the four usual 10% groups—90%-81%, 80%-71%, 70%-61%, and 60% and below.

With the assistance of parents or teachers, age assessment may be possible from documentary evidence, or the use of a local-events calendar, linked to the eruption of the permanent dentition (Table 5). While ages should ideally be determined to the nearest three months, the nearest year will, in fact, be adequate.

Where ages are unknown, it will be necessary to use weight-for-height figures alone. The disadvantage of this procedure is that it merely indicates whether the child is underweight for height; it does not reveal which children are both underweight and stunted (De Wijin, 1952). As the Baldwin-Wood data are not available in this form, figures derived from Harvard weight-for-height standards should be employed, although these are somewhat higher than the Baldwin-Wood measurements.

Low skin-fold measurements have been found in schoolchildren in developing regions (Wadsworth, 1963; Ferro-Luzzi & Ferro-Luzzi, 1962; Ferro-Luzzi, 1962a, b, c; Potgieter—personal communication, 1964; Robson, 1964b), possibly related to four factors—a lower calorie intake, greater physical exercise, genetic variation, and perhaps an adaptation to a warmer climate.

The arm circumference, as a measurement by itself, or as a means of calculating the muscle circumference, has not been much used, although Luyken & Luyken-Koning (1959, 1961), Kondakis, Maraelle & Kazungu

(1964), and Potgieter (personal communication, 1964) comment on its possible usefulness.

Malnutrition can also be assessed in a school-age population by repeated measurements to test the rate of growth. This can be done with individual children or with groups. As growth is relatively slow, a fairly prolonged interval is needed between weighings to allow for a significant and measurable increment. Probably the optimum time interval is one year, since this will also eliminate the effect of seasonal variations in growth and nutrition (Robson, 1964a). As an approximate index, it may be noted that between 5 and 10 years of age the weight increases by 10% and the height by 5 cm (2 in) annually.

Problems connected with the interpretation of growth in older school-children include variations between early and late maturers, the physiologically earlier puberty in girls, and the slowed growth that may precede the pubertal spurt. Also, in some less-well-fed parts of the world, growth is related to the availability of food and decreases during the hungry season.

Biochemical tests

Examination of the blood for haemoglobin levels should be included, together with stool examinations for ova and for occult blood, and a thick blood film for malaria, if relevant for the particular community.

Other biochemical tests may be carried out to cover a wide range of investigations or may be selected because of known or probable local problems.

Biophysical methods

Although usually not applicable, dark-adaptation tests or dynamometry may sometimes be practicable and indicated.

PREGNANT AND LACTATING WOMEN

Next to young children, pregnant and lactating women are nutritionally the most vulnerable group, especially in developing regions of the world, and yet comparatively little is known of their special nutritional needs (WHO Expert Committee on Nutrition in Pregnancy and Lactation, 1965).

In some areas, women may be in a constant state of nutritional stress from the time of an early marriage, before growth has ceased, until a premature death in their thirties. The whole of adult life may be continuously reproductive, as pregnancies and prolonged lactation follow one another without pause (Gopalan & Belvady, 1961).

Nutritional needs are high, particularly since, in some cultures, women may be responsible for much heavy work carried out with inefficient, clumsy tools (Phillips, 1954) and continued throughout pregnancy. Cultivation, carrying food to market, collecting water and wood, and pounding or hand-milling foods, as well as cooking for the family and carrying young children are commonly women's tasks.

Furthermore their nutritional status is frequently aggravated by food customs specifically applying to women, especially during pregnancy and the puerperium. For example, in some East African communities women are prohibited from eating chicken, eggs, mutton and certain types of fish, which are the main local sources of animal protein. It is rare for any dietary improvement to be made during pregnancy.

In such circumstances of continuous, cumulative nutritional drain, various types of what may be termed " maternal depletion syndrome " occur (Jelliffe & Maddocks, 1964). Probably the most common is protein-calorie malnutrition. This is usually insidious and undramatic, although oedema of nutritional origin can develop in extreme circumstances (Bailey, 1962). Even a kwashiorkor-like picture has—in rare cases—been described.

Lesser degrees of protein-calorie malnutrition in women of child-bearing age probably contribute to the low birth-weight of their neonates, to a failure to make the expected weight gain during pregnancy, and to a decrease in subcutaneous fat and muscle tissue. Ultimately, this cumulative process undoubtedly plays a part in the premature ageing and early death often seen among women in developing regions.

Specific maternal depletion syndromes can also occur, often becoming more marked with recurring pregnancies. These syndromes, which vary in different parts of the world, include osteomalacia, iron-deficiency (and megaloblastic) anaemias, and iodine-deficiency goitre.[1]

Surveys of pregnant women therefore have a place in public health activities because of the nutritional vulnerability of this group, because at least a sample are accessible at prenatal clinics, which are popular in many parts of the world, and because of the consequences of maternal malnutrition not only for the mother, but in relation to the health, nutrition and survival of her child. All prenatal clinical examinations in developing regions should give as much emphasis to the early detection of malnutrition and its prevention by dietary advice as to the more classical, mechanical aspects of pregnancy. While serial observations are ideal, from the nutritional viewpoint the optimum *single* time for examination is the sixth month, particularly since dietary correction is still feasible for the mother and hence for the foetus.

Nutritional assessment of pregnant and lactating women

Direct assessment

Clinical signs. Certain signs have a special importance in particular regions, depending upon the local nutritional problems. They include

---

[1] The interpretation of goitre in pregnancy in relation to dietary iodine lack is complicated by recent work showing that this occurs commonly in well-fed women, probably as a physiological response to a low plasma-inorganic-iodine level, attributable mainly to renal loss of iodine (Crooks et al., 1964).

angular cheilosis, pre-tibial oedema, conjunctival pallor, goitre, the bone pains of osteomalacia, and the " suggestive " signs of beriberi.

Nutritional anthropometry. In women seen at prenatal clinics, nutritional status, as regards protein-calorie malnutrition, can be assessed by weighing at intervals throughout pregnancy. Well-fed, healthy women gain about 15%-25% of their pre-gravid body-weight as a result of the developing foetus, placenta, uterus and amniotic fluid, together with breast enlargement and some increase in subcutaneous fat (Standard & Passmore, 1940; Leitch, 1957; Fish et al., 1960; Hytten & Leitch, 1964).

In poorly-fed communities, it is a common occurrence for weight gains in pregnancy to be inadequate, while in Ceylon 5% of a group of women studied showed a loss of weight (Clements, 1961).

It is suggested tentatively that, pending more precise information, a weight gain of less than 10% between " early pregnancy " and full-term pregnancy should be regarded as an indicator of protein-calorie malnutrition, and that low weights should be expressed according to the following grouping: more than 10%; 10%-5%; less than 5%-no gain; loss of weight.

If accurate prenatal records are available for past years, the incidence of progressive decrease of weight with successive pregnancies should be determined (Venkatachalam, 1962a).

The suggested use of serial measurements of triceps skin-fold and arm circumference as indicators of calorie and protein reserves in pregnancy requires further investigation.

Biochemical tests. The nutritional problems of local importance determine the nature and usefulness of these tests. Special standards are required for pregnant women, but since these are not usually available, ordinary adult standards must be used tentatively,

Biochemical tests may be helpful, as in India, where Venkatachalam, Belavady & Gopalan (1962) found that women of the lower socio-economic group had low serum-vitamin-A levels, which were less during pregnancy. Sometimes, however, little change occurs, as in Guatemala, where Beaton, Arroyave & Flores (1964) found no evidence of lower serum-protein levels in poorer women as a result of multiple pregnancies and prolonged lactation. As they point out, this may be due to unknown processes of adaptation, to unexpected dietary adequacy, or to lack of sensitivity of present methods.

Haemoglobin levels are of great practical value in the nutritional assessment of pregnant women, especially in regions where maternal deaths occur from anaemia alone, or combined with normal blood-loss during delivery. Haemoglobin determinations should be made at each prenatal attendance, above all at the sixth month of pregnancy.

The interpretation of haemoglobin levels in pregnancy must take into account the normal physiological fall in level of about 2 g/100 ml due to haemodilution. This pseudo-anaemia is associated with a decreased haematocrit reading, but no hypochromia.

Nutritional anaemia in pregnancy is sometimes caused by iron deficiency, or it may be megaloblastic, owing to an inadequate intake of folic acid and vitamin B_{12}, or possibly to increased excretion. Anaemia due to combined iron and folic-acid deficiency can occur.

If levels of haemoglobin are found below the standard for pregnant women, initial laboratory tests should include a haematocrit reading, a thin blood film (for cell morphology), a stool examination (for occult blood and hookworm ova), and a thick blood film for malarial parasites. If a diagnosis cannot be made with these simple tests, special investigations, such as bone-marrow and serum levels of iron, folic acid or vitamin B_{12}, are indicated (Annex 2).

Indirect assessment

For a number of complex reasons, maternal mortality and perinatal mortality are affected by the mother's socio-economic level, and figures should be collected, if practicable. A common source of these data is the biased samples attending prenatal clinics or admitted to hospital. Similar information should be sought concerning women seen in wards and clinics with various forms of maternal malnutrition, such as anaemia of pregnancy, osteomalacia, and beriberi.

Maternal malnutrition is among the causes of low birth-weights in both man (Wigglesworth, 1966) and livestock (Blaxter, 1957). In many parts of the world, the birth-weight in lower socio-economic groups is lower than in the well-to-do groups of the same genetic stock (Gopalan, 1957; Venkatacha-lam, 1962a; Udani, 1963).[1] At the same time, any study of birth-weights must also take account of a diversity of other factors (Jelliffe, 1966; Wiggles-worth, 1966): genetic influences, maternal ill-health and overwork, smoking habits, placental malarial infection (E. F. P. Jelliffe, in preparation), frequency of multiple births,[2] lack of prenatal supervision, obstetrical abnormalities.

As approximate indicators of maternal malnutrition, birth-weights of singleton neonates may be usefully compared (a) with the usual "general standard of reference" (2.5 kg or $5\frac{1}{2}$ lb), the so-called "prematurity" or "low birth weight" level (WHO Expert Committee on Maternal and Child Health, 1961); (b) with whatever has been calculated to be the local "special-care weight level" (e.g., in Kampala, 2 kg or $4\frac{1}{2}$ lb) (Jelliffe, 1966); and (c) with the birth-weights of the newborn of the well-fed, modern-living

---

[1] Low-birth-weight neonates are not a homogeneous group, but include at least two overlapping entities: the gestationally premature, expelled from the uterus before term, and the underweight full-term baby (Jelliffe, 1966).

[2] The incidence of dizygous twinning varies greatly. In Japan, it is 2.7 per 1000 births; in Ibadan, Nigeria, 39.9 per 1000 births. The reason for the difference is not clear: though presumed to be genetic, it may be connected with other factors, including nutrition.

élite of the same genetic stock, which may be expressed as a " socio-economic birth-weight quotient " (Bengoa, Jelliffe & Perez, 1959).

Hospital figures of birth-weights should be used with caution as they are often made by junior midwives with ill-checked scales and with variations in techniques, such as taking the measurement with large artery forceps still clamped to the cord.

Birth-weight figures must be based on large samples, preferably numbering at least 1000 of careful weighings of naked singleton babies, and made within 6 hours of delivery.

Attention will also have to be paid to minimizing sampling errors, since there is a likelihood of hospitals admitting a high proportion of primiparae (Morley & Knox, 1960).

ADULTS

With the exception of pregnant and lactating women, adults are the least vulnerable segment of a population in so far as undernutrition is concerned. Nevertheless, certain groups need special consideration—for example, old people and persons engaged in heavy labour. In any event, healthy well-nourished adults are important as productive supporters of the family and as actual or potential parents.

In adulthood, growth has ceased, and the only physiological changes in body dimensions are those that result from ageing or that are associated with constant physical exercise. Consequently, selected anthropometric measurements in adults have a useful place in assessing past or present protein-calorie malnutrition, or overnutrition from an excessive intake of calories, presenting clinically as obesity. They can be useful, if repeated in a community in successive generations, in revealing a positive or negative secular trend.

Standards

As stressed earlier, anthropometric data should, if possible, be compared both with local and with general standards of reference. Data on subcutaneous skin-folds and arm circumference are based on average measurements made on large samples of apparently healthy, well-fed Caucasian adults, and may therefore be inappropriate, for genetic reasons, in other ethnic groups.

The cited weight-for-height standards are not based on average figures, but derived mathematically from " desirable " levels calculated by American insurance companies on the basis of a large-scale study of body build, blood pressure, and other factors affecting longevity (Society of Actuaries, 1959; ICNND, 1963). The figures have been adjusted for people of average frame measured nude (E. Bridgforth—personal communication, 1965).[1]

---

[1] A system of applying different standards for men and women of " large ", " medium " and " small " frame-sizes suggested by the Society of Actuaries (1959) has not been followed, since, although it would be desirable to take due notice of the lateral aspect of human physique as a factor affecting body weight, no definition of the different frame-sizes exists at present.

Standards are given for each sex for " 25 years and over ", because it is currently considered that the increase in weight in middle age commonly seen in well-fed communities is probably undesirable from the viewpoint of health.

Undernutrition in adults

Surveys to assess the nutritional status of adults in poorly-fed communities are normally carried out by a combination of methods previously described. Anthropometric measurements should, as a matter of routine, include the weight, height, triceps skin-fold and arm circumference: jointly these give a useful guide to the general state of protein-calorie nutrition of adults (Fig. 55).

The clinical picture and anthropometric changes in adult protein-calorie malnutrition vary with its duration—classified as brief, prolonged, chronic and lifelong (World Health Organization, 1951)—the degree of deprivation, associated deficiences (e.g., vitamin B complex) and the presence of complicating infections. The malnutrition may also be seasonal, as in the endemic, recurring oedema seen in some regions during the " hungry season ".

Investigations of extreme cases of protein-calorie malnutrition seen in starvation during famines, in volunteer experiments (Keys et al., 1950) and among victims of concentration camps

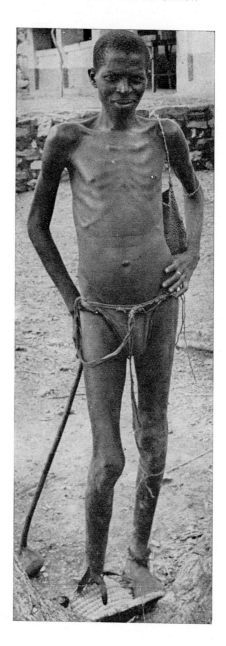

FIG. 55

MODERATE PROTEIN-CALORIE MALNUTRITION IN AN ADULT, SHOWING BODY DISPROPORTION

(Helweg-Larsen et al., 1952) have all shown severe weight loss with no alteration in height save for that produced by stooping. Body weights more than 50% below the original level were observed, and must, in fact, have been still lower, as water retention is a well-recognized feature, even in the absence of oedema. The skin in such circumstances is loose and inelastic. Muscle and fat wasting are strikingly obvious, and demonstrable quantitatively by the decrease in limb measurements, including the arm circumference. The head and the bony prominences appear to be enlarged because of the disappearance of muscle and fat " padding ". The general appearance is that of a person twenty or thirty years older than the real age.

To the paediatrician, the clinical picture, with the exception of the " famine oedema " of advanced cases, is identical with that of nutritional marasmus (inanition) in young children, even to the " little old man " faces. Accordingly—more particularly in view of the lack of a clinical label for this type of severe protein-calorie malnutrition in adults—the use of the same generic term, adult nutritional marasmus,[1] seems justified. The age-specificity normally attached to the word " marasmus " is not implicit in its original derivation; in fact, the term has been used for adult cases by previous workers (Helweg-Larsen et al., 1952).

Examples of severe adult marasmus are not common, except in famines and analogous disasters. However, less advanced protein-calorie malnutrition occurs among adults, particularly during the " hungry season ", and among women as a result of continuous maternal depletion.

Throughout the world, the elderly are susceptible to lesser degrees of protein-calorie malnutrition, as well as to vitamin deficiencies, because of lack of teeth, diminished earning power, solitude, inability to cultivate the land and collect or cook foods, diminished appetite, and apathy. The assessment of protein-calorie malnutrition in the elderly is complicated by uncertainty as to the " physiological " range of changes in weight, muscle atrophy, skin changes, and the decline in height associated with ageing (Trotter & Gleser, 1951).

Degrees of undernutrition can be expressed in four levels underweight (90%-80%, 80%-71%, 70%-61%, and 60% and lower), with recorded weights compared with " desirable " standards, or with previous weight levels in health, if these are known.

Meaning of measurements. Low body weights for heights may be related to a number of factors, e.g., a light bone structure. For practical purposes, however, they are principally a reflection of body thinness due to subnormal amounts of subcutaneous fat and muscle, the result either of poor development, or tissue wasting, or a combination of the two. Correction may be

---

[1] A clinical picture similar to that of kwashiorkor can be seen in adults, including oedema, dyspigmented hair and lightening in colour of the body skin, and can occur in association with chronic pancreatic damage, including calcification.

necessary to account for oedema or for grossly enlarged viscera (e.g., hepatomegaly) if present.

Calorie reserves are indicated by thickness of subcutaneous fat, usually measured, for convenience, at the triceps skin-fold (Skerlj, Brozek & Hunt, 1953); protein inadequacy is best reflected by thin musculature, due either to poor development or to wasting. This may be assessed by calculation of the arm-muscle circumference (Mason, Mundkur & Jacob, 1963).

The arm circumference is a simple measurement, requires no calculation, and provides a rough index of both protein and calorie reserves, probably with especial emphasis on protein stores as reflected by muscle tissue. This measurement has not been much used in nutritional assessment work among adults in developing regions, although it has been found to be of value in New Guinea (Bailey, 1963b). In the USA, Ohlson et al. (1956) found a relation between arm circumference and under-weightness in Michigan.

Overnutrition in adults

Certain diseases, including obesity, diabetes, hypertension, atheroma and caries, are associated with dietary patterns characterized by high intakes of calories, fat and cane sugar, although other factors undoubtedly come into play, such as genetic constitution, the psychological stress of urban life, amount of exercise, etc. Certainly it is in these communities that probably unphysiological increases in weight, subcutaneous fat, serum cholesterol and blood pressure occur with age.

Obesity, mainly associated with an excessive calorie intake, is widespread in children and adults in more privileged parts of the world. It affects a very small proportion of well-to-do persons in most countries. The cause is primarily over-eating. It results mainly from easy accessibility to foods, especially high-calorie fats, together with insufficient exercise. In some countries, obesity is culturally desired—in women as a mark of beauty, for example, among the Zulus (Abramson et al., 1961), or in either sex as a symbol of wealth and prestige, as in the rulers of ancient Hawaii (Jelliffe & Jelliffe, 1964).

Community surveys can use the chest/abdomen circumference ratio in males (Welham & Behnke, 1942), the weight-for-height measurements and the skin-fold thicknesses as screening tests. Abnormal levels are difficult to define, but Jolliffe (1962) suggests 10% over the " desirable " weight standard as a rough guide, if taken in conjunction with skin-fold measurements. Where subcutaneous fat is concerned, many authorities prefer a composite fat thickness, calculated by adding together results obtained at several sites. Jolliffe (1962) gives figures for combined readings from the triceps, subscapular and lateral chest sites. As a useful approximation, Mayer (1959) suggests that men should be considered obese if the triceps skin-fold exceeds 15 mm, and women if it exceeds 25 mm.

15

Obesity appears to be associated with a reduced expectation of life, as well as with a higher risk of hypertension and diabetes (Society of Actuaries, 1959). Screening tests for these conditions in field studies consist of blood-pressure measurements carefully taken under standard conditions, and urine examinations for sugar with easily transportable, chemically impregnated paper test-strips.

The etiology of atheroma is complex. Multiple factors are undoubtedly present, and they differ from one community to another. Field surveys are usually based on estimations of serum-cholesterol levels and electro-cardio-graphic tracings taken with a portable machine from men between 40 and 60 years of age. Results have to be correlated with height, weight and blood-pressure determinations, and considered together with the incidence figures of coronary-thrombosis cases in the area and such autopsy findings from adult hearts as may be available in adjacent hospitals.

The interpretation of serum-cholesterol levels is difficult, even though methods for comparing data from observers employing different techniques have been established. Levels can be raised or lowered in a short period by diets high in animal fat without in any way reflecting the presence or absence of any associated atheromatous deposits in the coronary arteries. However, on these premises, and subject to the reservation that the incidence of atheroma in a population has to be related to various aspects of the whole way of life, the probability of a community having a high rate of atheroma is greater if serum-cholesterol levels are " high " (250 ± 30 mg/100 ml) rather than " low " (120 ± 30 mg/100 ml).

Caries is also a disease of multiple causation, including the fluoride content of the drinking-water, genetic susceptibility, nutritional status and the oral effect of the diet itself. In particular, studies based on methods of geographical pathology have disclosed, among different peoples, a con-siderable incidence in groups whose diet is high in refined sugars and flours, as distinct from communities subsisting on unprocessed, natural animal and vegetable foods containing little free sugar and considerable cellulose fibre and roughage.

Caries is currently a major problem in technically developed parts of the world. It is also increasingly prevalent in children and adults in every part of the world, mainly because of dietary changes so often associated with urbanization and the cultural modifications it entails.

Caries should receive attention in general nutrition surveys, at least to the extent of determining its prevalence. The procedures recommended by the WHO Expert Committee on Dental Health (1962) and Wilson et al. (1964) are guides to more intensive, specialized community surveys.

ACKNOWLEDGEMENTS

The writer is deeply indebted to many colleagues working in all parts of the world, and in particular to the following, who have generously given their time and advice in the preparation of this monograph at various times:

Dr E. Bridgforth, Department of Preventive Medicine, University of Texas; Dr G. Briggs, Department of Food Science, Berkeley; Dr J. Brozek, Department of Psychology, Lehigh University, Pennsylvania; Dr Anne Burgess, Edinburgh; the late Professor R. F. A. Dean, Infant Malnutrition Research Unit, Kampala; Professor John Gordon, Massachusetts Institute of Technology, Cambridge, USA; Professor P. György, Pediatric Research Department, Philadelphia; Dr Ruth Huenemann, Department of Nutrition, School of Public Health, Berkeley; Professor D. S. McLaren, Department of Clinical Nutrition, American University of Beirut; Dr D. Morley, Department of Nutrition, London School of Tropical Medicine and Hygiene; Dr M. Robinow, Yellow Springs, Ohio; Dr G. Wadsworth, Department of Nutrition, Queen Elizabeth College, London; Professor Helen Wallace, Department of Maternal and Child Health, Berkeley; Professor C. Woodruff, School of Public Health, Ann Arbor; and Dr W. Unglaub, Department of Nutrition, Tulane University.

Grateful acknowledgement is also made to the following persons and institutes for kindly giving permission to reproduce illustrations:

Dr J. M. Bengoa, Fig. 51 (a), 51 (b); Burroughs Wellcome Museum of Tropical Medicine, London, Fig. 23 (a); Dr W. J. Darby, Vanderbilt University, Plates III A, IV C, IV D; Department of Pathology, University of Hong Kong, Fig. 27 and 29; Dr R. Duckworth, Dental School, London Hospital Medical College, Fig. 13, 14 and 15; FAO, Rome, Fig. 3, 45 (a), 45 (b), 52, 54 (c) and 55; Dr T. Gillmann, Fig. 2, 23 (b), and 24 (a); Professor D. Hubble, Birmingham University, Fig. 26; ICNND, Washington, Plates I A, II C and IV A and Fig. 6, 47 (a), 47 (b) and 48; INCAP, Guatemala, Fig. 11 and 12; Dr F. Lowenstein, Plates I C, III B and IV B; Dr D. McLaren, Plates II A and II B and Fig. 8, 9 and 10; National Institutes of Health, Washington, Plates III C and III D; Dr H. A. P. C. Oomen, Fig. 31; Professor B. S. Platt, Fig. 25; Dr G. Shaper, Fig. 1 (a), 20 and 30; UNICEF, New York, Fig. 45 (d); and Professor O. Wolff, Fig. 28.

The author is also very appreciative of the assistance given to him by the ICNND (Inter-departmental Committee on Nutrition for National Development) and would like to thank Dr A. Schaefer, Executive Director, and his colleagues for much valuable guidance, especially concerning questions of biochemical tests and anthropometric standards.

As will be apparent to the reader, the monograph is an elaboration of recommendations put forward by the 1963 WHO Expert Committee on the Medical Assessment of Nutrition, and is based in large measure on views put forward at this meeting. The author would then like to acknowledge his indebtedness to his fellow committee members and participants—Dr G. Arroyave, INCAP, Guatemala; Professor J. F. Brock, Department of Medicine, Cape Town; Dr D. M. Hegsted, Department of Nutrition, Harvard School of Public Health; Dr B. N. Nicol, Nutrition Division, FAO, Rome; Dr V. N. Patwardhan, Nutrition, WHO, Geneva; Dr A. Raoult, Marseilles; Dr P. S. Venkatachalam, Nutrition Research Laboratories, Hyderabad, India; and Dr G. R. Wadsworth, Queen Elizabeth College, London.

Lastly, sincere thanks are due for direction and stimulus given to the writer by all members of Nutrition, WHO, Geneva—including Dr V. N. Patwardhan, Dr F. Lowenstein, Dr J. P. Dustin and especially Dr J. M. Bengoa.

LIST OF REVIEWERS

Dr G. Arroyave, Chief, Division of Physiological Chemistry, INCAP, Guatemala City, Guatemala.

Dr M. F. Barakat, Professor of Public Health and Nutrition, Kasr El Ainy Faculty of Medicine, Cairo, UAR.

Dr R. Vivanco Bergamín, Chief, Nutrition Department, Instituto de la Concepción, Madrid, Spain.

Professor J. F. Brock, Department of Medicine, University of Cape Town, Republic of South Africa.

Dr R. C. Burgess, Department of Public Health and Social Medicine, University of Edinburgh, UK.

Dr F. W. Clements, Institute of Child Health, University of Sydney, Australia.

Dr H. D. Cremer, Director, Institut für Ernährungswissenschaft der Justus Liebig-Universität, Giessen, Germany.

Professor W. J. Darby, Director, Division of Nutrition, Vanderbilt University School of Medicine, Nashville, USA.

Dr H. Dupin, Director, Organisme de Recherches sur l'Alimentation et la Nutrition Africaine, Dakar, Senegal.

Professor G. Ferro-Luzzi, Divisione della Nutrizione, Ministero della Sanità, Rome, Italy.

Dr C. Gopalan, Director, Nutrition Research Laboratories, Hyderabad, India.

Professor R. H. Gounelle, 5, rue de l'Observatoire, Paris, France.

Dr D. M. Hegsted, Department of Nutrition, Harvard School of Public Health, Boston, USA.

Professor G. J. Janz, Instituto de Medicina Tropical, Lisbon, Portugal.

Dr J. Masek, Institute of Human Nutrition, Prague, Czechoslovakia.

Professor H. A. P. C. Oomen, Institute of Tropical Hygiene, Amsterdam, Holland.

Dr T. Oiso, Chief, Nutrition Section, Ministry of Health and Welfare, Tokyo, Japan.

Professor B. S. Platt, Director, Human Nutrition Research Unit, London, UK.

Dr R. Rueda Williamson, Director, National Institute of Nutrition, Bogota, Colombia.

Professor N. S. Scrimshaw, Head, Department of Food Science and Nutrition, Massachusetts Institute of Technology, Cambridge, USA.

Dr W. H. Sebrell, Director, Institute of Nutrition Sciences, Columbia University, New York, USA.

Professor R. Tarjan, Director of Nutrition, Budapest, Hungary.

Dr J. Tremolières, Director, Laboratoire de Nutrition Humaine, Paris, France.

Dr J. Waterlow, Tropical Metabolism Research Unit, Jamaica, West Indies.

Dr Cicely D. Williams, 167a, Bedford Hill, London, UK.

Annex 1

GENERAL ANTHROPOMETRIC STANDARDS OF REFERENCE

(1) WEIGHT FOR AGE, BIRTH TO 60 MONTHS, SEXES COMBINED *

Age (months)	Weight (kg)					Age (months)	Weight (kg)				
	Standard	9 % standard	80 % standard	70 % standard	60 % standard		Standard	90 % standard	80 % standard	70 % standard	60 % standard
0	3.4	3.0	2.7	2.4	2.0	31	13.7	12.4	11.0	9.7	8.2
						32	13.8	12.5	11.1	9.8	8.3
						33	14.0	12.65	11.2	9.9	8.4
1	4.3	3.7	3.4	2.9	2.5						
2	5.0	4.4	4.0	3.4	2.9						
3	5.7	5.1	4.5	4.0	3.4	34	14.2	12.8	11.3	10.0	8.5
						35	14.4	12.9	11.5	10.1	8.6
4	6.3	5.7	5.0	4.5	3,8	36	14.5	13.1	11.6	10.2	8.7
5	6.9	6.2	5.5	4.9	4,2						
6	7.4	6.7	5.9	5.2	4,5	37	14.7	13.2	11.8	10.3	8.8
						38	14.85	13.4	11.9	10.4	8.9
7	8.0	7.1	6.3	5.5	4.9	39	15.0	13.5	12.05	10.5	9.0
8	8.4	7.6	6.7	5.9	5.1						
9	8.9	8.0	7.1	6.2	5.3	40	15.2	13.6	12.2	10.6	9.1
						41	15.35	13.75	12.3	10.7	9.2
10	9.3	8.4	7.4	6.5	5.5	42	15.5	13.9	12.4	10.8	9.3
11	9.6	8.7	7.7	6.7	5.8						
12	9.9	8.9	7.9	6.9	6.0	43	15.7	14.0	12.6	10.9	9.4
						44	15.85	14.2	12.7	11.05	9.5
13	10.2	9.1	8.1	7.1	6.2	45	16.0	14.4	12.9	11.2	9.6
14	10.4	9.35	8.3	7.3	6.3						
15	10.6	9.5	8.5	7.4	6.4	46	16.2	14.6	12.95	11,3	9.7
						47	16.35	14.7	13.1	11.4	9.8
16	10.8	9.7	8.7	7.6	6.6	18	16.5	14.8	13.2	11.5	9.9
17	11.0	9.9	8.9	7.8	6.7						
18	11.3	10.1	9.0	7.9	6.8	49	16.65	15.0	13.35	11.6	10.0
						50	16.8	15.2	13.5	11.75	10.1
19	11.5	10.3	9.2	8.1	7.0	51	16.95	15.3	13.65	11.9	10.2
20	11.7	10.5	9.4	8.2	7.1						
21	11.9	10.7	9.6	8.3	7.2	52	17.1	15.45	13.8	12.0	10.3
						53	17.25	15.6	13.9	12.1	10.4
22	12.05	10.9	9.7	8.4	7.3	54	17.4	15.7	14.0	12.2	10.5
23	12.2	11.1	9.8	8.6	7.4						
24	12.4	11.2	9.9	8.7	7.5	55	17.6	15.85	14.2	12.3	00.6
						56	17.7	16.0	14.3	12.4	10.7
25	12.6	11.4	10.1	8.9	7.6	57	17.9	16.15	14.4	12.6	10.75
26	12.7	11.6	10.3	9.0	7.7						
27	12.9	11.8	10.5	9.2	7.8	58	18.05	16.3	14.5	12.7	10.8
						59	18.25	16.4	14.6	12.8	10.9
28	13.1	12.0	10.6	9.3	7.9	60	18.4	16.5	14.7	12.9	11.0
29	13.3	12.1	10.7	9.4	8.0						
30	13.5	12.2	10.8	9.5	8.1						

* Values derived from Harvard Standards—Stuart & Stevenson (1959).

(2) LENGTH FOR AGE, BIRTH TO 60 MONTHS, SEXES COMBINED*

Age (months)	Length (cm)				
	Standard	90 % standard	80 % standard	70 % standard	60 % standard
0	50.4	45.4	40.3	35.3	30.2
1	54.8	48.7	43.3	38.3	32.5
2	58.0	51.7	46.2	40.5	34.5
3	60.0	54.0	48.0	42.0	36.0
4	62.3	56.3	49.5	43.3	37.3
5	64.4	58.1	51.1	44.8	38.5
6	65.8	59.2	52.6	46.1	39.5
7	67.6	60.7	54.1	47.2	40.5
8	69.2	62.0	55.3	48.3	41.5
9	70.7	63.6	56.5	49.5	42.4
10	72.2	64.9	57.7	50.4	43.2
11	73.5	66.0	58.8	51.3	44.1
12	74.7	67.2	59.8	52.3	44.8
13	76.0	68.3	60.7	53.1	45.4
14	77.1	69.3	61.6	54.0	46.2
15	78.1	70.3	62.4	54.6	46.8
16	79.3	71.3	63.3	55.4	47.5
17	80.5	72.3	64.2	56.3	48.2
18	81.4	73.2	65.1	57.0	48.8
19	82.7	74.2	65.8	57.7	49.4
20	83.5	75.1	66.9	58.4	50.0
21	84.4	76.0	67.4	59.0	50.7
22	85.4	76.9	68.3	59.7	51.3
23	86.3	77.7	68.9	60.2	51.8
24	87.1	78.4	69.6	60.9	52.2
25	88.0	79.1	70.3	61.2	52.7
26	88.8	80.0	71.0	62.0	53.3
27	89.7	80.7	71.5	62.7	53.8
28	90.4	81.3	72.2	63.2	54.2
29	91.3	82.0	72.8	63.7	54.7
30	91.8	82.6	73.4	64.2	55.1
31	92.6	83.2	74.0	64.7	55.5
32	93.3	83.7	74.6	65.2	56.0

(2) LENGTH FOR AGE, BIRTH TO 60 MONTHS, SEXES COMBINED (continued)

Age (months)	Length (cm)				
	Standard	90 % standard	80 % standard	70 % standard	60 % standard
33	94.0	84.4	75.1	65.7	56.3
34	94.7	85.0	75.7	66.2	56.7
35	95.3	85.7	76.3	66.7	57.2
36	96.0	86.4	76.8	67.2	57.6
37	96.6	87.0	77.3	67.6	58.0
38	97.3	87.5	78.0	63.1	58.3
39	97.9	88.0	78.4	68.6	58.7
40	98.4	88.5	78.9	69.0	59.2
41	99.1	89.1	79.3	69.4	59.5
42	99.7	89.7	79.7	69.8	59.8
43	100.3	90.3	80.2	70.3	60.2
44	101.0	90.9	80.7	70.7	60.5
45	101.6	91.5	81.3	71.1	60.9
46	102.1	92.0	81.7	71.5	61.2
47	102.7	92.6	82.1	72.0	61.7
48	103.3	93.0	82.6	72.3	62.0
49	103.8	93.6	83.2	72.7	62.3
50	104.5	94.0	83.6	73.1	62.7
51	105.2	94.5	84.0	73.4	63.1
52	105.7	95.1	84.4	73.8	63.5
53	106.2	95.6	84.9	74.3	63.8
54	106.8	96.1	85.4	74.7	64.1
55	107.3	96.5	85.7	75.0	64.4
56	107.9	96.8	86.0	75.3	64.7
57	108.2	97.2	86.3	75.7	64.9
58	108.5	97.5	86.7	75.9	65.1
59	108.7	97.7	86.9	76.1	65.2
60	109.0	98.0	87.1	76.2	65.3

* Values derived from Harvard Standards—Stuart & Stevenson (1959).

(3) WEIGHT FOR LENGTH, YOUNG CHILDREN, SEXES COMBINED, 52-108 cm IN LENGTH*

Length (cm)	Weight (kg)				
	Standard	90 % standard	80 % standard	70 % standard	60 % standard
52	3.8	3.4	3.0	2.7	2.3
53	4.0	3.6	3.2	2.8	2.4
54	4.3	3.9	3.4	3.0	2.6
55	4.6	4.1	3.6	3.2	2.7
56	4.8	4.3	3.8	3.4	2.9
57	5.0	4.5	3.9	3.5	3.0
58	5.2	4.7	4.2	3.6	3.1
59	5.5	4.9	4.4	3.8	3.3
60	5.7	5.1	4.6	4.0	3.4
61	6.0	5.4	4.8	4.2	3.6
62	6.3	5.7	5.0	4.4	3.8
63	6.6	5.9	5.3	4.6	3.9
64	6.9	6.2	5.5	4.8	4.1
65	7.2	6.5	5.8	5.0	4.3
66	7.5	6.8	6.0	5.3	4.5
67	7.8	7.0	6.2	5.5	4.7
68	8.1	7.3	6.5	5.7	4.9
69	8.4	7.6	6.7	5.9	5.0
70	8.7	7.8	7.0	6.1	5.2
71	9.0	8.1	7.2	6.2	5.3
72	9.2	8,3	7.4	6.4	5.5
73	9.5	8.5	7.6	6.6	5.6
74	9.7	8.7	7.8	6.8	5.8
75	9.9	9.0	8.0	6.9	5.9
76	10.2	9.2	8.3	7.1	6.1
77	10.4	9.4	8.3	7.2	6.2
78	10.6	9.5	8.5	7.4	6.4
79	10.8	9.7	8.6	7.5	6.5
80	11.0	9.9	8.8	7.7	6.6
81	11.2	10.1	9.0	7.8	6.7
82	11.4	10.3	9.1	8.0	6.8
83	11.6	10.4	9.2	8.1	6.9
84	11.8	10.6	9.4	8.3	7.1

(3) WEIGHT FOR LENGTH, YOUNG CHILDREN, SEXES COMBINED, 52-108 cm IN LENGTH
(continued)

Length (cm)	Weight (kg)				
	Standard	90 % standard	80 % standard	70 % standard	60 % standard
85	12.0	10.7	9.6	8.4	7.2
86	12.2	11.0	9.8	8.5	7.3
87	12.4	11.1	9.9	8.6	7.4
88	12.6	11.3	10.1	8.8	7.6
89	12.8	11.5	10.2	9.0	7.7
90	13.1	11.8	10.5	9.2	7.9
91	13.4	11.9	10.7	9.3	8.0
92	13.6	12.2	10.9	9.5	8.2
93	13.8	12.4	11.0	9.6	8.3
94	14.0	12.6	11.2	9.8	8.4
95	14.3	12.8	11.4	10.0	8.5
96	14.5	13.1	11.6	10.2	8.7
97	14.7	13.3	11.8	10.3	8.8
98	15.0	13.5	12.0	10.5	9.0
99	15.3	13.7	12.3	10.7	9.2
100	15.6	14.0	12.5	10.9	9.4
101	15.8	14.2	12.6	11.1	9.5
102	16.1	14.5	12.9	11.3	9.7
103	16.4	14.7	13.2	11.5	9.8
104	16.7	15.0	13.4	11.7	10.0
105	17.0	15.3	13.6	11.9	10.1
106	17.3	15.6	13.8	12.1	10.4
107	17.6	15.9	14.0	12.3	10.5
108	18.0	16.2	14.4	12.6	10.8

* Values derived from Harvard Standards—Stuart & Stevenson (1959).

(4) WEIGHT FOR HEAD CIRCUMFERENCE, YOUNG CHILDREN, SEXES COMBINED *

Head circumfer-ence (cm)	Weight (kg)				
	Standard	90 % standard	80 % standard	70 % standard	60 % standard
35.0	3.4	3.1	2.7	2.6	2.0
35.5	3.6	3.3	2.9	2.6	2.1
36.0	3.8	3.4	3.0	2.7	2.3
36.5	4.0	3.6	3.2	2.8	2.4
37.0	4.2	3.8	3.4	2.9	2.5
37.5	4.4	3.9	3.5	3.1	2.6
38.0	4.6	4.1	3.7	3.2	2.8
38.5	4.8	4.3	3.8	3.3	2.9
39.0	5.0	4.5	4.0	3.5	3.0
39.5	5.2	4.7	4.2	3.7	3.1
40.0	5.5	5.0	4.4	3.9	3.3
40.5	5.7	5.2	4.6	4.0	3.4
41.0	6.0	5.4	4.8	4.2	3.6
41.5	6.3	5.6	5.0	4.4	3.8
42.0	6.6	5.9	5.3	4.6	4.0
42.5	6.9	6.2	5.5	4.8	4.2
43.0	7.2	6.5	5.8	5.0	4.3
43.5	7.5	6.8	6.0	5.2	4.5
44.0	7.9	7.1	6.3	5.5	4.7
44.5	8.2	7.4	6.6	5.7	5.0
45.0	8.6	7.7	6.9	6.0	5.2
45.5	9.0	8.1	7.2	6.3	5.4
46.0	9.4	8.5	7.5	6.6	5.6
46.5	9.8	8.9	7.8	6.9	5.9
47.0	10.3	9.3	8.2	7.2	6.2
47.5	10.9	9.8	8.7	7.6	6.5
48.0	11.4	10.3	9.1	8.0	6.8
48.5	11.9	10.7	9.5	8.3	7.1
49.0	12.6	11.3	10.1	8.8	7.6
49.5	13.6	12.3	10.9	9.5	8.2
50.0	15.1	13.6	12.1	10.6	9.1

* Calculated from Table (1) of this Annex and Table 6 of the text.

(5) TRICEPS SKIN-FOLD, BIRTH TO 60 MONTHS, SEXES SEPARATE *

Age (months)	Triceps skin-fold (mm)									
	Standard		90 % standard		80 % standard		70 % standard		60 % standard	
	M	F	M	F	M	F	M	F	M	F
Birth	6.0	6.5	5.4	5.9	4.8	5.2	4.2	4.6	3.6	3.9
6	10.0	10.0	9.0	9.0	8.0	8.0	7.0	7.0	6.0	6.0
12	10.3	10.2	9.3	9.2	8.2	8.2	7.2	7.1	6.2	6.1
18	10.3	10.2	9.3	9.2	8.2	8.2	7.2	7.1	6.2	6.1
24	10.0	10.1	9.0	9.1	8.0	8.1	7.0	7.1	6.0	6.1
36	9.3	9.7	8.4	8.7	7.5	7.8	6.5	6.8	5.6	5.8
48	9.3	10.2	8.4	9.2	7.5	8.2	6.5	7.2	5.6	6.1
60	9.1	9.4	8.2	8.5	7.3	7.5	6.4	6.6	5.5	5.7

* Adapted from Hammond (1955a); Tanner & Whitehouse (1962).

(6) ARM CIRCUMFERENCE, 1-60 MONTHS, SEXES SEPARATE *

Age (months)	Arm circumference (cm)									
	Standard		90 % standard		80 % standard		70 % standard		60 % standard	
	M	F	M	F	M	F	M	F	M	F
1	11.5	11.1	10.3	10.0	9.2	8.9	8.0	7.8	6.9	6.7
2	12.5	12.0	11.2	10.8	10.0	9.6	8.7	8.4	7.5	7.2
3	12.7	13.3	11.4	12.0	10.2	10.6	8.9	9.3	7.6	8.0
4	14.6	13.5	13.2	12.1	11.7	10.8	10.2	9.4	8.8	8.1
5	14.7	13.9	13.2	12.5	11.7	11.1	10.3	9.7	8.8	8.3
6	14.5	14.3	13.1	12.9	11.6	11.5	10.2	10.0	8.7	8.6
7	15.0	14.6	13.5	13.2	12.0	11.7	10.5	10.2	9.0	8.8
8	15.5	15.0	14.0	13.5	12.4	12.0	10.9	10.5	9.3	9.0
9	15.8	15.3	14.2	13.7	12.6	12.2	11.0	10.7	9.5	9.2
10	15.8	15.4	14.2	13.8	12.6	12.3	11.1	10.8	9.5	9.2
11	15.8	15.5	14.3	14.0	12.7	12.4	11.1	10.9	9.5	9.3
12	16.0	15.6	14.4	14.0	12.8	12.5	11.2	10.9	9.6	9.4
15	16.1	15.7	14.5	14.1	12.9	12.5	11.3	11.0	9.7	9.4
18	15.7	16.1	14.1	14.5	12.5	12.9	11.0	11.3	9.4	9.7
21	16.2	15.9	14.6	14.3	13.0	12.7	11.4	11.1	9.7	9.6
24	16.3	15.9	14.7	14.4	13.0	12.8	11.4	11.2	9.8	9.6
27	16.6	16.4	15.0	14.7	13.3	13.1	11.7	11.5	10.0	9.8
30	16.4	16.4	14.8	14.8	13.1	13.1	11.5	11.5	9.9	9.8
33	16.4	16.1	14.8	14.5	13.1	12.9	11.5	11.3	9.8	9.7
36	16.2	15.9	14.6	14.3	13.0	12.7	11.3	11.1	9.7	9.6
39	16.9	17.4	15.2	15.7	13.5	14.0	11.8	12.2	10.1	10.5
42	16.5	16.3	15.0	14.7	13.2	13.1	11.6	11.4	9.9	9.8
45	16.7	16.8	15.0	15.1	13.4	13.5	11.7	11.8	10.0	10.1
48	16.9	16.9	15.2	15.2	13.5	13.5	11.8	11.8	10.1	10.2
51	17.2	16.8	15.5	15.1	13.8	13.4	12.0	11.7	10.3	10.1
54	17.5	16.6	15.7	15.0	14.0	13.3	12.2	11.7	10.5	10.0
57	17.2	16.8	15.5	15.1	13.8	13.4	12.1	11.7	10.4	10.1
60	17.0	16.9	15.3	15.2	13.6	13.5	11.9	11.8	10.2	10.1

* From Wolanski (personal communication, 1964).

(7) MID-ARM-MUSCLE CIRCUMFERENCE, 6-60 MONTHS, SEXES SEPARATE *

Age (months)	Mid-arm-muscle circumference (cm)									
	Standard		90 % standard		80 % standard		70 % standard		60 % standard	
	M	F	M	F	M	F	M	F	M	F
6	11.4	11.2	10.3	10.1	9.1	9.0	8.0	7.8	6.8	6.7
12	12.7	12.4	11.4	11.2	10.2	9.9	8.9	8.7	7.6	7.4
18	12.9	12.5	11.6	11.3	10.3	10.1	9.0	8.8	7.7	7.6
24	13.1	12.8	11.8	11.5	10.5	10.2	9.2	9.0	7.9	7.7
36	13.3	12.9	12.0	11.6	10.3	10.3	9.3	9.0	8.0	7.7
48	14.0	13.7	12.6	12.3	11.2	11.0	9.8	9.6	8.4	8.2
60	14.1	13.9	12.7	12.5	11.3	11.1	9.9	9.7	8.5	8.3

* Calculated from Tables (5) and (6) of this Annex.

(8) WEIGHT FOR HEIGHT FOR AGE, 6-19 YEARS, BOYS

Translated and extended from the Baldwin-Wood tables in the English system of measurement by B. T. Baldwin. Issued by the Iowa Child Welfare Research Station, State University of Iowa, September 1924 (Baldwin, 1925; Baldwin & Wood, 1923

Height (cm)	6 years	7 years	8 years	9 years	10 years	11 years	12 years	13 years	14 years	15 years	16 years	17 years	18 years	19 years	Height (cm)
97	*15.0														97
98	*15.1														98
99	*15.3														99
100	*15.5														100
101	*15.7														101
102	*15.9														102
103	*16.1														103
104	16.6														104
105	16.8	*16.8													105
106	17.0	*17.0													106
107	17.2	*17.2	*17.2												107
108	17.5	*17.6	*17.4												108
109	17.8	*17.9	*17.7												109
110	18.3	*18.4	*18.2												110
111	18.9	*18.9	*18.8												111
112	19.4	19.4	*19.4												112
113	19.7	19.7	19.7												113
114	20.0	20.0	*20.0												114
115	20.4	20.4	*20.4	*20.3											115
116	20.7	20.8	20.7	*20.6											116
117	21.1	21.5	21.1	*21.2											117
118	21.5	21.8	21.4	*21.4											118
119	21.9	21.9	21.8	*21.7											119
120	22.3	22.4	22.2	*22.2	*22.2										120
121	22.5	22.8	22.7	*22.7	*22.7										121
122	22.9	23.2	23.1	23.2	*23.2										122
123	23.4	23.6	23.6	23.6	*23.5										123
124	23.9	23.8	24.1	24.0	*23.8										124
125	24.3	24.3	24.5	24.4	24.2	*24.4									125
126	*24.6	24.9	24.9	24.9	24.8	*24.9									126
127	*25.0	25.3	25.3	25.3	25.4	*25.4	*25.4								127
128		25.9	25.9	25.7	25.9	*25.9	*25.9								128
129		26.4	26.5	26.2	26.4	26.4	26.4								129
130		26.9	27.0	26.7	26.8	27.0	26.9								130
131		27.2	27.4	27.3	27.3	27.5	*27.3								131
132		27.5	27.9	27.8	27.8	28.0	27.7								132
133		*28.0	28.4	28.4	28.3	28.5	28.3	*28.5							133
134		*28.5	28.9	28.9	28.8	28.9	29.0	*29.3							134
135			29.4	29.4	29.3	29.4	29.6	29.9							135
136			30.0	29.9	29.7	29.8	30.3	*30.3							136
137			30.6	30.4	30.2	30.2	30.9	*30.7							137
138			*30.9	30.8	30.9	30.8	31.3	31.2	*31.7						138
139			*31.2	31.1	31.5	31.5	31.9	31.8	*32.0						139

Height (cm)	1	2	3	4	5	6	7	8	9	10	11	12
140	*31.6	31.6	32.2	32.2	32.4	32.4	*32.5					
141	*32 1	32.3	32.9	32.8	32.9	33.2	*33.1					
142	*32.6	33.1	33.7	33.5	33.4	34.0	*33.7					
143		*33.6	34.1	34.2	34.1	34.7	34.5					
144		*34.1	34.4	35.0	34.7	35.2	35.5					
145		*3.56	34.9	35.7	35.4	35.8	36.3					
146		*3.63	35.7	36.2	36.2	36.5	36.9					
147		*3.40	36.5	36.7	36.9	37.1	37.4					
148			37.0	37.2	37.6	37.8	38.0	*35.3				
149			37.5	37.8	38.2	38.4	38.6	*35.8				
150			38.1	38.5	39.0	39.1	39.3	*36.3	39.2			
151			*38.7	39.2	39.5	39.7	40.0	*37.0	40.3			
152			*39.4	39.9	40.0	40.3	40.7	*37.7	41.5			
153				40.5	40.6	41.1	41.6	38.2	42.6			
154				41.0	41.4	41.9	42.5	38.7	43.7			
155				*41.5	42.1	42.7	43.4	39.3	44.8	*46.3		
156				*42.3	42.9	43.4	44.0	40.3	45.5	*47.2		
157				*43.2	43.8	44.1	44.7	41.3	46.3	48.1		
158				*44.0	44.6	44.9	45.5	42.1	47.3	49.2	*51.3	
159				*44.9	45.4	45.8	46.4	42.8	48.6	50.3	*52.6	
160				*45.8	46.2	46.7	47.4	43.5	49.8	51.5	53.9	*55.4
161					47.4	47.3	48.1	44.2	50.2	52.0	54.4	*55.9
162					48.7	48.0	48.8	44.9	50.6	52.5	54.9	*56.4
163					49.4	48.8	49.6	45.8	51.2	53.2	55.5	*57.0
164					*49.6	49.9	50.5	46.9	52.1	54.1	56.3	*57.7
165					*49.7	50.9	51.4	48.0	53.1	55.1	57.1	58.3
166						51.4	52.1	48.8	54.1	56.1	57.9	59.3
167						51.8	52.9	49.6	55.1	57.0	58.7	60.3
168						52.3	53.7	50.5	56.1	57.8	59.4	61.0
169						*53.1	54.7	51.4	57.1	58.5	60.0	61.4
170						*53.9	55.6	52.3	58.1	59.1	60.5	61.7
171							56.7	53.2	58.8	59.9	61.2	62.5
172							57.8	54.0	59.5	60.9	62.0	63.4
173							58.7	54.8	60.2	61.8	62.8	64.2
174							59.2	55.7	61.1	62.7	63.8	65.1
175							59.7	56.5	61.9	63.5	64.7	65.9
176							60.5	57.3	62.5	64.0	65.3	66.5
177							61.4	58.0	62.9	64.3	65.7	67.2
178							62.4	58.7	63.4	64.7	66.1	67.8
179							*63.3	59.6	64.5	65.4	66.6	68.4
180							*64.2	60.4	65.7	66.1	67.1	68.8
181								61.2	66.4	66.7	67.7	69.6
182								62.0	67.0	67.3	68.3	70.4
183								62.8	67.6	68.0	69.0	71.2
184								63.9	68.6	69.1	70.1	71.8
185								*68.2	69.5	70.3	71.3	72.5
186								*68.8	70.3	71.3	72.2	73.2
187								*69.3	71.0	72.3	73.1	73.8
188								*69.8	71.7	73.3	73.9	74.4

Starred (*) figures represent values based on theoretical computations rather than on exact averages. Age is taken at the nearest birthday, height at the nearest centimetre, weight at the nearest tenth of a kilogramme.

(9) WEIGHT FOR HEIGHT FOR AGE, 6-18 YEARS, GIRLS

Translated and extended from the Baldwin-Wood tables in the English system of measurement by B. T. Baldwin.
Issued by the Iowa Child Welfare Research Station, State University of Iowa, September 1924 (Baldwin, 1925; Baldwin & Wood, 1923)

Height (cm)	Weight (kg) 6 years	7 years	8 years	9 years	10 years	11 years	12 years	13 years	14 years	15 years	16 years	17 years	18 years	Height (cm)
100	15.3													100
101	15.7													101
102	16.0	*16.0												102
103	16.1	*16.1												103
104	16.3	*16.3												104
105	16.6	*16.6												105
106	16.8	*16.8												106
107	17.1	17.1												107
108	17.6	17.5												108
109	18.0	17.8												109
110	18.2	18.1	*18.2											110
111	18.4	18.5	*18.4											111
112	18.6	18.8	*18.6											112
113	19.2	19.3	*19.1											113
114	19.7	19.8	*19.7											114
115	20.2	20.1	20.2											115
116	20.6	20.3	20.8											116
117	21.0	20.5	21.3											117
118	21.4	21.1	21.5											118
119	21.8	21.8	21.8											119
120	22.3	22.3	22.2	*22.3	*22.3									120
121	22.7	22.7	22.7	*22.9	*22.9									121
122	23.1	23.1	23.1	23.2	23.4	*23.4								122
123	23.3	23.4	23.5	23.6	23.8	*23.7								123
124	23.4	23.7	23.8	24.2	24.1	24.0								124
125	23.7	24.1	24.3	24.7	24.6	*24.7								125
126	*24.2	24.4	24.8	25.2	25.3	25.8								126
127	*24.7	24.8	25.4	25.8	26.0	26.9	26.9							127
128		25.2	25.8	26.2	26.4	27.2	*27.1							128
129		25.7	26.2	26.6	26.7	27.5	*27.3							129
130		*26.3	26.7	27.0	27.1	27.9	27.3							130
131		*27.1	27.4	27.5	27.7	28.2	28.4							131
132		*27.8	28.1	28.0	28.2	28.6	29.5							132
133		*28.4	28.6	28.6	28.8	29.1	29.9							133
134		*28.9	29.1	29.2	29.5	29.6	30.3							134
135			29.6	29.8	30.1	30.1	30.7	*31.5						135
136			30.0	30.4	30.5	30.7	31.0	*31.9						136
137			30.4	31.0	31.0	31.3	31.4	*32.2						137

Height	C1	C2	C3	C4	C5	C6	C7	C8	C9	C10	C11
138		31.6	31.6	31.9	32.0	*32.8					
139		32.3	32.3	32.5	32.6	*33.4					
140	*30.9	32.9	32.9	33.1	33.2	34.1	*34.8				
141	*31.4	33.3	33.6	33.7	34.0	34.9	*35.6				
142		33.6	34.4	34.3	34.8	35.8	*36.5				
143		*34.2	35.1	35.0	35.5	36.3	*37.4				
144		*34.9	35.9	35.6	36.0	36.7	*38.4				
145			36.6	36.4	36.6	37.2	39.3	*41.1			
146			36.8	37.3	37.3	38.0	40.3	*42.0			
147			37.1	38.2	37.9	38.8	41.4	*42.8			
148			37.6	38.9	38.6	39.5	42.0	*43.5	*45.1		
149			38.2	39.5	39.2	40.3	42.5	*44.0	*45.5		
150			38.8	40.2	39.9	41.1	43.0	44.6	*45.9	*46.4	
151			*39.5	41.0	40.8	41.9	43.8	45.5	*46.8	*47.3	
152			*40.2	41.8	41.7	42.7	44.6	46.4	*47.7	48.1	
153				42.6	42.7	43.5	45.4	47.1	48.6	48.9	*49.9
154				43.4	43.8	44.2	46.2	47.6	49.4	49.7	50.7
155				44.0	44.8	45.0	47.0	48.1	50.2	50.4	51.4
156				*44.1	45.5	45.7	47.5	48.9	50.7	51.1	51.7
157				*44.2	46.2	46.5	48.1	49.8	51.1	51.8	52.0
158					47.0	47.4	48.7	50.5	51.4	52.2	52.4
159					47.9	48.3	49.2	51.0	51.7	52.5	52.7
160					48.9	49.2	49.8	51.5	51.9	52.8	53.1
161					*49.6	49.9	50.7	52.1	52.6	53.3	53.6
162					*50.3	50.6	51.5	52.7	53.2	53.7	54.0
163					*51.0	51.4	52.3	53.3	53.8	54.2	54.6
164					*51.7	52.2	53.2	53.7	54.3	54.8	55.3
165					*52.4	53.1	54.0	54.2	54.8	55.4	55.9
166						54.0	54.5	54.6	55.7	56.1	56.6
167						54.9	54.9	55.0	56.6	56.9	57.4
168						*55.6	55.5	55.7	57.4	57.6	58.2
169						*56.2	56.6	56.9	58.2	58.2	59.2
170						*56.8	57.6	58.0	58.9	58.9	60.1
171						*57.2	58.2	58.8	59.5	59.7	60.7
172						*57.8	58.7	59.5	60.0	60.7	61.1
173							59.1	60.1	60.5	61.4	61.6
174							*59.6	*60.5	*60.9	*61.8	*62.3
175							*60.0	*60.8	*61.2	*62.1	*62.9
176							*60.2	*61.0	*61.6	*62.5	*63.4
177							*60.4	*61.2	*62.0	*62.8	*63.7
178							*60.6	*61.5	*62.4	*63.2	*64.0
179							*60.9	*61.8	*62.7	*63.5	*64.2
180							*61.3	*62.2	*63.0	*63.9	*64.4

Starred (*) figures represent values based on theoretical computations rather than on exact averages. Age is taken at the nearest birthday, height at the nearest centimetre, weight at the nearest tenth of a kilogramme.

(10) WEIGHT FOR HEIGHT, BOYS *

Height (cm)	Weight (kg)				
	Standard	90 % standard	80 % standard	70 % standard	60 % standard
112	19.7	17.7	15.8	13.8	11.8
114	20.6	18.5	16.5	14.4	12.4
116	21.3	19.2	17.0	14.9	12.8
118	22.1	19.9	17.7	15.5	13.3
120	22.9	20.6	18.3	16.0	13.7
122	23.7	21.3	19.0	16.6	14.2
124	24.5	22.1	19.6	17.2	14.7
126	25.4	22.9	20.3	17.8	15.2
128	26.4	23.8	21.1	18.5	15.8
130	27.3	24.6	21.8	19.1	16.4
132	28.2	25.4	22.6	19,7	16.9
134	29.2	26.3	23.4	20.4	17.5
136	30.2	27.2	24.2	21.1	18.1
138	31.4	28.3	25.1	22.0	18.8
140	32.5	29.3	26.0	22.8	19.5
142	33.7	30.3	27.0	23.6	20.2
144	35.1	31.6	28.1	24.6	21.1
146	36.2	32.6	29.0	25.3	21.7
148	37.4	33.7	29.9	26.2	22.4
150	38.6	34.7	30.9	27.0	23.2
152	40.0	36.0	32.0	28.0	24.0
154	41.4	37.4	33.1	29.0	24.8
156	43.1	38.8	34.5	30.2	25.9
158	44.7	40.2	35.8	31.3	26.8
160	46.5	41.9	37.2	32.6	27.9
162	48.2	43.4	38.6	33.7	28.9
164	50.2	45.2	40.2	35.1	30.1
166	52.5	47.3	42.0	36.8	31.5
168	54.8	49.3	43.8	38.4	32.9
170	57.0	51.3	45.6	40,0	34.2
172	59.4	53.5	47.5	41.6	35.6
174	62.2	56.0	49.8	43.6	37.3

* Values derived from Harvard Standards—Stuart & Stevenson (1959).

(11) WEIGHT FOR HEIGHT, GIRLS *

Height (cm)	Weight (kg)				
	Standard	90 % standard	80 % standard	70 % standard	60 % standard
110	18.8	16.9	15.0	13.2	11.3
112	19,6	17.6	15.7	13.7	11.8
114	20.4	18.4	16.3	14.3	12.2
116	21.2	19.1	17.0	14.8	12.7
118	22.0	19.8	17.6	15.4	13.2
120	22.8	20.5	18.2	16.0	13.7
122	23.6	21.2	18.9	16.5	14.2
124	24.5	22.1	19.6	17.2	14.7
126	25.4	22.9	20.3	17.8	15.3
128	26.4	23.8	21.1	18.5	15.8
130	27.4	24.7	21.9	19.2	16.4
132	28.5	25.7	22.8	20.0	17.1
134	29.5	26.6	23.6	20.7	17.7
136	30.6	27.5	24.5	21.4	18.4
138	31.6	28.4	25.3	22.1	19.0
140	32.8	29.5	26.2	23.0	19.7
142	34.0	30.6	27.2	23.8	20.4
144	35.3	31.8	28.2	24.7	21.2
146	36.5	32.9	29.2	25.6	21.9
148	37.7	33.9	30.2	26.4	22.6
150	38.7	34.8	31.0	27.1	23.2
152	39.8	35.8	31.8	27.9	23.9
154	42.0	37.8	33.6	29.4	25.2
156	43.9	39.5	35.1	30.7	26.3
158	46.4	41.8	37.1	32.5	27.8
160	49.7	44.7	39.8	34.8	29.8
162	52.7	47.4	42.2	36.9	31.6

* Values derived from Harvard Standards—Stuart & Stevenson (1959).

(12) TRICEPS SKIN-FOLD, 5-15 YEARS, SEXES SEPARATE *

Age (years)	Triceps skin-fold (mm)									
	Standard		90 % standard		80 % standard		70 % standard		60 % standard	
	M	F	M	F	M	F	M	F	M	F
5	9.1	9.4	8.2	8.5	7.3	7.5	6.4	6.6	5.5	5.7
6	8.2	9.6	7.4	8.6	6.6	7.7	5.8	6.7	4.9	5.8
7	7.9	9.4	7.1	8.5	6.3	7.5	5.5	6.6	4.7	5.7
8	7.6	10.1	6.8	9.1	6.1	8.1	5.3	7.1	4.5	6.1
9	8.2	10.3	7.4	9.2	6.6	8.2	5.8	7.2	4.9	6.2
10	8.2	10.4	7.4	9.3	6.6	8.3	5.7	7.3	4.9	6.2
11	8.9	10.6	8.1	9.6	7.2	8.5	6.3	7.5	5.4	6.4
12	8.5	10.1	7.6	9.1	6.8	8.1	5.9	7.0	5.1	6.0
13	8.1	10.4	7.3	9.4	6.5	8.3	5.7	7.3	4.9	6.2
14	7.9	11.3	7.1	10.1	6.3	9.0	5.5	7.9	4.8	6.8
15	6.3	11.4	5.7	10.2	5.0	9.1	4.4	8.0	3.8	6.8

* Adapted from Hammond (1955a).

(13) ARM CIRCUMFERENCE, 6-17 YEARS, SEXES SEPARATE *

Age (years)	Arm circumference (cm)									
	Standard		90 % standard		80 % standard		70 % standard		60 % standard	
	M	F	M	F	M	F	M	F	M	F
6	17.3	17.3	15.6	15.5	13.8	13.8	12.1	12.1	10.4	10.4
7	17.8	17.8	16.0	16.0	14.2	14.2	12.5	12.5	10.7	10.7
8	18.4	18.4	16.5	16.6	14.7	14.7	12.9	12.9	11.0	11.1
9	19.0	19.1	17.1	17.2	15.2	15.3	13.3	13.4	11.4	11.5
10	19.7	19.9	17.7	17.9	15.8	15.9	13.8	13.9	11.8	11.9
11	20.4	20.7	18.4	18.6	16.3	16.5	14.3	14.5	12.2	12.4
12	21.2	21.5	19.1	19.3	16.9	17.2	14.8	15.0	12.7	12.9
13	22.2	22.4	20.0	20.2	17.7	17.9	15.5	15.7	13.3	13.4
14	23.2	23.2	20.9	20.9	18.6	18.5	16.3	16.2	13.9	13.9
15	25.0	24.4	22.5	22.0	20.0	19.5	17.5	17.1	15.0	14.6
16	26,0	24.7	23.4	22.2	20.8	19.7	18.2	17.3	15.6	14.8
17	26.8	24.9	24.1	22.3	21.4	19.9	18.8	17.4	16.1	14.9

* Adapted from O'Brien, Girshik & Hunt (1941).

(14) MUSCLE CIRCUMFERENCE, 6-15 YEARS, SEXES SEPARATE *

Age (years)	Muscle circumference (cm)									
	Standard		90 % standard		80 % standard		70 % standard		60 % standard	
	M	F	M	F	M	F	M	F	M	F
6	14.7	14.2	13.2	12.8	11.8	11.4	10.3	9.9	8.8	8.5
7	15.3	14.8	13.8	13.3	12.2	11.8	10.7	10.4	9.2	8.9
8	16.0	15.3	14.4	13.8	12.8	12.2	11.2	10.7	9.6	9.2
9	16.5	15.9	14.9	14.3	13.2	12.7	11.6	11.1	9.9	9.5
10	17.1	16.6	15.4	14.9	13.7	13.3	12.0	11.6	10.3	10.0
11	17.6	17.3	15.8	15.6	14.1	14.1	12.3	12.1	10.6	10.4
12	18.5	18.3	16.6	16.5	14.8	14.6	12.9	12.8	11.1	11.0
13	19.6	19.1	17.6	17.2	15.7	15.3	13.7	13.4	11.8	11.5
14	20.8	19.6	18.7	17.6	16.6	15.7	14.6	13.7	12.5	11.8
15	23.0	20.8	20.7	18.7	18.4	16.6	16.1	14.6	13.8	12.5

* Calculated from Tables (12) and (13) of this Annex.

(15) WEIGHT FOR HEIGHT, ADULT MALES *

Weight ranges (kg), corresponding to the percentages given in the first column, for the heights shown

Percentage of standard weight	145 cm	146 cm	147 cm	148 cm	149 cm	150 cm	151 cm	152 cm	153 cm	154 cm	155 cm
50-54	26.0-28.5	26.2-28.7	26.5-29.0	26.8-29.4	27.0-29.6	27.3-29.9	27.5-30.2	27.8-30.5	28.1-30.8	28.3-31.1	28.6-31.4
55-59	28.6-31.1	28.8-31.4	29.1-31.7	29.5-32.0	29.7-32.3	30.0-32.6	30.3-32.9	30.6-33.3	30.9-33.6	31.2-33.9	31.5-34.3
60-64	31.2-33.7	31.5-34.0	31.8-34.3	32.1-34.7	32.4-35.0	32.7-35.4	33.0-35.7	33.4-36.1	33.7-36.4	34.0-36.7	34.4-37.1
65-69	33.8-36.3	34.1-36.6	34.4-37.0	34.8-37.4	35.1-37.7	35.5-38.1	35.8-38.4	36.2-38.9	36.5-39.2	36.8-39.6	37.2-40.0
70-74	36.4-38.9	36.7-39.2	37.1-39.6	37.5-40.1	37.8-40.4	38.2-40.8	38.5-41.2	39.0-41.6	39.3-42.0	39.7-42.4	40.1-42.8
75-79	39.0-41.5	39.3-41.9	39.7-42.3	40.2-42.7	40.5-43.1	40.9-43.5	41.3-43.9	41.7-44.4	42.1-44.8	42.5-45.2	42.9-45.7
80-84	41.6-44.1	42.0-44.5	42.4-44.9	42.8-45.4	43.2-45.8	43.6-46.3	44.0-46.7	44.5-47.2	44.9-47.6	45.3-48.1	45.8-48.6
85-89	44.2-46.7	44.6-47.1	45.0-47.6	45.5-48.1	45.9-48.5	46.4-49.0	46.8-49.4	47.3-50.0	47.7-50.4	48.2-50.9	48.7-51.4
90-94	46.8-49.3	47.2-49.7	47.7-50.2	48.2-50.8	48.6-51.2	49.1-51.7	49.5-52.2	50.1-52.8	50.5-53.2	51.0-53.7	51.5-54.3
95-99	49.4-51.8	49.8-52.3	50.3-52.8	50.9-53.4	51.3-53.9	51.8-54.4	52.3-54.9	52.9-55.5	53.3-56.0	53.8-56.5	54.4-57.1
100-104	**59.1-54.4**	**52.4-55.0**	**52.9-55.5**	**53.5-56.1**	**54.0-56.7**	**54.5-57.2**	**55.0-57.7**	**55.6-58.3**	**56.1-58.9**	**56.6-59.4**	**57.2-60.0**
105-109	54.5-57.0	55.1-57.6	55.6-58.1	56.2-58.8	56.8-59.3	57.3-59.9	57.8-60.5	58.4-61.1	59.0-61.7	59.5-62.2	60.1-62.9
110-114	57.1-59.6	57.7-60.2	58.2-60.8	58.9-61.5	59.4-62.1	60.0-62.6	60.6-63.2	61.2-63.9	61.8-64.5	62.3-65.0	63.0-65.7

Percentage of standard weight	156 cm	157 cm	158 cm	159 cm	160 cm	161 cm	162 cm	163 cm	164 cm	165 cm	166 cm
50-54	29.0-31.8	29.3-32.2	29.7-32.5	30.0-32.9	30.3-33.2	30.6-33.5	30.9-33.9	31.2-34.2	31.5-34.5	31.8-34.9	32.0-35.1
55-59	31.9-34.7	32.3-35.1	32.6-35.5	33.0-35.9	33.3-36.2	33.6-36.6	34.0-36.9	34.3-37.3	34.6-37.7	35.0-38.0	35.2-38.3
60-64	34.8-37.6	35.2-38.0	35.6-38.5	36.0-38.9	36.3-39.3	36.7-39.6	37.0-40.0	37.4-40.4	37.8-40.8	38.1-41.2	38.4-41.5
65-69	37.7-40.5	38.1-41.0	38.6-41.4	39.0-41.9	39.4-42.3	39.7-42.7	40.1-43.1	40.5-43.5	40.9-44.0	41.3-44.4	41.6-44.7
70-74	40.6-43.4	41.1-43.9	41.5-44.4	42.0-44.9	42.4-45.3	42.8-45.8	43.2-46.2	43.6-46.7	44.1-47.1	44.5-47.6	44.8-47.9
75-79	43.5-46.3	44.0-46.8	44.5-47.4	45.0-47.9	45.4-48.3	45.9-48.8	46.3-49.3	46.8-49.8	47.2-50.3	47.7-50.7	48.0-51.1
80-84	46.4-49.1	46.9-49.7	47.5-50.3	48.0-50.9	48.4-51.4	48.9-51.9	49.4-52.4	49.9-52.9	50.4-53.4	50.8-53.9	51.2-54.3
85-89	49.2-52.1	49.8-52.7	50.4-53.3	51.0-53.9	51.5-54.4	52.0-54.9	52.5-55.5	53.0-56.0	53.5-56.5	54.0-57.1	54.4-57.5
90-94	52.2-54.9	52.8-55.6	53.4-56.3	54.0-56.9	54.5-57.4	55.0-58.0	55.6-58.8	56.1-59.1	56.6-59.7	57.2-60.3	57.6-60.7
95-99	55.0-57.8	55.7-58.5	56.4-59.2	57.0-59.8	57.5-60.4	58.1-61.0	58.9-61.6	59.2-62.2	59.8-62.8	60.4-63.4	60.8-63.9
100-104	**57.9-60.7**	**58.6-61.5**	**59.3-62.2**	**59.9-62.8**	**60.5-63.5**	**61.1-64.1**	**62.3-65.4**	**62.3-65.4**	**62.9-66.0**	**63.5-66.6**	**64.0-67.1**
105-109	60.8-63.6	61.6-64.4	62.3-65.2	62.9-65.8	63.6-66.5	64.2-67.2	64.8-67.8	65.5-68.5	66.1-69.1	66.7-69.8	67.2-70.3
110-114	63.7-66.5	64.5-67.3	65.3-68.1	65.9-68.8	66.6-69.5	67.3-70.2	67.9-70.9	68.6-71.6	69.2-72.3	69.9-73.0	70.4-73.6

	167 cm	168 cm	169 cm	170 cm	171 cm	172 cm	173 cm	174 cm	175 cm	176 cm
50-54	32.3-35.5	32.6-35.8	33.0-36.2	33.3-36.5	33.7-36.9	34.0-37.3	34.4-37.7	34.7-38.1	35.1-38.5	35.4-38.9
55-59	35.6-38.7	35.9-39.1	36.3-39.5	36.6-39.9	37.0-40.3	37.4-40.7	37.8-41.1	38.2-41.6	38.6-42.0	39.0-42.4
60-64	38.8-41.9	39.2-42.3	39.6-42.8	40.0-43.2	40.4-43.7	40.8-44.1	41.2-44.6	41.7-45.0	42.1-45.5	42.5-45.9
65-69	42.0-45.2	42.4-45.6	42.9-46.1	43.3-46.5	43.8-47.0	44.2-47.5	44.7-48.0	45.1-48.5	45.6-49.0	46.0-49.5
70-74	45.3-48.4	45.7-48.8	46.2-49.4	46.6-49.9	47.1-50.4	47.6-50.9	48.1-51.5	48.6-52.0	49.1-52.5	49.6-53.0
75-79	48.5-51.6	48.9-52.1	49.5-52.7	50.0-53.2	50.5-53.8	51.0-54.3	51.6-54.9	52.1-55.5	52.6-56.0	53.1-56.6
80-84	51.7-54.9	52.2-55.4	52.8-56.0	53.3-56.5	53.9-57.1	54.4-57.7	55.0-58.3	55.6-58.9	56.1-59.5	56.7-60.1
85-89	55.0-58.1	55.5-58.6	56.1-59.3	56.6-59.9	57.2-60.5	57.8-61.1	58.4-61.8	59.0-62.4	59.6-63.0	60.2-63.7
90-94	58.2-61.3	58.7-61.9	59.4-62.5	60.0-63.2	60.6-63.9	61.2-64.5	61.9-65.2	62.5-65.9	63.1-66.5	63.8-67.2
95-99	61.4-64.5	62.0-65.1	62.6-65.8	63.3-66.5	64.0-67.2	64.6-67.9	65.3-68.6	66.0-69.3	66.6-70.0	67.3-70.7
100-104	**64.6-67.8**	**65.2-68.4**	**65.9-69.1**	**66.6-69.9**	**67.3-70.6**	**68.0-71.3**	**68.7-72.1**	**69.4-72.8**	**70.1-73.6**	**70.8-74.3**
105-109	67.9-71.0	68.5-71.7	69.2-72.4	70.0-73.2	70.7-74.0	71.4-74.7	72.2-75.5	72.9-76.3	73.7-77.1	74.4-77.8
110-114	71.1-74.2	71.8-74.9	72.5-75.7	73.3-76.5	74.1-77.3	74.8-78.2	75.6-79.0	76.4-79.8	77.2-80.6	77.9-81.4

	177 cm	178 cm	179 cm	180 cm	181 cm	182 cm	183 cm	184 cm	185 cm	186 cm
50-54	35.8-39.3	36.2-39.7	36.7-40.2	37.1-40.7	37.5-41.2	37.9-41.6	38.3-42.0	38.9-42.4	39.1-42.9	39.5-43.3
55-59	39.4-42.9	39.8-43.4	40.3-43.9	40.8-44.5	41.3-44,9	41.7-45.4	42.1-45.8	42.5-46.3	43.0-46.8	43.4-47.3
60-64	43.0-46.5	43.5-47.0	44.0-47.6	44.6-48.2	45.0-48.7	45.5-49.2	45.9-49.7	46.4-50.2	46.9-50.7	47.4-51.2
65-69	46.6-50.1	47.1-50.6	47.7-51.2	48.3-51.9	48.8-52.4	49.3-53.0	49.8-53.5	50.3-54.0	50.8-54.6	51.3-55.2
70-74	50.2-53.6	50.7-54.2	51.3-54.9	52.0-55.6	52.5-56.2	53.1-56.8	53.6-57.3	54.1-57.9	54.7-58.5	55.3-59.1
75-79	53.7-57.2	54.3-57.9	55.0-58.6	55.7-59.3	56.3-59.9	56.9-60.6	57.4-61.1	58.0-61.8	58.6-62.4	59.2-63.1
80-84	57.3-60.8	58.0-61.5	58.7-62.2	59.4-63.0	60.0-63.7	60.7-64.4	61.2-65.0	61.9-65.6	62.5-66.3	63.2-67.0
85-89	60.9-64.4	61.6-65.1	62.3-65.9	63.1-66.7	63.8-67.4	64.5-68.2	65.1-68.8	65.7-69.5	66.4-70.2	67.1-70.9
90-94	64.5-68.0	65.2-68.7	66.0-69.6	66.8-70.4	67.5-71.2	68.3-71.9	68.9-72.6	69.6-73.4	70.3-74.1	71.0-74.9
95-99	68.1-71.5	68.8-72.3	69.7-73.2	70.5-74.1	71.3-74.9	72.0-75.7	72.7-76.4	73.5-77.2	74.2-78.0	75.0-78.8
100-104	**71.6-75.1**	**72.4-76.0**	**73.3-76.9**	**74.2-77.9**	**75.0-78.7**	**75.8-79.5**	**76.5-80.3**	**77.3-81.1**	**78.1-81.9**	**78.9-82.8**
105-109	75.2-78.7	76.1-79.6	77.0-80.6	78.0-81.6	78.8-82.5	79.6-83.3	80.4-84.1	81.2-84.9	82.0-85.9	82.9-86.7
110-114	78.8-82.3	79.7-83.2	80.7-84.3	81.7-85.3	82.6-86.2	83.4-87.1	84.2-87.9	85.0-88.9	86.0-89.8	86.8-90.7

* Adapted by permission from Society of Actuaries (1959)—modified for average frame size and nude measurements (ICNND, 1963; Bridgforth—personal communication, 1965).

(16) WEIGHT FOR HEIGHT, ADULT FEMALES *

Weight ranges (kg), corresponding to the percentages given in the first column, for the heights shown

Percentage of standard weight	140 cm	141 cm	142 cm	143 cm	144 cm	145 cm	146 cm	147 cm	148 cm	149 cm
50-54	22.5-24.6	22.7-24.9	23.0-25.2	23.2-25.4	23.5-25.8	23.8-26.1	24.0-26.3	24.3-26.7	24.6-27.0	24.9-27.3
55-59	24.7-26.9	25.0-27.2	25.3-27.5	25.5-27.8	25.9-28.1	26.2-28.4	26.4-28.7	26.8-29.1	27.1-29.5	27.4-29.8
60-64	27.0-29.1	27.3-29.4	27.6-29.8	27.9-30.1	28.2-30.5	28.5-30.8	28.8-31.1	29.2-31.5	29.6-31.9	29.9-32.3
65-69	29.2-31.4	29.5-31.7	29.9-32.1	30.2-32.4	30.6-32.8	30.9-33.2	31.2-33.5	31.6-33.9	32.0-34.4	32.4-34.8
70-74	31.5-33.6	31.8-34.0	32.2-34.4	32.5-34.7	32.9-35.2	33.3-35.6	33.6-35.9	34.0-36.4	34.5-36.8	34.9-37.3
75-79	33.7-35.9	34.1-36.3	34.5-36.7	34.8-37.1	35.3-37.5	35.7-37.9	36.0-38.3	36.5-38.8	36.9-39.3	37.4-39.8
80-84	36.0-38.1	36.4-38.5	36.8-39.0	37.2-39.4	37.6-39.9	38.0-40.3	38.4-40.7	38.9-41.3	39.4-41.8	39.9-42.3
85-89	38.2-40.3	38.6-40.8	39.1-41.3	39.5-41.7	40.0-42.2	40.4-42.7	40.8-43.1	41.4-43.7	41.9-44.2	42.4-44.8
90-94	40.4-42.6	40.9-43.1	41.4-43.5	41.8-44.0	42.3-44.6	42.8-45.1	43.2-45.5	43.8-46.1	44.3-46.7	44.9-47.3
95-99	42.7-44.8	43.2-45.3	43.6-45.8	44.1-46.3	44.7-46.9	45.2-47.4	45.6-47.9	46.2-48.5	46.8-49.1	47.4-49.7
100-104	**44.9-47.1**	**45.4-47.6**	**45.9-48.1**	**46.4-48.7**	**47.0-49.3**	**47.5-49.8**	**48.0-50.3**	**48.6-51.0**	**49.2-51.6**	**49.8-52.2**
105-109	47.2-49.3	47.7-49.9	48.2-50.4	48.8-51.0	49.4-51.7	49.9-52.2	50.4-52.7	51.1-53.4	51.7-54.1	52.3-54.7
110-114	49.4-51.6	50.0-52.2	50.5-52.7	51.1-53.3	51.8-54.0	52.3-54.6	52.8-55.2	53.5-55.8	54.2-56.5	54.8-57.2

Percentage of standard weight	150 cm	151 cm	152 cm	153 cm	154 cm	155 cm	156 cm	157 cm	158 cm	159 cm
50-54	25.2-27.6	25.5-28.0	25.8-28.3	26.0-28.5	26.3-28.8	26.6-29.1	26.9-29.5	27.7-29.8	27.5-30.1	27.8-30.5
55-59	27.7-30.2	28.1-30.5	28.4-30.8	28.6-31.1	28.9-31.4	29.2-31.8	29.6-32.1	29.9-32.5	30.2-32.9	30.6-33.2
60-64	30.3-32.7	30.6-33.1	30.9-33.4	31.2-33.7	31.5-34.1	31.9-34.4	32.2-34.8	32.6-35.2	33.0-35.6	33.3-36.0
65-69	32.8-35.2	33.2-35.6	33.5-36.0	33.8-36.3	34.2-36.7	34.5-37.1	34.9-37.5	35.3-37.9	35.7-38.4	36.1-38.8
70-74	35.3-37.7	35.7-38.2	36.1-38.8	36.4-38.9	36.8-39.3	37.2-39.8	37.6-40.2	38.0-40.7	38.5-41.1	38.9-41.6
75-79	37.8-40.3	38.3-40.7	38.9-41.1	39.0-41.5	39.4-41.9	39.9-42.4	40.3-42.9	40.8-43.4	41.2-43.9	41.7-44.3
80-84	40.4-42.8	40.8-43.3	41.2-43.7	41.6-44.1	42.0-44.6	42.5-45.1	43.0-45.6	43.5-46.1	44.0-46.6	44.4-47.1
85-89	42.9-45.3	43.4-45.8	43.8-46.3	44.2-46.7	44.7-47.2	45.2-47.7	45.7-48.3	46.2-48.8	46.7-49.3	47.2-49.9
90-94	45.4-47.8	45.9-48.4	46.4-48.9	46.8-49.3	47.3-49.8	47.8-50.4	48.4-51.4	48.9-51.5	49.4-52.1	50.0-52.7
95-99	47.9-50.3	48.5-50.9	49.0-51.4	49.4-51.9	49.9-52.4	50.5-53.0	51.5-53.6	51.6-54.2	52.2-54.8	52.8-55.4
100-104	**50.4-52.9**	**51.0-53.5**	**51.5-54.0**	**52.0-54.5**	**52.5-55.1**	**53.1-55.7**	**53.7-56.3**	**54.3-57.0**	**54.9-57.6**	**55.5-58.2**
105-109	53.0-55.4	53.6-56.1	54.1-56.6	54.6-57.1	55.2-57.7	55.8-58.4	56.4-59.0	57.1-59.7	57.7-60.3	58.3-61.0
110-114	55.5-57.9	56.2-58.6	56.7-59.2	57.2-59.8	57.8-60.3	58.5-61.0	59.1-61.7	59.8-62.4	60.4-63.1	61.1-63.8

	160 cm	161 cm	162 cm	163 cm	164 cm	165 cm	166 cm	167 cm	168 cm	169 cm
50-54	28.1-30.8	28.5-31.2	28.8-31.6	29.2-32.0	29.5-32.3	29.8-32.7	30.1-33.0	30.4-33.3	30.7-33.7	31.1-34.1
55-59	30.9-33.7	31.3-34.1	31.7-34.5	32.1-34.9	32.4-35.3	32.8-35.6	33.1-36.0	33.4-36.3	33.8-36.8	34.2-37.2
60-64	33.8-36.5	34.2-36.9	34.6-37.4	35.0-37.8	35.4-38.2	35.7-38.6	36.1-39.0	36.4-39.4	36.9-39.8	37.3-40.3
65-69	36.6-39.3	37.0-39.8	37.5-40.3	37.9-40.7	38.3-41.2	38.7-41.6	39.1-42.0	39.5-42.4	39.9-42.9	40.4-43.4
70-74	39.4-42.1	39.9-42.6	40.4-43.1	40.8-43.7	41.3-44.1	41.7-44.6	42.1-45.0	42.5-45.5	43.0-46.0	43.5-46.5
75-79	42.2-44.9	42.7-45.5	43.2-46.0	43.8-46.6	44.2-47.1	44.7-47.5	45.1-48.0	45.6-48.5	46.1-49.1	46.6-49.6
80-84	45.0-47.7	45.6-48.3	46.1-48.9	46.7-49.5	47.2-50.0	47.6-50.5	48.1-51.0	48.6-51.5	49.2-52.1	49.7-52.7
85-89	47.8-50.5	48.4-51.1	49.0-51.8	49.6-52.4	50.1-52.9	50.6-53.5	51.1-54.0	51.6-54.6	52.2-55.2	52.8-55.8
90-94	50.6-53.3	51.2-54.0	51.9-54.7	52.5-55.3	53.0-55.9	53.6-56.5	54.1-57.0	54.7-57.6	55.3-58.3	55.9-58.9
95-99	53.4-56.1	54.1-56.8	54.8-57.5	55.4-58.2	56.0-58.8	56.6-59.4	57.1-60.0	57.7-60.6	58.4-61.3	59.0-62.0
100-104	**56.2-59.0**	**56.9-59.7**	**57.6-60.4**	**58.3-61.2**	**58.9-61.8**	**59.5-62.4**	**60.1-63.1**	**60.7-63.7**	**61.4-64.4**	**62.1-65.1**
105-109	59.1-61.8	59.8-62.5	60.5-63.3	61.3-64.1	61.9-64.7	62.5-65.4	63.2-66.1	63.8-66.7	64.5-67.5	65.2-68.3
110-114	61.9-64.6	62.6-65.4	63.4-66.2	64.2-67.0	64.8-67.7	65.5-68.4	66.2-69.1	66.8-69.8	67.6-70.6	68.4-71.4

* Adapted by permission from Society of Actuaries (1959)—modified for average frame size and nude measurements (ICNND, 1963; Bridgforth—personal communication, 1965).

(17) TRICEPS SKIN-FOLD, ADULTS, SEXES SEPARATE

Sex	Triceps skin-fold (mm)				
	Standard	90 % standard	80 % standard	70 % standard	60 % standard
Male	12.5	11.3	10.0	8.8	7.5
Female	16.5	14.9	13.2	11.6	9.9

(18) ARM CIRCUMFERENCE, ADULTS, SEXES SEPARATE *

Sex	Arm circumference (cm)				
	Standard	90 % standard	80 % standard	70 % standard	60 % standard
Male	29.3	26.3	23.4	20.5	17.6
Female	28.5	25.7	22.8	20.0	17.1

* Adapted from O'Brien & Shelton (1941); Hertzberg et al. (1963).

(19) MUSCLE CIRCUMFERENCE, ADULTS, SEXES SEPARATE *

Sex	Muscle circumference (cm)				
	Standard	90 % standard	80 % standard	70 % standard	60 % standard
Male	25.3	22.8	20.2	17.7	15.2
Female	23.2	20.9	18.6	16.2	13.9

* Calculated from Tables (17) and (18) of this Annex.

Annex 2

FURTHER BIOCHEMICAL TESTS

Selected, more complicated biochemical tests, listed in Table 7 as category 2 tests, are given below. They may be indicated for research purposes.

Protein

J. Edozien (personal communication, 1965) has suggested that the total plasma alpha-amino acids may be assessed and that low levels suggest an inadequate dietary intake of protein.

The possibility of analysis of hair for amino-acid composition, including cystine content, has been suggested, as have various other chemical and physical tests (Ishikawa, Takanohashi & Wako, 1965; Godwin, 1962; Jelliffe & Welbourn, 1963).

Ascorbic acid

Actual tissue levels of ascorbic acid can be more easily measured in white blood cells (WBC), and it has been shown that disappearance of ascorbic acid from these cells closely parallels the development of scurvy (Lowry, 1952). The WBC ascorbic-acid level is, then, a good index of vitamin-C intake and tissue concentrations.

The dietary intake of ascorbic acid can also be assessed by measuring a 24-hour urinary excretion, or, in field circumstances, by estimating the ratio of ascorbic acid to creatinine in a random sample of urine, preferably fasting. Load tests will usually not be practicable in field surveys unless special circumstances permit careful observation of those tested for a period of 24 hours.

Thiamine

Various thiamine load tests have been described, but they are impracticable for field surveys. Similarly, diagnosin of thiamine deficiency by assessment of metabolic alterations that occur (e.g., increased blood levels of lactate and pyruvate) are of limited value in estimating mild degrees of deficiency, and are too elaborate for survey work. Recently, Brin (1962) has introduced a method that tests transketolase activity of a haemolysate of red blood cells. This appears to be a specific test for thiamine inadequacy, as it seems to be related to early metabolic change and not merely to thiamine intake. At present, this method is too complicated tor non-specialized laboratories and in any case awaits trial in nutrition survey work.

Riboflavin

Of various possible blood tests, the most consistent and significant appears to be the red blood cell (RBC) riboflavin content. Deficient groups showed values of 10.0-13.1 mcg/100 ml, and those with an adequate ribo-flavin intake 20.2-27.6 mcg (Bessey, Horwitt & Love, 1956). For usual field purposes, this test is too complicated, and standards for children are not known.

Similarly, load tests have been used for evaluating riboflavin nutrition, and the four-hour urinary excretion following parenteral administration of 1 mg of the vitamin has been advocated. As with other load tests, it cannot, for practical reasons, have wide application in rural surveys.

Niacin

Load tests have been employed to assess the state of niacin nutrition. Thus, 10 mg of niacinamide may be given by mouth followed by urine collection for 12 hours. These tests are aimed at estimating the state of tissue depletion, but are impracticable under field conditions.

Iron and folates

In more elaborate haematological surveys, the serum iron may be estimated, and in iron-deficiency anaemia will be found to be below 50 mcg per 100 ml. According to a recent study, the percentage saturation of plasma transferrin may be a most useful test for iron deficiency—a figure of 16% or less indicating an inadequate supply of iron being delivered to the marrow (Bainton & Finch, 1964). However, in young children, due attention must be paid to the fact that hypoproteinaemia may result in a decrease of the specific iron-binding beta-globulin.

Serum levels of B_{12} and *L. casei* folate levels may be required (see tables below).

SERUM VITAMIN B_{12} CONCENTRATIONS IN MAN

Serum B_{12} level [a] ($\mu\mu$g/ml)	Interpretation
200-960	Range in normal healthy subjects
140-200	Diagnostically indeterminate
80-140	Equivocal; in non-anaemic patients such levels probably indicate early B_{12} deficiency
<80	Levels in anaemic patients with B_{12} deficiency and in patients with neurological complications of B_{12} deficiency

[a] Assayed with *Euglena gracilis*.

INTERPRETATION OF SERUM *L. CASEI* FOLATE LEVELS

Level ($\mu\mu$g/ml)	Interpretation
<3	Folate deficiency
3-6	Probable folate deficiency
6-20	Normal
>25	Elevated

Iodine

In more detailed investigations, the urinary iodine in a urine sample can give an indication of dietary intake. Tests of thyroid function may also be carried out in special research circumstances, especially the PBI (protein-bound iodine). Follis (1964) has recently reported his own extensive results and commented on problems of interpretation.

REFERENCES

Abramson, J. H. (1959) Observations on the growth and maturation of Indian boys in Durban, South Africa. *Brit. J. prev. soc. Med.*, **13**, 67

Abramson, J. H., Gampel, B., Slome, C. & Scotch, N. (1961) Sex variations in the nutritional state of urban Zulu adults. *Amer. J. clin. Nutr.*, **9**, 217

André, J. & Holemans, K. (1955) Signification des cheveux roux chez le nourrisson noir du Kwange. *Ann. Soc. belge Méd. trop.*, **35**, 467

Archibald, R. M. (1945) *J. biol. Chem.*, **157**, 507

Arroyave, G. (1961) Biochemical evaluation of nutritional status in man. *Fed. Proc.*, **20**, 39

Arroyave, G., Jansen, A. A. J. & Torrico, M. Urinary urea: creatinine ratio as an indication of relative protein nutrition (in preparation)

Arroyave, G. & Wilson, D. (1961) Urinary excretion of creatinine of children under different nutritional conditions. *Amer. J. clin. Nutr.*, **9**, 170

Arroyave, G., Wilson, D., Couteras, C. & Behar, M. (1965) Alterations in serum concentration of vitamin A associated with the hypoproteinemia of severe protein malnutrition. *J. Pediat.*, **62**, 920

Asenjo, C. F. (1962) Variations in the nutritive values of foods. *Amer. J. clin. Nutr.*, **11**, 368

Ashcroft, M. T. & Lovell, H. G. (1964) Heights and weights of Jamaican children of various racial origins. *Trop. geogr. Med.*, **4**, 346

Ashcroft, M. T. & Lovell, H. G. (1965) Changes in mean size of children in some Jamaican schools. *W. Indian med. J.*, **14**, 48

Ashcroft, M. T., Lovell, H. G., George, M. & Williams, A. (1965) Heights and weights of infants and children in a rural community in Jamaica. *J. trop. Pediat.*, **11**, 56

Aykroyd, W. R. (1965) Nutrition in the Caribbean. *J. Hyg. (Lond.)*, **63**, 137

Aykroyd, W. R. & Doughty, J. (1964) *Legumes in human nutrition*, Rome, Food and Agriculture Organization (FAO nutritional studies, No. 19)

Aykroyd, W.R . & Krishnan, B. G. (1941) Infantile mortality in the beriberi area of the Madras presidency. *Ind. J. med. Res.*, **29**, 703

Bailey, K. V. (1962) Rural nutrition in Indonesia. VI—Field surveys of lactating women. *Trop. geogr. Med.*, **14**, 11

Bailey, K. V. (1963a) Dental development of New Guinean infants. *J. Pediat.*, **64**, 97

Bailey, K. V. (1963b) Nutritional status in east New Guinean populations. *Trop. geogr. Med.*, **15**, 389

Bainton, D. F. & Finch, C. A. (1964) *The diagnosis of iron deficiency anaemia. Amer. J. Med.*, **37**, 62

Bakwin, H. & McLaughlin, S. M. (1964) Secular increase in height—is the end in sight ? *Lancet*, **2**, 1195

Baldwin, B. T. (1925) Weight-height-age standards in metric units for American-born children. *Amer. J. phys. Anthrop.*, **8**, 1

Baldwin, B. T. & Wood, T. D. (1923) Weight-height-age tables. *Mother and Child*, July 23rd Supplement

Barness, L. A. & György, P. (1962) *Wld Rev. Nutr. Diet.*, **3**, 1

Beaton, G. H. (1964) Inter-relationships of nutrients. *Proc. Nutr. Soc.*, **23**, 30

Beaton, G. H., Arroyave, G. & Flores, M. (1964) Alternations in serum proteins during pregnancy and lactation in urban and rural populations in Guatemala. *Amer. J. clin. Nutr.*, **14**, 269

Bell, Q. (1964) Convergence: an accelerated longitudinal approach. *Child Develop.*, **24**, 145

Bengoa, J. M. (1940) *Medicina social en el medio rural venezolano*, Caracas, Litografía del comercio

Bengoa, J. M., Jelliffe, D. B. & Perez, C. (1959) Some indicators for the broad assessment of the magnitude of protein-calorie malnutrition in young children in population groups, *Amer. J. clin. Nutr.*, **7**, 714

Bessey, O. A., Horwitt, M. K. & Love, R. H. (1956) Dietary deprivation of riboflavin and blood riboflavin levels in man. *J. Nutr.*, **58**, 37

Best, E. W. R. (1953) *An improved caliper for measurement of skinfold thickness*, Chicago, US Army Medical Nutrition Laboratory, Report No. 113

Best, E. W. R. (1954) An improved caliper for measurement of skinfold thickness, *J. Lab. clin. Med.*, **43**, 967

Bigwood, E. J. (1939) *Directives pour les enquêtes sur la nutrition des populations*, Série de Publications de la Société des Nations, III Hygiène, III.I., Geneva

Bisht, D. & Singh, S. S. (1962) Pigmented bands on the nails: a new sign in malnutrition, *Lancet*, **1**, 507

Blankhart, D. M. (1958) The association of growth retardation and endemic enlarged liver in schoolchildren in the island of Sangir, Indonesia. *Trop. geogr. Med.*, **10**, 1

Blankhart, D. M. (1965) Measured food intakes in young children in Indonesia. *J. trop. Pediat.*, **8**, 18

Blaxter, K. L. (1957) The effects of defective nutrition during pregnancy in farm livestock. *Proc. Nutr. Soc.*, **16**, 52

Brin, M. (1962) Erythrocyte transketolase in early thiamine deficiency. *Ann. N.Y. Acad. Sci.*, **98**, 528

British Medical Journal, 1965, **1**, 645. Standardization in haemoglobinometry

Brožek, J. (1956) Physique and nutritional status of adult men. *Hum. Biol.*, **28**, 124

Burch, H. B., Bressy, O. A., Love, R. H. & Lorry, O. H. (1952) The determination of thiamine and thiamine phosphate in small quantities of blood and blood cells. *J. biol. Chem.*, **198**, 477

Burgess, A. & Dean, R. F. A., ed. (1962) *Malnutrition and food habits*, London, Tavistock Publications, p. 94

Burgess, H. J. L. & Dean, R. F. A. (1962) Protein-calorie malnutrition in Uganda. 1—General. *E. Afr. med. J.*, **39**, 357

Cannon, R. K. (1958) Hemoglobin standard. *Science*, **127**, 1376

Carpenter, K. J. & Kodicek, E. (1950) The fluorometric estimation of *N*-methylnicotinamide and its differentiation from coenzyme I. *Biochem. J.*, **46**, 421

Catzel, P. & Basson, H. (1956) Muehrcke's lines in kwashiorkor and other nutritional disorders. *S. Afr. J. Lab. clin. Med.*, **2**, 336

Chagula, W. K. (1960) The age of eruption of third permanent molars in male East Africans. *Amer. J. phys. Anthrop.*, **18**, 77

Chatfield, C. (1954) *Food composition tables—minerals and vitamins (for international use)*, Rome, FAO Nutritional Studies, No. 11

Cheraskin, E., Ringsdorf, W. M. & El-Ashiry, G. (1964) A lingual vitamin-C test. *Int. Z. Vitamin-forsch.*, **34**, 31

Clark, L. C. jr, Thompson, H. L., Beck, E. I. & Jacobsen, W. (1951) Excretion of creatine and creatinine by children. *Amer. J. Dis. Child.*, **81**, 774

Clements, E. B. (1953) Changes in mean stature and weight of British children in the past seventy years. *Brit. med. J.*, **2**, 897

Clements, F. W. (1961) Nutrition in infant and maternal feeding. *Fed. Proc.*, **20**, 165

Collis, W. R. F., Dema, I. & Lesi, F. E. A. (1962) Transverse survey of health and nutrition, Pankshim Division, Northern Nigeria. *W. Afr. med. J.*, **11**, 131

Collis, W. R. F., Dema, I. & Omolulu, A. (1962a) On the ecology of child health and nutrition in Nigerian villages. 1—Environment, population and resources. *Trop. geogr. Med.*, **14**, 140

Collis, W. R. F., Dema, I. & Omolulu, A. (1962b) On the ecology of child health and nutrition in Nigerian villages. 2—Dietary and medical surveys. *Trop. geogr. Med.*, **14**, 201

Committee on Nutritional Anthropometry of the Food and Nutrition Board of the National Research Council (1956) Recommendations concerning body measurements for the characterization of nutritional status. *Hum. Biol.*, **28**, 111

Consolazio, C. F., Johnson, R. E. & Marck, E. (1951) *Metabolic methods*, St Louis, C. V. Mosby

Consolazio, C. F., Johnson, R. E. & Pecora, L. J. (1963) *Physiological measurements of metabolic functions in man*, New York, McGraw-Hill

Crooks, J., Aboul-Kheir, S. A., Turnbull, A. C. & Hytten, F. E. (1964) The incidence of goitre during pregnancy, *Lancet*, **2**, 334

Cruickshank, E. K. (1947) Experiences in the military camp at Singapore. *Proc. Nutr. Soc.*, **5**, 121

Cruickshank, E. K. (1961) Neuromuscular disease in relation to nutrition. *Fed. Proc.*, **20**, suppl. 7, 345

Darby, W. J., McGanity, W. J., McLaren, D. S., Paton, D., Alemu, A. Z. & Medhew, A. M. G. (1960) Bitot's spots and vitamin-A deficiency. *Publ. Hlth Rep. (Wash.)*, **75**, 738

Darby, W. J. et al. (1953) The Vanderbilt cooperative study of maternal and infant nutrition. *J. Nutr.*, **51**, 539

Davidson, S. & Passmore, R. (1963) *Human nutrition and dietetics*, 2nd ed., Edinburgh, Livingstone

Dean, H. T. (1934) Classification of mottled dental enamel. *J. Amer. dent. Assoc.*, **21**, 1421

Dean, H. T. (1942) *The investigation of physiological effects by the epidemiological method.* In: *Fluorine and Dental Health*, Washington, D.C., American Association for the Advancement of Science

Dean, R. F. A. (1960) Treatment of kwashiorkor with moderate amounts of protein. *J. Pediat.*, **56**, 675

Dean, R. F. A. (1961) Kwashiorkor in Malaya: the clinical evidence, part I. *J. trop. Pediat.*, **7**, 3

Dean, R. F. A. (1964) *Kwashiorkor.* In: Gairdner, D. (ed.) *Recent advances in pediatrics*, London, Churchill, p. 234

Dean, R. F. A. (1965) Effects of malnutrition, especially of slight degree, on the growth of young children. *Courrier*, **15**, 73

Dean, R. F. A. & Jelliffe, D. B. (1960) The diagnosis and treatment of protein-calorie malnutrition. *Courrier*, **10**, 429

Dean, R. F. A. & Schwartz, R. (1953) The serum chemistry in uncomplicated kwashiorkor. *Brit. J. Nutr.*, **7**, 131

Dean, R. F. A. & Skinner, M. (1957) A note on the treatment of kwashiorkor. *J. trop. Pediat.*, **2**, 215

De Silva, C. C. (1964) *Common nutritional disorders of childhood in the tropics.* In: Levine, S. (ed.) *Advances in Pediatrics*, vol. 13, Year Book Medical Publishers

De Wijin, J. F. (1952) Errors in the evaluation of the nutritional condition of schoolchildren. *Doc. Med. geogr. trop. (Amst.)*, **4**, 273

Downs, E. F. (1964) Nutritional dwarfing, a syndrome of early protein-calorie malnutrition. *Amer. J. clin. Nutr.*, **15**, 275

Dugdale, A. E. & Edkins, E. (1964) Urinary urea/creatinine ratio in healthy and malnourished children. *Lancet*, **1**, 1062

Edwards, D. A. W., Hammond, W. H., Healy, M. J. R., Tanner, J. M. & Whitehouse, R. (1955) Design and accuracy of calipers for measuring subcutaneous tissue thickness. *Brit. J. Nutr.*, **9**, 133

Falkner, F. (1960) *The somatic investigations.* In: *Modern problems in pediatrics*, Basle and New York, S. Karger, p. 70

Falkner, F. (1962a) The physical development of children. *Pediat.*, **29**, 448

Falkner, F. (1962b) Some physical growth standards for white North American children. *Pediat.*, **29**, 467

FAO, Committee on Calorie Requirements (1957) *Calorie requirements*, Rome, Food and Agriculture Organization (FAO Nutritional Studies No. 15)

FAO, Committee on Protein Requirements (1957) *Protein requirements*, Rome, Food and Agriculture Organization (FAO Nutritional Studies No. 16)

Ferro-Luzzi, A. & Ferro-Luzzi, G. (1962) Study on skinfold thickness of schoolchildren in some developing countries. 1—Skinfold thickness of Libyan boys. *Metabolism*, **11**, 1064

Ferro-Luzzi, G. (1962a) Study on skinfold thickness of schoolchildren in some developing countries. 2—Skinfold thickness in Moroccan boys. *Metabolism*, **11**, 1072

Ferro-Luzzi, G. (1962b) Study on skinfold thickness of Polynesians. *Quad. Nutr.*, **22**, Nos. 5-6

Ferro-Luzzi, G. (1962c) Study on skinfold thickness of Mauritanian children. *Quad. Nutr.*, **22**, Nos. 5-6

Fish, J. S., Bartholomew, R. A., Colvin, E. D., Grimes, W. H. jr, Lester, W. M. & Galloway, W. H. (1960) The relationship of pregnancy weight gain to toxemia. *Amer. J. Obstet. Gynec.*, **78**, 743

Flores, M. (1962) Dietary studies for assessment of the nutritional status of populations in non-modernized societies. *Amer. J. clin. Nutr.*, **11**, 344

Flores, M. & García, B. (1960) The nutritional status of children of pre-school age in the Guatemalan community of Amatitlan. 1—Comparison of family and child diets. *Brit. J. Nutr.*, **14**, 207

Flores, M., García, B., Flores, Z. & Lara, M. Y. (1964) Annual patterns of family and children's diet in three Guatemalan Indian communities. *Brit. J. Nutr.*, **18**, 281

Folin, O. & Wu, H. (1919) A system of blood analysis: determination of creatinine and creatine, *J. biol. Chem.*, **38**, 98

Follis, R. H. (1964) Patterns of urinary iodine excretion in goitrous and non-goitrous areas. *Amer. J. clin. Nutr.*, **14**, 253

Food and Agriculture Organization (1964a) *Program of food consumption surveys*, Rome

Food and Agriculture Organization (1964b) *Bibliography of food consumption surveys*, Rome

Forbes, G. (1962) Methods for determining composition of the human body. *Pediat.*, **29**, 477

Ford, F. J. (1964) Can a standard for " malnutrition " in childhood be devised ? *J. trop. Pediat.*, **10**, 47

Foster, G. M. (1952) Relationships between theoretical and applied anthropology: a public health program analysis. *Hum. Org.*, **11**, 5

Foster, G. M. (1966) *Social anthropology and nutrition of the pre-school child.* In: *Proceedings of the International Conference on the Prevention of Malnutrition in the Pre-School Child*, Washington, National Academy of Sciences (in press)

Frenk, S., Metcoff, J., Gomez, F., Ramos-Galvan, R., Cravioto, J. & Antonowicz, I. (1957) Intracellular composition and homeostatic mechanisms in chronic infantile malnutrition. 2—Composition of tissues. *Pediat.*, **20**, 105

Garn, S. M. (1957) Selection of body sites for fat measurements. *Science*, **126**, 550

Garn, S. M. (1962) Anthropometry in clinical appraisal of nutritional status. *Amer. J. clin. Nutr.*, **11**, 418

Garn, S. M. (1966) *Malnutrition and skeletal development in the pre-school child*. In: *Proceedings of International Conference on the Prevention of Malnutrition in the Pre-School Child*, Washington, National Academy of Sciences (in press)

Garn, S. M. & Clark, L. C. (1955) Creatinine weight coefficient as an index of obesity. *J. appl. Physiol.*, **8**, 135

Garn, S. M., Lewis, A. B. & Kerensky, R. S. (1964) *Genetic, nutritional and maturational correlates of dental development*, Yellow Springs, Ohio, Fels Research Institute

Garrow, J. S., Fletcher, K. & Halliday, D. (1965) Body composition in severe infantile malnutrition. *J. clin. Invest.*, **44**, 417

Gilles, H. M. (1964) *Akufo : an environmental study of a Nigerian village community*, Ibadan, University Press

Godwin, K. O. (1962) *Wld Rev. Nutr. Diet.*, **3**, 103

Goldsmith, G. A. (1959) *Nutritional diagnosis*, Springfield, Ill., Charles C. Thomas

Gomez, F., Galvan, R. R., Craviato, J. & Frenk, S. (1955) *Malnutrition in infancy and childhood with special reference to kwashiorkor*. In: Levine, S. (ed.) *Advances in Pediatrics*, New York, Year Book Publishers, vol. 7, p. 131

Gongora, J. & McFie, J. (1959) Malnutrition, malaria and mortality: the use of a simple questionnaire in an epidemiological study. *Trans. roy. Soc. Trop. Med. Hyg.*, **53**, 238

Gopalan, C. (1957) Malnutrition in infants and young children in India. *J. trop. Pediat.*, **3**, 3

Gopalan, C. (1961) *A report on some recent studies on protein malnutrition in India*. In: *Meeting protein needs of infants and children*, Washington, National Academy of Sciences (National Research Council Publication 843), p. 211

Gopalan, C. & Belvady, B. (1961) Nutrition and lactation. *Fed. Proc.*, **20**, 177

Gordon, J. E. (1963) Field epidemiology. *Amer. J. med. Sci.*, **246**, 132

Gordon, J. E., Chitkara, I. D. & Wyon, J. B. (1963) Weanling diarrhoea. *Amer. J. med. Sci.*, **245**, 129

Gordon, J. E., Jansen, A. A. J. & Ascoli, W. (1964) Measles in rural Guatemala. *J. Pediat.*, **66**, 779

Gounelle, H. (1952) Un nouveau signe de la dénutrition: parotidite par carence azotée élective. *Bull. Soc. méd. Hôp. Paris*, **22**, 866

Gounelle, H., Vallette, A. & Moine, M. (1942) Enquête sur le poids et la taille des écoliers parisiens en 1941. *Bull. Acad. nat. Méd. (Paris)*, **126**, 272

Graham, G. G. (1966) *Programs for combating malnutrition in the pre-school child in Chile*. In: *Proceedings of International Conference on the Prevention of Malnutrition in the Pre-School Child*, Washington, National Academy of Sciences (in press)

Graham, G. G. & Morales, E. (1963) Studies in infantile nutrition. 1—Nature of the problem in Peru. *J. Nutr.*, **79**, 479

Grandon, J. H., Lund, C. & Dill, D. (1940) Experimental human scurvy. *New Engl. J. Med.*, **223**, 353

Grech, P. & Latham, M. C. (1964) Fluorosis in the northern regions of Tanganyika. *Trans. roy. Soc. trop. Med. Hyg.*, **58**, 566

Greulich, W. W. (1957) A comparison of the physical growth and development of American-born and native Japanese children. *Amer. J. phys. Anthrop.*, **15**, 489

Grounds, J. G. (1964) Mortality and wastage rates for East African children in Kenya. *E. Afr. med. J.*, **41**, 333

Guest, E. M. & Siler, V. E. (1934) A centrifuge method for the determination of the volume of cells in the blood. *J. Lab. clin. Med.*, **19**, 757

Hammond, W. H. (1955a) Body measurements of pre-school children. *Brit. J. prev. soc. Med.*, **9**, 152

Hammond, W. H. (1955b) Measurement and interpretation of subcutaneous fat with norms for children and young adult males. *Brit. J. prev. soc. Med.*, **9**, 201

Hansen, A. L., Stewart, R. A., Hughes, G. & Söderhjelm, L. (1962) The relation of linoleic acid to infant feeding. *Acta paediat. (Uppsala)*, **5**, Suppl. 137, p. 1

Harland, P. S. E. G. & Brown, R. E. Tuberculin sensitivity following BCG vaccination in undernourished children (in preparation)

Harney, L. (1958) The effect of additional dietary skimmed milk on the nutrition of children of the colony of St Kitts-Nevis-Anguilla, using deaths from 1-4 years as indicator. *W. Indian med. J.*, **7**, 211

Harris, R. S. (1960) Reliability of nutrient analyses and food tables. *Amer. J. clin. Nutr.*, **11**, 377

Harrison, G. A., Weiner, J. S., Tanner, J. M. & Barnicot, N. A. (1964) *Human Biology*, London, Oxford University Press

Hassan, M. M. (1960) Kwashiorkor in Sudanese children: clinical notes. *J. trop. Pediat.*, **6**, 98

Helweg-Larsen, P. et al. (1952) Famine disease in German concentration camps: complications and sequelae. *Acta med. scand.*, supplement 247

Hertzberg, H. T. E., Churchill, E., Dupertius, C. W., White, R. M. & Damon, A. (1963) *Anthropometric survey of Turkey, Greece and Italy*, Oxford, Pergamon Press

Hollingsworth, D. F. (1961) Dietary determination of nutritional status. *Fed. Proc.*, **20**, 50

Holt, L. E., Snyderman, S. E., Norton, P. M., Roitman, E. & Finch, J. (1963) The plasma aminogram in kwashiorkor. *Lancet*, **2**, 1343

Hytten, F. & Leitch, I. (1964) *The physiology of human pregnancy*, Oxford, Oxford University Press

ICNND (1959a) *Alaska : an appraisal of the health and nutritional status of the Eskimo*, Washington, US Government Printing Office

ICNND (1959b) *Ethiopia : nutrition survey*, Washington, US Government Printing Office

ICNND (1960a) *Ecuador : nutrition survey*, Washington, US Government Printing Office

ICNND (1960b) *Republic of Viet Nam : nutrition survey*, Washington, US Government Printing Office

ICNND (1961a) *Chile : nutrition survey*, Washington, US Government Printing Office

ICNND (1961b) *Colombia : nutrition survey*, Washington, US Government Printing Office

ICNND (1961c) *Kingdom of Thailand : nutrition survey (preliminary)*, Washington, US Government Printing Office

ICNND (1962a) *Kingdom of Thailand : nutrition survey*, Washington, US Government Printing Office

ICNND (1962b) *Republic of Lebanon : nutrition survey*, Washington, US Government Printing Office

ICNND (1962c) *The Hashemite Kingdom of Jordan : nutrition survey*, Washington, US Government Printing Office

ICNND (1962d) *The West Indies : nutrition survey*, Washington, US Government Printing Office

ICNND (1963) *Manual for nutrition surveys*, Washington, US Government Printing Office

Ishikawa, K., Takanohashi, T. & Wako, H. (1965) Compulsory milk feeding and the cystine content of the hair in children as a subclinical standard of nutritional status. *Indones. J. Pediat.*, **2**, 535

Jackson, C. M. (1925) *The effects of inanition and malnutrition upon growth and structure*, Philadelphia, Blakiston

Jadhav, M., Webb, J. K. G., Vaishnava, S. & Baker, S. J. (1962) Vitamin B_{12} deficiency in Indian infants. *Lancet*, **2**, 903

Jelliffe, D. B. (1955a) Hypochromotrichia and malnutrition in Jamaican infants. *J. trop. Pediat.*, **1**, 25

Jelliffe, D. B. (1955b) *Infant nutrition in the subtropics and tropics*, Geneva (*World Health Organization : Monograph Series*, No. 29)

Jelliffe, D. B. (1957) Cultural blocks and protein malnutrition of early childhood in rural West Bengal. *J. Pediat.*, **20**, 128

Jelliffe, D. B. (1959) Protein-calorie malnutrition in tropical pre-school children: a review of recent knowledge. *J. Pediat.*, **54**, 277

Jelliffe, D. B. (1962) Culture, social change and infant feeding. *Amer. J. clin. Nutr.*, **10**, 19

Jelliffe, D. B. (1963) The incidence of protein-calorie malnutrition of early childhood. *Amer. J. publ. Hlth.*, **53**, 912

Jelliffe, D. B. (1964) *Cultural and anthropological factors in infant and maternal nutrition.* In: *Proceedings of Ross Laboratories Pediatric Research Conference on International Child Health*, Columbus, Ohio, Ross Laboratories, p. 52

Jelliffe, D. B. (1966) *Prematurity.* In: Stewart, D. & Lawson, J., ed., *Obstetrics and gynaecology in the tropics*. London, Arnold

Jelliffe, D. B. & Bennett, F. J. (1961) Cultural and anthropological factors in infant and maternal feeding. *Fed. Proc.*, **20**, 185

Jelliffe, D. B. & Bennett, F. J. (1962a) Worldwide care of the mother and newborn child. *Clin. Obstet. Gynec.*, **5**, 64

Jelliffe, D. B. & Bennett, F. J. (1962b) Cultural problems and technical assistance. *Children*, **9**, 171

Jelliffe, D. B., Bennett, F. J., Jelliffe, E. F. P. & White, R. H. R. (1964) Ecology of childhood disease in the Karamojong of Uganda. *Arch. environm. Hlth.*, **9**, 25

Jelliffe, D. B., Bennett, F. J., Stroud, C. E., Novotny, M. E., Karrach, H. A., Musoke, L. K. & Jelliffe, E. F. P. (1961a) Field survey of the health of Bachiga children in the Kayonza District of Kigezi, Uganda. *Amer. J. trop. Med. Hyg.*, **10**, 435

Jelliffe, D. B., Bennett, F. J., Stroud, C. E., Welbourn, H. F. & Jelliffe, E. F. P. (1963) The health of Acholi children. *Trop. geogr. Med.*, **14**, 33

Jelliffe, D. B., Bennett, F. J., White, R. H. R., Cullinan, T. R. & Jelliffe, E. F. P. (1962a) The children of the Lugbara. *Trop. geogr. Med.*, **14**, 33

Jelliffe, D. B., Bras, G. & Stuart, K. L. (1954) Kwashiorkor and marasmus in Jamaican infants. *W. Indian med. J.*, **3**, 43

Jelliffe, D. B. & Dean, R. F. A. (1959) Protein-calorie malnutrition in early childhood: practical notes. *J. trop. Pediat.*, **5**, 96

Jelliffe, D. B. & Jelliffe, E. F. P. (1960) The prevalence of protein-calorie malnutrition of early childhood in Haiti. *Amer. J. publ. Hlth.*, **50**, 1355

Jelliffe, D. B. & Jelliffe, E. F. P. (1961) The nutritional status of Haitian children. *Acta trop. (Basel)*, **18**, 1

Jelliffe, D. B. & Jelliffe, E. F. P. (1963) *The assessment of protein-calorie malnutrition of early childhood as a community problem.* In: *Proceedings of the Båstad Conference*, Swedish Nutrition Foundation, 1962

Jelliffe, D. B., Jelliffe, E. F. P., Garcia, L. & De Barrios, C. (1961b) The children of the San Blas Indians of Panama. *J. Pediat.*, **59**, 271

Jelliffe, D. B. & Maddocks, I. (1964) Ecologic malnutrition in the New Guinea Highlands. *Clin. Pediat.*, **3**, 432

Jelliffe, D. B., Symonds, B. E. R. & Jelliffe, E. F. P. (1960) The pattern of malnutrition in early childhood in Southern Trinidad. *J. Pediat.*, **57**, 922

Jelliffe, D. B. & Welbourn, H. F. (1963) *Clinical signs of mild moderate-protein calorie malnutrition of early childhood.* In: *Proceedings of the Båstad Conference*, Swedish Nutrition Foundation, 1962

Jelliffe, D. B., Woodburn, J., Bennett, F. J. & Jelliffe, E. F. P. (1962b) The children of the Hadza hunters. *J. Pediat.*, **50**, 907

Jelliffe, E. F. P. Malarial infection of the placenta and low birth weight (in preparation)

Jelliffe, E. F. P. & Jelliffe, D. B. (1964) Children in ancient Polynesian Hawaii. *Clin. Pediat.*, **3**, 604

Jolliffe, N. ed. (1962) *Clinical nutrition*, 2nd ed., New York, Harper and Bros.

Jolliffe, N., Goodhart, R. S., Archer, M., López, H. & Díaz, F. G. (1958) Nutrition status survey of the sixth grade school population in Cuba. *J. Nutr.*, **64**, 355

Jones, P. R. M. & Dean, R. F. A. (1956) The effects of kwashiorkor on the development of the bones of the hand. *J. trop. Pediat.*, **2**, 51

Journal of Tropical Pediatrics, 1963, **9**, 65, Pre-school protection programme (editorial article)

Jyothi, K. K., Dhakshayani, R., Swaminathan, M. C. & Venkatachalam, P. S. (1963) A study of the socio-economic diet and nutritional status of a rural community near Hyderabad. *Trop. geogr. Med.*, **15**, 403

Kark, S. L. & Steuart, G. W. (1962) *A practice of social medicine*, Edinburgh, Livingstone

Keys, A., Brozek, J., Henschel, A., Michelsen, O. & Taylor, H. L. (1950) *The biology of human starvation*, Minneapolis, University of Minnesota Press, vols. I and II

King, K. W., Faucauld, J., Fougere, W. & Severinghaus, E. L. (1963) Height and weight of Haitian children. *Amer. J. clin. Nutr.*, **13**, 106

Kinney, T. D. & Follis, R. H. (1958) Hypovitaminosis A in nutritional diseases. *Fed. Proc.*, **17**, 103

Kondakis, X. G., Maraelle, A. L. D. & Kazungu, M. (1964) Cross-sectional study of protein-calorie malnutrition in Tanganyika. *J. trop. Med. Hyg.*, **67**, 224

Krehl, W. A. & Hodges, R. E. (1965) The interpretation of nutritional survey data. *Amer. J. clin. Nutr.*, **17**, 191

Lange, K. O. & Brozek, J. (1961) A new model of skinfold calipers. *Amer. J. phys. Anthrop.*, **19**, 98

Laporte, M. (1946) Effect of war-imposed dietary limitations on growth of Paris school children. *Amer. J. Dis. Child.*, **71**, 244

Latham, M. C. (1964) Nutritional aetiology of a neuropathy found in Tanganyika. *Brit. J. Nutr.*, **18**, 129

Leitch, I. (1957) Changing concepts in the physiology of human pregnancy. *Proc. Nutr. Soc.*, **16**, 38

Leitch, I. (1963) The assessment of nutritional status in man. *Proc. Nutr. Soc.*, **22**, 47

Lewis, H. E., Masterton, J. P. & Ferres, H. M. (1958) Selection of representative sites for measuring changes in human subcutaneous tissue thickness. *Clin. Sci.*, **17**, 369

Lewis, S. M. & Carne, S. J. (1965) Clinical haemoglobinometry: an evaluation of a modified grey-wedge photometer. *Brit. med. J.*, **2**, 1167

Lowry, O. H. (1952) Biochemical evidence of nutritional status. *Physiol. Rev.*, **32**, 431

Lowry, O. H., Lopez, J. A. & Bessey, O. A. (1945) The determination of ascorbic acid in small amounts of blood serum. *J. biol. Chem.*, **160**, 609

Luyken, R. & Luyken-Koning, F. W. M. (1959) Nutrition research in the Windward Islands. 2—Medical examination of the population. *Trop. geogr. Med.*, **11**, 103

Luyken, R. & Luyken-Koning, F. W. M. (1960) Studies on the physiology of nutrition in Surinam. 3—Urea excretion. *Trop. geogr. Med.*, **12**, 37

Luyken, R. & Luyken-Koning, F. W. M. (1961) Studies on the physiology of nutrition in Surinam. 9—Somatometrical data. *Trop. geogr. Med.*, **13**, 123

McArthur, J. (1958) A new concept in microscope design for tropical medicine. *Amer. J. trop. Med.*, **7**, 382

McCance, F. R. (1964) Some effects of undernutrition. *J. Pediat.*, **65**, 1008

MacDonald, I. (1961) Ambient fat and depot fat iodine number in children. *Nature (Lond.)*, **192**, 393

McFie, J. & Welbourn, H. F. (1962) Effect of malnutrition in infancy on the development of bone, muscle and fat. *J. Nutr.*, **76**, 97

McGregor, I. A. (1964) The Sukuta project. *Trans. roy. Soc. trop. Med. Hyg.*, **58**, 483

McGregor, I. A., Billewicz, W. Z. & Thomson, A. M. (1961) Growth and mortality in children in an African village. *Brit. med. J.*, **2**, 1661

McLaren, D. S. (1956) A study of the factors underlying the special incidence of kerato-malacia in Oriya children in the Phulbani and Ganjam districts of Orissa, India. *J. trop. Pediat.*, **2**, 135

McLaren, D. S. (1963) *Malnutrition and the eye*, New York and London, Academic Press

McLaren, D. S. (1966) *Prevention of vitamin A deficiency in the pre-school child*. In: *Proceedings of International Conference on the Prevention of Malnutrition in the Pre-School Child*, Washington, National Academy of Sciences (in press)

McLaren, D. S., Ammoun, C. & Houri, G. (1964) The socio-economic background to marasmus in Lebanon. *J. méd. Liban.*, **17**, 85

McLaren, D. S., Kamel, W. W. & Ayyoub, N. (1965) Plasma amino-acids and the detection of protein-calorie malnutrition. *Amer. J. clin. Nutr.*, **17**, 152

McLaren, D. S., Oomen, H. A. P. C. & Escapini, H. (1966). The ocular manifestations of vitamin A deficiency in man. *Bull. Wld Hlth Org.*, **34**, 357

McLaren, D. S. & Read, W. W. C. (1962) Fatty acid composition of adipose tissue. *Clin. Sci.*, **23**, 247

Majaj, A. S., Dinning, J. S., Azzam, S. A. & Darby, W. J. (1963) Vitamin E responsive megaloblastic anaemia in infants with protein-calorie malnutrition. *Amer. J. clin. Nutr.*, **12**, 374

Mannheimer, E. (1966) *Programs for combating malnutrition in the pre-school child in Ethiopia*. In: *Proceedings of International Conference on the Prevention of Malnutrition in the Pre-School Child*, Washington, National Academy of Sciences (in press)

Marsden, P. D. (1964) The Sukuta project: a longitudinal study of health of Gambian children from birth to 18 months. *Trans. roy. Soc. trop. Med. Hyg.*, **58**, 455

Mason, E. D., Mundkur, V. & Jacob, M. (1963) Basal energy metabolism and heights, weights, arm skinfold and muscle of young Indian women in Bombay, with prediction standards for B.M.R. *Indian J. med. Res.*, **51**, 925

Massler, M. & Schour, I. (1944) *Atlas of the mouth and adjacent parts in health and disease*, Chicago, American Dental Association

Mayer, J. (1959) Obesity: diagnosis. *Postgrad. Med.*, **25**, 469

Mead, M., ed. (1953) *Cultural pattern and technical change*, Paris, Unesco

Meredith, H. V. (1941) Stature and weight of private-school children in two successive decades. *Amer. J. phys. Anthrop.*, **28**, 1

Mickelson, O. & Yamamoto, R. (1958) Methods for the determination of thiamine. *Meth. bioch. Anal.*, **6**, 191

Miller, F. J. W., Court, S. D. M., Walton, W. S. & Knox, E. G. (1960) *Growing up in Newcastle upon Tyne*, London, Oxford University Press

Mitchell, H. S. (1962) Nutrition in relation to stature. *J. Amer. diet. Ass.*, **40**, 52

Moncada, G. B. (1963) *Estudios sobre alteraciones del crecimiento y del desarrollo psicológico del síndrome pluricarencial o kwashiorkor*, Caracas, Editora Grafos

Mönckeburg, F. (1966) *Programs for combating malnutrition in the pre-school child in Chile*. In: *Proceedings of International Conference on the Prevention of Malnutrition in the Pre-School Child*, Washington, National Academy of Sciences (in press)

Money, G. L. (1959) Endemic neuropathies in Epe District of Southern Nigeria. *W. Afr. med., J.*, **8**, 3

Morell, D. B. & Slater, E. C. (1946) The fluorimetric determination of riboflavin in urine. *Biochem. J.*, **40**, 652

Morley, D. C. (1963) A health service for under fives in Nigeria. *Trans. roy. Soc. trop. Med. Hyg.*, **57**, 79

Morley, D. C. (1962) Measles in Nigeria. *Amer. J. Dis. Child.*, **103**, 230

Morley, D. C. & Knox, G. (1960) The birth weights of Yoruba babies. *J. Obstet. Gynaec. Brit. Cwlth*, **67**, 975

Morley, D., Woodland, M. & Martin, W. J. (1966) Whooping cough in Nigerian children. *J. Pediat.* (in press)

Muehrcke, R. C. (1956) The fingernails in chronic hypo-albuminaemia. *Brit. med. J.*, **1**, 1327

Musoke, L. K. (1961) Analysis of admissions to the padiaetric division, Mulage Hospital, 1959. *Arch. Dis. Childh.*, **36**, 305

Nelson, G. K. & Dean, R. F. A. (1959) The electroencephalogram in African children. *Bull. Wld Hlth Org.*, **21**, 779

Norris, T. (1949) *Dietary surveys—their technique and interpretation*, Washington, Food and Agriculture Organization (FAO Nutritional Studies No. 4)

O'Brien, R., Girshik, M. A. & Hunt, E. P. (1941) *Body measurements of American boys and girls for garment and pattern construction*, Washington, United States Department of Agriculture (Miscellaneous Publication No. 366)

O'Brien, R. & Shelton, W. C. (1941) *Women's measurements for garment and pattern construction*, Washington, United States Department of Agriculture (Miscellaneous Publication No. 454)

Ohlson, M. A., Biester, A., Brewer, W. D., Hawthorne, B. E. & Hutchinson, M. B. (1956) Anthropometry and the nutritional status of adult women. *Hum. Biol.*, **28**, 189

Oomen, H. A. P. C. (1955) The external pattern of malnutrition in Djarkarta toddlers. *Doc. Med. geogr. trop. (Amst.)*, **7**, 1

Oomen, H. A. P. C. (1957a) The relationship between liver size and diet in Papuan children. *Doc. Med. geogr. trop. (Amst.)*, **9**, 84

Oomen, H. A. P. C. (1957b) The incidence of xerophthalmia in Java in relation to age and sex. *Doc. Med. geogr. trop. (Amst.)*, **9**, 357

Oomen, H. A. P. C. & Malcolm, S. H. (1958) *Nutrition and the Papuan child*, Noumea, New Caledonia (South Pacific Commission, Technical Paper No. 118)

Oomen, H. A. P. C., McLaren, D. S. & Escapini, H. (1964) Epidemiology and public health aspects of hypovitaminosis A: a global survey of xerophthalmia. *Trop. geogr. Med.*, **4**, 271

Oomen, H. A. P. C., Prawirowinoto, R. & Latuasan, L. E. (1954) Food, health, and nutritional state in toddlers. *Berita Kementerian (Kesehatan, Indonesia)*, **3**, 3

Orr, J. B. & Gilks, J. L. (1931) Studies of nutrition: the physique and health of two African tribes. *Spec. Rep. Ser. med. Res. Coun. (Lond.)*, No. 155

Patton, R. C., Gardner, L. I. & Richmond, J. B. (1963) *Growth failure in maternal deprivation*, Springfield, Ill., Charles C. Thomas

Patwardhan, V. N. (1961) *Nutrition in India*, 2nd ed., Bombay, *Indian Journal of Medical Sciences*

Pearson, W. N. (1962) Biochemical appraisal of nutritional status in man. *Amer. J. clin. Nutr.*, **11**, 462

Perez, C. Scrimshaw, N. S. & Munoz, J. A. (1960) *Technique of endemic goitre surveys*. In: *Endemic goitre*, Geneva (*World Health Organization : Monograph Series*, No. 44)

Pett, L. B. & Ogilvie, G. F. (1956) *The Canadian weight height survey*. In: *Body measurements and human nutrition*, Detroit, Wayne University Press, p. 67

Phadke, M. V. & Pande, S. S. (1965) Pitfalls and difficulties in field studies in children. *Indian Pediat.*, **2**, 121

Pharaon, H. M., Darby, W. J., Shammout, H. A., Bridgforth, E. B. & Wilson, C. S. (1965) A longitudinal nutrition survey of infants and pre-school children in Jordan. *J. Trop. Pediat.*, **11**, suppl., p. 1

Phillips, P. G. (1954) The metabolic cost of common West African agricultural activities. *J. trop. Med. Hyg.*, **57**, 12

Picou, D., Alleyne, O., Waterlow, J. C. & Seakins, A. (1965) Hydroxyproline and creatinine excretion in protein depleted infants. *Biochem. J.*, **95**, 18

Platt, B. S. (1958) Malnutrition and the pathogenesis of disease. *Trans. roy. Soc. trop. Med. Hyg.*, **52**, 189

Platt, B. S. (1962) Tables of representative values of food commonly used in tropical countries. *Spec. Rep. Ser. med. Res. Coun. (Lond.)*, No. 302

Platt, B. S., Miller, D. S. & Payne, P. R. (1961) *Recent advances in human nutrition*, London, Churchill, chapter 28

Platt, B. S. & Stewart, R. J. C. (1962) Transverse trabeculae and osteoporosis in bones in experimental protein calorie deficiency. *Brit. J. Nutr.*, **16**, 483

Plough, I. C. (1962) Clinical evaluation of nutritional status under field conditions. *Amer. J. clin. Nutr.*, **11**, 413

Powell, R. C., Plough, I. C. & Baker, E. M. (1961) The use of nitrogen to creatinine ratios in random urine specimens to estimate dietary protein. *J. Nutr.*, **73**, 47

Prinsloo, J. G. (1964) The selection and recording of body measurements in nutrition work: review of the literature. *S. Afr. J. Lab. clin. Med.*, **10**, 11

Puyet, J., Downs, E. F. & Budeir, R. (1963) Nutritional and growth characteristics of Arab refugee children in Lebanon. *Amer. J. clin. Nutr.*, **13**, 147

Ramos-Galván, R. (1965) *Manual de Somatometría Aplicada a la Evaluación del Estado de Nutrición en los Niños*, Washington, Pan-American Health Organization

Ramos-Galván, R. (1966) *Malnutrition in the pre-school child in Mexico—prevalence and programs.* In: *Proceedings of International Conference on the Prevention of Malnutrition in the Pre-School Child*, Washington, National Academy of Sciences (in press)

Rao, K. S., Swaminathan, M. C., Swarup, S. & Patwardhan, V. N. (1959) Protein malnutrition in South India, *Bull. Wld Hlth Org.*, **20**, 603

Rao, M. V. R. (1961) Clinical evaluation of vitamin and mineral status in man. *Fed. Proc.*, **20**, 32

Raoul, Y. (1947) Microdosage de la vitamine C. *Bull. Soc. clin. Biol.*, **29**, 728

Raoult, A., Thomas, J., Thierry, A., Perrin, G. & Perrelton, G. (1957) Les parotidoses de malnutrition en A.O.F. *Bull. méd. A.O.F.*, **2**, 5

Raper, A. B. (1948) Pigmentation of the tongue. *E. Afr. med. J.*, **25**, 245

Reh, E. (1962) *Manual on household food consumption surveys*, Rome, Food and Agriculture Organization (FAO Nutritional Studies No. 18)

Robinow, M. & Jelliffe, D. B. The field assessment of protein-calorie malnutrition of early childhood in Busoga, Uganda (in preparation)

Robson, J. R. K. (1964a) Seasonal influence on height and weight increments of boys and girls in Tanganyika. *J. trop. Med. Hyg.*, **67**, 46

Robson, J. R. K. (1964b) Skinfold thickness in apparently normal African adolescents. *J. trop. Med. Hyg.*, **67**, 209

Rodger, F. C., Saiduzzafar, H., Grover, A. D. & Fazal, A. (1963) A reappraisal of the ocular lesion known as Bitot's spot. *Brit. J. Nutr.*, **17**, 475

Russell, A. L. (1961) The differential diagnosis of fluoride and non-fluoride enamel opacities. *Publ. Hlth Dent.*, **21**, 145

Schaefer, A. E. (1961) Sampling, organization and general plan for the evaluation of nutritional status in man. *Fed. Proc.*, **20**, 11

Schendel, H. E., Hansen, J. D. L. & Brock, J. F. (1960) A comparative study of biochemical indices used in evaluating dietary protein in children. *S. Afr. med. J.*, **34**, 791

Schorr, E. (1941) *Science*, **94**, 545

Scrimshaw, N. S. (1964) Ecological factors in nutritional disease. *Amer. J. clin. Nutr.*, **14**, 112

Scrimshaw, N. S., Taylor, C. E. & Gordon, J. E. (1959) Interactions of nutrition and infection. *Amer. J. med. Sci.*, **237**, 367

Scrimshaw, N. S., Taylor, C. E. & Gordon, J. E. Interactions of nutrition and infection, Geneva (*World Health Organization : Monograph Series* (in press)

Sebrell, W. H., Smith, S. C., Severinghaus, E. L., Delva, H., Reid, B. L., Olcott, H. S., Bernadotte, J., Fougere, W., Barron, G. P., Nicolas, G., King, K., Brinkman, G. L. & French, C. E. (1959) Appraisal of nutrition in Haiti. *Amer. J. clin. Nutr.*, **7**, 538

Sénécal, J. & Aubry, L. (1958) Etude des malnutritions frustes chez l'enfant africain. *Bull. méd. A.O.F.*, **3**, 9

Sénécal, J., Masse, G. & Moreigne, F. (1959) L'évolution dentaire de l'enfant africain durant les trois premières années de la vie. *Bull. Soc. méd. Afr. noire Langue franç.*, **4**, 483

Shevalev, V. E. (1962) *Cicatritial xerosis of the eye*, New York, Consultants Bureau

Simpson, I. A. & Chow, A. Y. (1956) The thiamine content of human milk in Malaya. *J. trop. Pediat.*, **2**, 69

Sinclair, H. M. (1948) The assessment of human nutriture. *Vitam. and Horm.*, **6**, 110

Sinclair, H. M. (1964) *The assessment of nutriture.* In: Witts, L. J., ed., *Medical surveys and clinical trials*, London, Oxford University Press

Skerlj, B., Brozek, J. & Hunt, E. E. (1953) Subcutaneous fat and age changes in body build and body form in women. *Amer. J. phys. Anthrop.*, **11**, 577

Smythe, P. M. (1958) Changes in intestinal bacterial flora and the role of infection in kwashiorkor. *Lancet*, **2**, 274

Society of Actuaries (1959) *Build and blood pressure study*, Chicago, vols. I and II

Spence, J., Walton, W. S., Miller, F. J. W. & Court, S. D. M. (1954) *A thousand families in Newcastle upon Tyne*, London, Oxford University Press

Squires, B. T. (1965) Differential staining of buccal epithelium smears as an indicator of poor nutritional status due to protein-calorie deficiency. *J. Pediat.*, **66**, 891

Standard, H. J. & Passmore, J. B. (1940) Weight and changes during pregnancy and the puerperium. *Amer. J. Obstet. Gynec.*, **39**, 928

Standard, K. L., Lovell, H. G. & Garrow, J. S. (1966) The validity of certain signs as indices of generalised malnutrition in young children. *J. trop. Pediat.* (in press)

Standard, K. L. & Miall, W. E. (1965) Studies on weight gain in the first year of life. *W. Indian med. J.*, **14**, 131

Standard, K. L., Wills, V. G. & Waterlow, J. C. (1959) Indirect indicators of muscle mass in malnourished infants. *Amer. J. clin. Nutr.*, **7**, 271

Stearns, G., Newman, J. K., McKinley, J. B. & Jeans, P. C. (1958) The protein requirements of children from one to ten years of age. *Ann. N.Y. Acad. Sci.*, **69**, 857

Stewart, A. & Acheson, R. (1964) *Child health and development.* In: Witts, L. J., ed., *Medical surveys and clinical trials*, London, Oxford University Press

Stewart, R. J. C. (1965) Bone pathology in experimental malnutrition. *Wld Rev. Nutr. Diet.*, **5**, 275

Stoch, M. B. & Smythe, P. M. (1963) Does undernutrition during infancy inhibit brain growth and subsequent intellectual development ? *Arch. Dis. Childh.*, **38**, 546

Stott, G. (1960) Anaemia in Mauritius. *Bull. Wld Hlth Org.*, **23**, 781

Stuart, H. C. & Stevenson, S. S. (1959) *Physical growth and development.* In: Nelson, W., ed., *Textbook of pediatrics*, 7th ed., Philadelphia, Saunders, pp. 12-61

Sundharagiati, B. & Harinasuta, C. (1964) Determination of haemoglobin in dry blood on filter paper. *Trans. roy. Soc. trop. Med. Hyg.*, **58**, 579

Swaminathan, M. C., Jyothi, K. K., Singh, R., Madhavan, S. & Gopalan, C. (1964) A semi-longitudinal study of growth of Indian children and related factors. *Ind. J. Pediat.*, **1**, 255

Swaroop, S. (1966) *Statistical methods in malaria eradication*, Geneva (*World Health Organization : Monograph Series*, No. 51)

Talbot, N. B. (1938) Measurement of obesity by the creatinine coefficient. *Amer. J. Dis. Child.*, **55**, 42

Tanner, J. M. (1959) The measurement of body fat in man. *Proc. Nutr. Soc.*, **18**, 148

Tanner, J. M. & Whitehouse, R. H. (1962) Standards for subcutaneous fat in British children. *Brit. med. J.*, **1**, 446

Thomson, F. A. (1960) Child nutrition: a survey of the Parit district of Parak, Federation of Malaya. *Bull. Inst. med. Res. Malaya*, No. 10

Toal, J. N. & Daniel, E. P. (1950) Simple digestion unit, with notes on the microdetermination of nitrogen by direct nesslerization. *J. Lab. clin. Med.*, **36**, 950

Trimmer, M. (1965) Child malnutrition in Jogjakarta, Java. *Trop. geogr. Med.*, **17**, 126

Trotter, M. & Gleser, G. (1951) The effect of ageing on stature. *Amer. J. phys. Anthrop.*, **9**, 311

Trowell, H. C., Davis, J. N. P. & Dean, R. F. A. (1954) *Kwashiorkor*, London, Arnold

Tukei, P. M. (1963) A calendar for the assessment of the ages of young Baganda child en. *J. trop. Med. Hyg.*, **65**, 42

Udani, P. M. (1963) Physical growth of children in different socio-economic groups in Bombay. *Ind. J. Child Hlth*, **12**, 593

United States, National Research Council (1964) *Recommended daily dietary allowances*, 6th rev. ed., Washington, National Academy of Sciences

Uttley, K. H. (1963) The death-rate in the age-group 1-4 years as an index of malnutrition in tropical countries. *Trans. roy. Soc. trop. Med. Hyg.*, **57**, 41

Van Niekerk, B. D. H., Reid, J. T., Bensadoun, A. & Paladines, O. L. (1963) Urinary creatinine as an index of body composition. *J. Nutr.*, **79**, 463

Venkatachalam, P. S. (1962a) Maternal nutritional status and its effect on the newborn. *Bull. Org. mond. Santé*, **26**, 193

Venkatachalam, P. S. (1962b) *A study of the diet, nutrition and health of the people of the Chimbu area, New Guinea Highlands*, Port Moresby, Territory of Papua and New Guinea, Department of Public Health (Monograph No. 42)

Venkatachalam, P. S., Belavady, B. & Gopalan, C. (1962) Studies on vitamin A: nutritional status of poor communities in India. *J. Pediat.*, **61**, 262

Voors, A. W. & Metselaar, D. (1958) The reliability of dental age as a yardstick to assess unknown calendar age. *Trop. geogr. Med.*, **10**, 175

Wadsworth, G. R. (1959) Nutritional factors in anaemia. *Wld Rev. Nutr. Diet.*, **1**, 149

Wadsworth, G. R. (1963) Nutrition surveys: clinical signs and biochemical measurements. *Proc. Nutr. Soc.*, **22**, 72

Walters, J. H. & McGregor, I. A. (1960) The mechanism of malarial hepatomegaly and its relationship to hepatic fibrosis. *Trans. roy. Soc. trop. Med. Hyg.*, **54**, 135

Waterlow, J. C. (1948) Fatty liver disease in infants in the British West Indies. *Spec. Rep. med. Res. Coun. (Lond.)*, No. 263

Waterlow, J. C. (1963) The assessment of marginal protein malnutrition. *Proc. Nutr. Soc.*, **22**, 66

Waterlow, J. C. & Mendes, C. B. (1957) The protein content of liver and muscle in malnourished human infants. *Nature (Lond.)*, **180**, 1361

Waterlow, J. C. & Scrimshaw, N. S. (1957) The concept of kwashiorkor from a public health point of view. *Bull. Wld Hlth Org.*, **16**, 458

Watson, E. H. & Lowrey, G. H. (1958) *Growth and development of children*, 3rd ed., Chicago, Year Book Medical Publishers

Welbourn, H. F. (1954) Signs of malnutrition among Baganda children attending child welfare clinics. *E. Afr. med. J.*, **31**, 332

Welbourn, H. F. (1956) The teeth of children attending Kampala child welfare clinics and schools. *E. Afr. med. J.*, **33**, 181

Welham, W. C. & Behnke, A. K. (1942) The specific gravity of healthy man. *J. Amer. med. Assoc.*, **118**, 498

Whitehead, R. G. (1964) Rapid determination of some plasma amino-acids in subclinical kwashiorkor. *Lancet*, **1**, 250

Whitehead, R. G. (1965) Hydroxyproline creatinine ratio as an index of nutritional status and rate of growth. *Lancet*, **2**, 567

Whitehead, R. G. & Dean, R. F. A. (1964) Serum amino-acids in kwashiorkor. 2—An abbreviated method of estimation and its application. *Amer. J. clin. Nutr.*, **14**, 320

WHO Expert Committee on Dental Health (1962) Standardization of reporting of dental diseases and conditions. *Wld Hlth Org. techn. Rep. Ser.*, **242**

WHO Expert Committee on Maternal and Child Health (1961) Public health aspects of low birth weight. *Wld Hlth Org. techn. Rep. Ser.*, **217**

WHO Expert Committee on Medical Assessment of Nutritional Status (1963) *Wld Hlth Org. techn. Rep. Ser.*, **258**

WHO Expert Committee on Nutrition and Infection (1965) *Wld Hlth Org. techn. Rep. Ser.*, **314**

WHO Expert Committee on Nutrition in Pregnancy and Lactation (1965) *Wld Hlth Org. techn. Rep. Ser.*, **302**

WHO Study Group on Iron Deficiency Anaemia (1959) *Wld Hlth Org. techn. Rep. Ser.*, **182**

Widdowson, E. M. & McCance, R. A. (1963) The effect of finite periods of undernutrition at different ages on the composition and subsequent development of the rat. *Proc. roy. Soc.*, **158**, 329

Wigglesworth, J. S. (1966) Foetal growth retardation. *Brit. med. Bull.*, **22**, 13

Williams, C. D. (1933) A nutritional disease of children associated with a maize diet. *Arch. Dis. Childh.*, **8**, 434

Williams, C. D. (1964) The Sukuta project. *Trans. roy. Soc. trop. Med. Hyg.*, **58**, 485

Wills, V. G. & Waterlow, J. C. (1958) The death-rate in the age-group 1-4 years as an index of malnutrition. *J. trop. Pediat.*, **3**, 167

Wilson, C. S., Schaefer, A. E., Darby, W. J., Bridgforth, E. B., Pearson, W. N., Combs, G. F., Leatherwood, E. C., Greene, J. C., Teply, L. J., Plough, I. C., McGanity, W. J., Hand, D. B., Kertesz, Z. I. & Woodruff, C. W. (1964) A review of methods used in nutrition surveys conducted by the Inter-departmental Committee on Nutrition for National Development (ICNND). *Amer. J. clin. Nutr.*, **15**, 29

Winter, S. T. (1954) The incidence of rickets in Israeli infants: a clinical and radiological study. *Acta med. orient. (Tel-Aviv)*, **13**, 91

Witts, L. J. ed. (1964) *Medical surveys and clinical trials*, London, Oxford University Press

Woodruff, A. W. & Pettitt, L. E. (1965) Plasma proteins in Tristan da Cunha islanders. *Trans. roy. Soc. trop. Med. Hyg.*, **59**, 356

Woodruff, C. W. (1966) *Analysis of the ICNND data in physical growth in the pre-school child.* In: *Proceedings of International Conference on the Prevention of Malnutrition in the Pre-School Child*, Washington, National Academy of Sciences (in press)

Woodruff, C. W. & Hoerman, K. (1960) Nutrition of infants and pre-school children in Ethiopia. *Publ. Hlth Rep. (Wash.)*, **75**, 724

Woolsey, T. D., Cochran, W. G., Mainland, D., Martin, M. P., Moore, F. E. & Patton, R. E. (1954) On the use of sampling in the field of public health. *Amer. J. publ. Hlth.*, **44**, 719

World Health Organization (1951) Prevention and treatment of severe malnutrition in times of disaster. *Wld Hlth Org. techn. Rep. Ser.*, **45**

INDEX

INDEX

Action, remedial, on results of survey data, 164, 174
Adults, nutritional assessment of, 214
  overnutrition, 217
  standards of reference, 214
  undernutrition, 215
Age assessment in nutritional anthropometry, 58
  average eruption time of deciduous teeth, 62
  average eruption time of permanent teeth, 63
  of young Baganda children, events-calendar for, 60, 61
  standard visual coding of deciduous dentition in, 59
Age considerations in analysis of survey data, 165
  abbreviation, 166
  estimation, 165
  groups, 166
  standards, 165
Age significance in clinical signs produced by nutrient deficiency, 42
Amino acids, test for imbalance of, 86
Anaemia, community surveys for, 93
  in kwashiorkor, 185
  in pregnant and lactating women, 211
  in young children, 207
Analysis of survey data, 164, 165
  age considerations, 165
  expression of results, 166
  grouping of results, 165
Anthropometry, 50-78
  age assessment, 58
  chest circumference, 70
  head circumference, 69
    weight for, in young children, 226
  in protein-calorie malnutrition in early childhood, 194
  linear measurements, 67
    height (or length), 68
    standards of reference, 69, 222-225, 230-235, 238-241
  photography in, 64
  radiological methods, 72

Anthropometry (*continued*)
  results of survey data, mathematical reporting of, 167
    presentation of, 173
    reporting in relation to standards of reference, 167
  soft-tissues, 71-78
    muscle, 75
      standards of reference, 78, 228, 229, 236, 237, 242
    subcutaneous fat, 72
      standards of reference, 75, 227, 236, 242
    subscapular (infrascapular, back) skin-fold, 74
    triceps (upper arm, dorsal arm, arm) skin-fold, 74
  standardization of techniques, 52
  standards of reference, 53-57
    general, 56, 168, 221-242
    actuaries, 57
    Baldwin-Wood, 57
    Harvard, 56
    local, 54
    reporting, 167
  weight, 64
    standards of reference, 67, 221, 224-226, 230-234, 238-241
Arm circumference, in anthropometric measurement, 76
  mid-arm-muscle circumference, 76
  standards of reference, 78
    arm circumference, 228, 236, 242
    mid-arm-muscle circumference, 229
    muscle circumference, 237, 242
Ascorbic acid, biochemical tests for, 90
  research tests, 243
Atheroma, associated with overnutrition, 217
  etiology of, 218
Attrition, dental, 28
Avitaminosis A in young children, 177, 178, 205
  assessment in community, 205
  ecological assessment, 205
  etiology of, 205